Qualitative Research
IN NURSING

Advancing
the Humanistic
Imperative

Qualitative Research
IN NURSING

Advancing the Humanistic Imperative

third edition

Helen J. Streubert Speziale, EdD, RN

Professor
Department of Nursing
College Misericordia
Dallas, Pennsylvania

Dona R. Carpenter, EdD, RN, CS

Professor
Department of Nursing
University of Scranton
Scranton, Pennsylvania

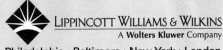

LIPPINCOTT WILLIAMS & WILKINS
A Wolters Kluwer Company

Philadelphia • Baltimore • New York • London
Buenos Aires • Hong Kong • Sydney • Tokyo

Acquisitions Editor: Margaret Zuccarini
Managing Editor: Barclay Cunningham
Editorial Assistant: Helen Kogut
Production Editor: Debra Schiff
Senior Production Manager: Helen Ewan

Art Director: Doug Smock
Manufacturing Manager: William Alberti
Indexer: Nancy Newman
Printer: Maple Binghamton

3rd Edition

Library of Congress Cataloging-in-Publication Data
Speziale Streubert, Helen J.
  Qualitative research in nursing : advancing the humanistic imperative / Helen J. Streubert Speziale, Dona R. Carpenter.--3rd ed.
    p. cm
  Includes bibliographical references and index.
  ISBN 0-7817-3483-5
  1. Nursing--Research--Methodology. 2. Sociology--Research--Methodology. I. Carpenter, Dona Rinaldi. II. Title.
RT81.5 .S78 2002
610.73'072--dc21

                                                                2002069375

Care has been taken to confirm the accuracy of the information presented and to describe generally accepted practices. However, the authors, editors, and publisher are not responsible for errors or omissions or for any consequences from application of the information in this book and make no warranty, express or implied, with respect to the content of the publication.

The authors, editors, and publisher have exerted every effort to ensure that drug selection and dosage set forth in this text are in accordance with the current recommendations and practice at the time of publication. However, in view of ongoing research, changes in government regulations, and the constant flow of information relating to drug therapy and drug reactions, the reader is urged to check the package insert for each drug for any change in indications and dosage and for added warnings and precautions. This is particularly important when the recommended agent is a new or infrequently employed drug.

Some drugs and medical devices presented in this publication have Food and Drug Administration (FDA) clearance for limited use in restricted research settings. It is the responsibility of the health care provider to ascertain the FDA status of each drug or device planned for use in his or her clinical practice.

This book is dedicated to my father, who has taught me more about perseverance in the shadow of extreme hardship than any person ever could have. He is truly my inspiration on a daily basis. I would also like to acknowledge the love and constant support of my husband, Michael, and my sons, Michael and Matthew.

HJS

This book is dedicated to my children, Emily Joy and Brian Wells, Jr., and my husband, Brian Wells Carpenter, Sr. Without their love, support and encouragement, this 3rd edition would not have been possible

DRS

ABOUT THE AUTHORS

Helen J. Streubert Speziale, EdD, RN, is Professor of Nursing and Director of the Service Leadership Center at College Misericordia, Dallas, Pennsylvania, where she teaches nursing research and wellness to undergraduates and nursing theory and the integration of nursing knowledge courses to graduate students. Her research interests focus on nursing education and the implementation of qualitative research methods. Dr. Streubert Speziale has authored and co-authored articles and book chapters on qualitative research and nursing education. She presents her work in national and international forums.

Dona Rinaldi Carpenter, EdD, RN, CS, is Professor of Nursing and Director of the RN-BS Track at the University of Scranton, Scranton, Pennsylvania, where she teaches medical-surgical nursing and nursing research to undergraduate and graduate students. Her research interests focus on doctoral education in nursing, professional commitment, and quality of life. She has authored and co-authored several articles and book chapters and has presented her work at national and international meetings.

Sandra Beth Lewenson, EdD, RN, FAAN, is Associate Dean of Academic Affairs at the Lienhard School of Nursing at Pace University, Pleasantville, New York. She teaches in both the undergraduate and graduate programs. Her areas of expertise include community health, history of managed care, and history of political activism in nursing. Her research focus is nursing's historical relationship with the women's suffrage movement at the beginning of the 20th century. She has published several books and articles on the topic.

TERESA APRIGLIANO, EdD, RN

Assistant Professor, Coordinator for Center for Nursing Research
Molloy College
Rockville Centre, New York

CAROL J. CORNWELL, PhD, MS, RN, CS

Assistant Professor of Nursing
Georgia Southern University School of Nursing
Statesboro, Georgia

JEAN BURLEY MOORE, PhD, RN

Associate Professor
George Mason University
College of Nursing and Health Sciences
Fairfax, Virginia

NANCY L. OLEN, EdD, MSN, RN

Associate Professor of Nursing
Bethel College
Roseville, Minnesota

LOIS B. TAFT, DNSc, RN, CS

Associate Professor, Department of Nursing Systems
University of Wisconsin–Eau Claire
Eau Claire, Wisconsin

The third edition of *Qualitative Research in Nursing: Advancing the Humanistic Imperative* presents an updated view of the essentials of qualitative research that have been published in the last two editions. Added to this edition is a more complete and expansive look at the actual process of conducting a qualitative research study, writing a qualitative research proposal, dealing with ethical issues, and clinical application of qualitative methods. We have worked diligently to bring to you the latest in qualitative thinking by nurses and those who have supported nurses' work. This edition includes the same strong philosophical and methodological principles that have been important to our readers over the past 7 years.

This book is intended to assist those new to qualitative inquiry to discover the fundamental characteristics of a set of methods that have been very important to us in advancing nursing's scientific base. We believe that those who open this text and begin to read will find it to be a strong reference for understanding qualitative methodology. We believe strongly, however, that it is only through engagement in the methods that those new to qualitative inquiry will begin to appreciate the value of the methods (approaches) for studying the human condition as it is revealed in nursing practice.

We have been most impressed with the place that qualitative research has attained since writing our first edition. One of our most vivid recollections in the "early days" was being the lone qualitative researchers on a research program. Today, you will find a significant number of journal pages and conference time allotted to the results of qualitative inquiry. Although there is still a long way to go in the ability to attract and garner research funds for qualitative research, we are heartened by the fact that there are more qualitative researchers who are able to become panel members of grant review teams. It is our belief that in the near future, qualitative research will secure the research dollars warranted for this exciting and enlightening research paradigm.

Those of you familiar with our text know that our original work arose from our own experiences with trying to develop a qualitative research agenda based on reading the works of, and studying with, those outside of the nursing discipline. Although it was our way of discovering a set of methods relatively new to nursing, we were interested in sharing some of the research and references that we found valuable during our personal journeys. This text builds on our experience and shares with the reader the expansion of our own thinking but also the works of those who have been significant in opening our collective vision in the field of qualitative study.

Our personal lives as nurses, nurse educators, and nurse researchers are built on the common understanding that individuals are integrated wholes who share in common experiences with other individuals. It is for this reason that qualitative inquiry supports our commitment to understanding the human condition. We fully believe that we live lives that recognize the interconnectedness of our humanness and we strive to assist others to join in the mutual understanding that we derive from being part of the human experience. The skills for understanding the human experience are found in the pages of this text. We believe that the understanding that is gleaned from participating in qualitative inquiry gives each nurse the opportunity to see his or her practice through a unique lens. To fully realize the skills of a qualitative researcher, we believe that fundamental understanding of the history, elements, context, and outcomes of each approach presented in the text is essential. Further, those who find qualitative inquiry supportive of their personal research philosophy are encouraged to use the primary references documented in the text to explore more deeply the basic ideologies that were responsible for the development of the qualitative research paradigm.

As in our previous editions, the text introduces the historical background of each approach, shares the fundamental elements, how one decides whether to use a particular approach, and the expected outcomes. Knowing these "parts" will help the reader begin to integrate and synthesize the research paradigm that we have found so successful in bring about an understanding of a whole and authentic human experience.

ORGANIZATION

The text is organized to facilitate the reader's comprehension of each approach and to provide examples of how the approaches have been used in nursing practice, education, and administration.

In Chapter 1, Philosophy and Theory: Foundations of Qualitative Research, the reader is introduced to the traditions of science, the interpretations of what constitutes science, perceptions of reality, and the influences of critical and feminist theory on the discipline of qualitative research.

In Chapter 2, The Conduct of Qualitative Research: Common Essential Elements, the development of a qualitative study is examined. The characteristics common to all qualitative studies are offered, including selection of the method, understanding the philosophic underpinnings of the approach selected, use of a literature review, explicating the researcher's beliefs, choosing a setting, selecting the informants, and achieving saturation.

Chapter 3 is new, representing an expansion of Chapter 2 from the second edition. In this chapter, Designing Data Generation and Management Strategies, the reader is offered ideas about how to select and use specific data collection strategies including interviews, focus groups, narratives, chat rooms, participant observation, and field notes. In addition, an explanation is provided for managing data including the common elements of data analysis, demonstrating trustworthiness, and presentation of the findings.

Chapter 4, Writing a Qualitative Research Proposal, is also a new chapter. In this chapter, the reader is introduced to the concept of developing a qualitative research agenda, as well as the elements of developing a qualitative research proposal.

Chapter 5, Phenomenology as Method, offers an in-depth description of philosophic and methodologic conceptualizations of this approach to qualitative inquiry. An overview of the phenomenological perspective, with descriptive and interpretive views of the process, is offered. The reader is given an exceptional guide to the process of phenomenological inquiry, including an expansion of previously presented hermeneutics. Table 5-1 lists the procedural steps for implementing a phenomenological study from the perspective of six phenomenologists. It is an exceptional reference for the would-be phenomenological researcher.

Chapter 6, Phenomenology in Practice, Education, and Administration, as in previous editions, offers the reader the opportunity to understand the presentation of the method offered in Chapter 5 by giving examples of published phenomenological research from practice, education, and administration. Critique guidelines and formal critique by the chapter author also are provided to assist in understanding the application and quality of the work that is published. To facilitate the integration of the information presented, a reprint of one of the critiqued studies is included. Finally, a table of recently published phenomenological research gives the reader a ready reference of work using this specific approach.

Chapter 7, Grounded Theory as Method; Chapter 9, Ethnography as Method; Chapter 11, Historical Research Method; and Chapter 13, Action Research Method, follow the format found in Chapter 5. This includes in-depth discussion of the philosophic and methodologic issues specific to the approach. Data generation and treatment as well as ethical issues specific to the particular approach are discussed in detail.

Chapters 8, 10, 12, and 14 repeat the format found in Chapter 6, incorporating a detailed examination of published studies that illustrate a particular approach followed by guidelines for critiquing the approach used. These chapters include tables that offer a substantial resource list of recent studies completed in the areas of education, administration, and practice. Finally, each of these chapters includes a reprinting of a selected study that illustrates the qualitative method discussed in that particular chapter.

Chapter 15, Triangulation as a Qualitative Research Strategy, expands on information related to data, investigator, theory, and methodological triangulation. It is intended to enhance the reader's understanding of the different ways triangulation can be used in a qualitative research study.

Chapter 16, Ethical Considerations in Qualitative Research, represents a major revision to the information presented in the last edition. A significant amount of literature has been published since the last edition with regard to ethical issues in qualitative research. This information is offered to assist the reader in fully understanding the unique and sensitive relationship that occurs in the process of a qualitative study and suggests ways to maximize protection of human subjects while engaged in the relationship.

Chapter 17, A Practical Guide for Sharing Qualitative Research Results, provides a full description of issues related to funding qualitative research projects and dissemination of qualitative research findings. It details for the reader the potential triumphs and the pitfalls in moving qualitative research into a public forum. An example of a funded grant and critique is included in the chapter.

KEY FEATURES AND BENEFITS

The following features are included in the philosophical and methodological framework.

- Description of the philosophical underpinnings of each approach. This description provides more than the "how" of the approach; it presents the underlying assumptions of the approaches.
- Detailed description of procedural steps used in each of the approaches. This offers the reader the opportunity to learn step by step how the approach is implemented.
- Tables profiling studies conducted using each of the approaches. These tables offer the reader an excellent resource for further exploring the existing body of knowledge specific to the approach being discussed.
- In-depth discussion of published research studies that have used the approaches under discussion. This examination shares with the reader not only what has been published but also the strengths and weaknesses of the studies reviewed.
- Specific critiquing guidelines available in all companion chapters for each of the approaches. These guidelines help the reader understand the specific questions that should be asked of research studies that have used or will be using the approach.
- Inclusion of chapters on action research. This methodology used in other disciplines is gaining increasing acceptance in nursing. Readers will benefit from having this cutting-edge information available to them.
- Inclusion of companion chapters. Comparison chapters describing application of each of the approaches included in this text provide strong evidence of the impact these qualitative research methods are having on the discipline of nursing, and the potential benefits they will continue to have. These chapters all provide neophyte qualitative researchers with clear descriptions of what is expected from the researchers who will evaluate their work.
- Inclusion of a sample of a funded qualitative research grant including the critique offered by the grant review panel.
- Chapters on Ethical Considerations in Qualitative Research and Triangulation.
- Tables highlighting the methods described as they have been used to study nursing practice issues.
- Two new chapters, one that expands on the use of data generation and analysis strategies and the other that details the development of a qualitative research proposal and outlines the development of a qualitative research agenda.

We hope that this book will serve as both a starting point for the new researcher and a reference for more experienced nurses. It is expected that each approach detailed will offer the reader a sound understanding of qualitative research methods.

Helen J. Streubert Speziale
Dona Rinaldi Carpenter

ACKNOWLEDGMENTS

The third edition of this textbook continues to be an outcome of our life experiences with friends and colleagues who have supported and valued our work. Our commitment to another voice and another way of creating meaning remains, and we are grateful to those who continue to care about and influence our lives. We wish to acknowledge all those people who continue to shape our thinking and our way of being in the world...our friends, our families, our teachers, our students, and our colleagues.

Specifically, we wish to acknowledge those who have been most closely involved in the production of the third edition of this text. The authors are grateful for the editorial direction and assistance of Margaret Zuccarini, Helen Kogut, Barclay Cunningham, and Debra Schiff; the research support of Joan Pastorelli, College Misericordia librarian; and the research assistance of Ann M. Kutney, Jessica A. Patterson, Julie Robbins, Kim Sullivan, and Erin M. Walsh, University of Scranton nursing students.

CONTENTS

5

Phenomenology as Method 51

DONA RINALDI CARPENTER

6

Phenomenology in Practice, Education, and Administration 75

DONA RINALDI CARPENTER

7

Grounded Theory as Method 107

DONA RINALDI CARPENTER

8

Grounded Theory in Practice, Education, and Administration 123
DONA RINALDI CARPENTER

9

Ethnography as Method 153
HELEN J. STREUBERT SPEZIALE

10

Ethnography in Practice, Education, and Administration 181
HELEN J. STREUBERT SPEZIALE

Philosophy and Theory: Foundations of Qualitative Research

Since the first edition of this book, there has been much written about qualitative research. There have been debates about its rigor, its value, its utility. There have been still other debates about the qualifications necessary to conduct qualitative research, how it is funded, and its place in advancing nursing science. Through all of the debates, there appears to be one pervasive and ongoing reality. Qualitative research is an accepted, meaningful, and important methodological approach to the development of a substantive body of nursing knowledge. This conclusion is based primarily on its regular appearance in highly regarded nursing research journals. Thus, it appears important to look at the foundations of qualitative research so that those new to its purpose understand its roots.

Not new to most readers is the fact that the tradition of science is uniquely quantitative. The quantitative approach to research has been justified by its success in measuring, analyzing, replicating, and applying knowledge gained from this paradigm. The inability to quantitatively measure some phenomena and the dissatisfaction with the results of measurement of other phenomena have led to an intense interest in using other approaches to study particularly human phenomena. This interest has led to an acceptance of qualitative research approaches as another way to discover knowledge. One cannot help but be struck by the "success of qualitative research methods in the marketplace of academic ideas" (Atkinson, 1995, p. 117). The use of qualitative methods to discover knowledge is far more commonplace in nursing today than 10 years ago.

The tradition of using qualitative methods to study human phenomena is grounded in the social sciences. The tradition arose because aspects of human values, culture, and relationships were unable to be described fully using quantitative research methods. Krasner (2000) states that the early philosophers "argued that human phenomena could not and should not be reduced to mathematical formulas" (p. 70). The practice of qualitative research has expanded to clinical settings because "empirical approaches have proven to be of limited service in answering some of the challenging and pressing clinical questions, especially where human subjectivity and interpretation are involved" (Thorne, 1997, p. 288). The appeal for nurses is that qualitative research methods attempt to describe and interpret perplexing human phenomena: phenomena that are not easily quantifiable (Krasner, 2000, p. 70). Nurses and other health care professionals clearly want to grasp the lived experience of their clients, to enter into the world their clients inhabit, and to understand the basic social processes that illuminate human health and illness events (Thorne, 1997).

This chapter shares with the reader the foundations of qualitative research. Its purpose is to present qualitative knowledge structure and generate excitement for the qualitative research approach as an alternative to quantitative inquiry.

PHILOSOPHIC UNDERPINNINGS OF QUALITATIVE RESEARCH

From a philosophic viewpoint, the study of humans is deeply rooted in descriptive modes of science. Human scientists have been concerned with describing the fundamental patterns of human thought and behavior since early times. Descartes' view of science was long held as the only approach to new knowledge. His ideas were grounded in an objective reality, a position that supported the idea that cause and effect could explain all things. Kant is attributed with questioning the fundamental nature of reality as seen through a Cartesian lens. He opened discussion about human rationality. Kant proposed that perception was more than the act of observation. For him, all reality was not explainable by cause and effect. He raised issues supporting the notion that nature was not independent of thought or reason (Hamilton, 1994). What was observed, therefore, was not the only reality.

The concept of scientific versus practical reason was born of Kant's ideas about nature, specifically as the concept relates to perception (Ermath, 1978; Hamilton, 1994). Later existentialists advanced Kant's ideas to explore reality as it is perceived rather than as an observed phenomenon only. Kant's ideas about freedom and practical reasoning emancipated science. Scientists questioned whether empiricism was the only way to gain knowledge. Later philosophers such as Husserl furthered Kant's propositions, and, eventually, the German school of philosophy developed and expanded the ideas about self, self-consciousness, reality, and freedom.

The early debates about science and reality established the foundations of the qualitative paradigm that many social scientists use today. Qualitative research offers the opportunity to focus on finding answers to questions centered on social experience, how it is created, and how it gives meaning to human life (Denzin & Lincoln, 1994). Knowing how social experiences construct an individual's reality is an important criterion for developing science. Based on this idea, an exploration of ways of knowing is appropriate.

If one takes the ontologic position that reality is apprehensible, then the positivist or empiricist framework becomes one's reference point. However, it seems inconceivable that individuals can believe they are able to fully apprehend reality. According to Denzin and Lincoln (1994), post-positivists believe there is a reality to be known but have conceded that this reality only will be "imperfectly or probabilistically apprehendable [sic]" (p. 109). Critical theorists and constructivists see reality from a dynamic standpoint. The critical theorist perspective is that reality is "shaped by social, political, cultural, economic, ethnic, and gender values" (Denzin & Lincoln, 1994, p. 109). Further, feminist critical theorists believe that knowledge is co-created by researcher and those researched. The constructivist, however, sees reality as "relativism—local and specific" (Denzin & Lincoln, 1994, p. 109). Therefore, "reality is actually realities" (Lincoln, 1992, p. 379). Clearly, it is a post-positivist viewpoint that supports the notion of a dynamic reality.

According to Cheek (1996), "the qualitative research enterprise is about allowing multiple readings of the same reality to surface" (p. 503). In a human enterprise such as nursing, it is imperative that nurses embrace a research tradition that provides for the most meaningful way to describe and understand human experiences. Recognizing that reality is dynamic is the first step in establishing a truly humanistic perspective of research.

WAYS OF KNOWING

Belenky, Clinchy, Goldberger, and Tarule's (1986) viewpoint on knowing has provided a lens to question why objective science has been accepted as the predominant route to truth. Their exploration of the way women come to know supports a feminist ideology. However, holders of this viewpoint sometimes view feminist ideas as subjective and, therefore, less valuable than traditional positivist science. This way of thinking is changing as scientists become increasingly comfortable with the diversity in society and the richness of exploring and using multiple methods of inquiry to discover particular phenomena.

The idea of *received knowledge* is an important premise set forth by Belenky et al. (1986). Individuals learn usually by being told—by receiving knowledge. All too frequently, though, the act of being told limits the opportunity to engage the self in a dialogue about what is real. When presented with received knowledge, the receiver of the knowledge should ask, "What are my perceptions about this knowledge as it is presented to me?"

From the time individuals are young, they are told by people who "know"—usually adults they view as authority figures—the beliefs or knowledge they should retain. These authority figures present most of the knowledge they share as truths. These truths are usually facts that, in some way, have been passed on or proven to be correct. The proof of correctness often occurs as a direct result of an objective manipulation of factors or variables.

Empirical scientists who support a Cartesian framework believe that if objective measurement cannot be assigned to a phenomenon, then the importance and thus the existence of the phenomenon may be in question. Many contemporary scientists and philosophers question the value of this system, particularly in situations that include humans and their interactions with other humans. Little available objectively derived measurement exists that is meaningful when one studies human phenomena within a social context. The concepts of objectivity, reduction, and manipulation, which are fundamental to empirical science, defy the authentic fiber of humans and their social interactions. Too many intervening or confounding variables can raise objections to empirical science when the focus is human social context or interaction.

With the belief that science should inform the lives of people who interact and function in society, researchers need to examine all parts of reality—subjective reality as well as its objective counterpart. Researchers should acknowledge knowing in the subjective sense and value it equally so that scientific knowledge will represent the views of people who experience life. The early phenomenologists believed that the only reality was the one that is perceived. Thus, the measurement of perception challenges the empirical scientist. Perception is not objective; rather, perception is a way of observing and processing those things that are present to the self. For example, two individuals may observe the same lecture and leave the classroom with different interpretations of what the lecturer said. Each individual's interpretation is based on what that person perceived to be reality—a reality that is developed and constructed over a lifetime of receiving, processing, and interpreting information, as well as engaging in human interaction. The internalization of what becomes known as belief systems comes from perception and construction of what is real for the individual.

WAYS OF KNOWING IN NURSING

In her seminal work on ways of knowing in nursing, Carper (1978) identified four fundamental patterns that emerge as the way nurses come to know: empirical knowing, aesthetic knowing, personal knowing, and moral knowing. *Empirical knowing* represents the traditional, objective, logical, and positivist tradition of science. Empirical knowing and thus empirical science is committed to providing explanations for phenomena and then controlling them. An example of empirical knowing is the knowledge derived from the biologic sciences that describes and explains human function. Through this description and explanation, biologic scientists have been able to predict and control certain aspects of human structure and function. Treatment of diabetes mellitus is an example of empirical research being applied in the health care field. From their empirical studies, biologic scientists know that providing insulin to individuals with diabetes mellitus controls the symptoms created by the nonfunctioning pancreas. The nursing profession's alignment with empirical knowing and its subsequent pursuit of this mode of inquiry follows the positivist paradigm, which believes that objective data, measurement, and generalizability are essential to the generation and dissemination of knowledge.

Aesthetic knowing is the art of nursing. The understanding and interpretation of subjective experience and the creative development of nursing care are based on an appreciation of subjective expression. Aesthetic knowing is abstract and defies a formal description and measurement. According to Carper (1978),

The aesthetic pattern of knowing in nursing involves the perception of abstract particulars as distinguished from the recognition of abstracted universals. It is the knowing of the unique particular rather than an exemplary class (p. 16).

Aesthetic knowing in nursing provides the framework for the exploration of qualitative research methodologies. Qualitative research calls for recognition of patterns in phenomena rather than the explication of facts that will be controllable and generalizable. An example of aesthetic knowing is the way a nurse would provide care differently for two elderly women who are preparing for cataract surgery, based on the nurse's knowledge of each woman's particular life patterns.

Wainwright (2000) states "a nursing aesthetic can provide us with an essential set of tools to help answer the question of what amounts to good nursing. It may also provide us with additional insights into the nature of nursing ethics" (p. 755). "Nursing knowledge as defined in nursing theories and when lived by nurses creates the art of nursing" (Mitchell, 2001, p. 207).

Personal knowing requires that the individual—in this case, the nurse—know the self. The degree to which an individual knows oneself is determined by his or her abilities to self-actualize. Movement toward knowledge of the self and self-actualization requires comfort with ambiguity and a commitment to patience in understanding. Personal knowing is a commitment to authentication of relationships and a *presencing* with others, that is, the enlightenment and sensitization people bring to genuine human interactions. Personal knowing deals with the fundamental *existentialism* of humans, that is, the capacity for change and the value placed on becoming.

Personal knowing also supports the qualitative research paradigm. In the conduct of qualitative inquiry, researchers are obligated by the philosophic underpinnings of the methodologies they use to accept the self as part of the research enterprise and to approach research participants in a genuine and authentic manner. An awareness of one's beliefs and understandings is essential to fully discover the phenomena studied in a qualitative research inquiry. Furthermore, qualitative researchers believe there is always subjectivity in their pursuit of the truth. The very nature of human interactions is based on subjective knowledge. In the most objective research endeavor, subjective realities will affect what is studied. "Scientific research, as a human endeavor to advance knowledge, is influenced by the sociocultural and historical context in which it takes place and is considered neither value free, objective, nor neutral" (Henderson, 1995, p. 59).

Moral knowing reflects our ethical obligations in a situation or our ideas about what should be done in a given situation. Through the moral way of knowing, individuals come to a realization of what is right and just. As with personal knowing and aesthetic knowing, moral knowing is another abstract dimension of how it is that individuals come to know a situation. Moral knowing is based on traditional principles and codes of ethics or conduct. This type of knowing becomes most important when humans face situations in which decisions of right and wrong are blurred by differences in values or beliefs. Moral knowing requires an openness to differences in philosophic positions. Ethics and logic are required to examine the intricacies of human situations that do not fit standard formulas for conduct.

Munhall (2001) states "all of the foregoing patterns are rich and essential sources of nursing knowledge that can be studied from various perspectives of science" (p. 41). The importance of sharing these ways of knowing is to offer the reader a context in which to judge the appropriateness of nursing knowledge and the way that nurses develop that knowledge. It is only through examinations of current belief structures that people are able to achieve their own standards of what will be best in a given situation. Moreover, when we select our research methods, we should choose them based on the questions we are asking (Burnard & Hannigan, 2000) within the context of what is known and what we believe.

May (1994) and Sandelowski (1994) expanded on the idea of knowing as it relates to nursing knowledge. May (1994) used the term *abstract knowing* to describe the analytic experience of knowing:

> The rigorous implementation and explication of method alone never explains the process of abstract knowing, regardless of which paradigm the scientist espouses and which method is chosen. Method does not produce insight or understanding or the creative leap that the agile mind makes in the struggle to comprehend observation and to link them together. Regardless of the paradigmatic perspective held by the scientist, the process of knowing itself cannot be observed and measured directly, but only by its product (p. 13).

May (1994) further suggested that knowledge is "shaped *but not completely defined* by the process through which it is created" (p. 14). Based on her ideas about knowing, she gave credibility to what she called "magic," which is similar to the intuitive connections discussed in Benner's (1984) work on expert clinical judgment. Based on her conversations with and observations of qualitative researchers, May (1994) determined that, at a certain point, pattern recognition creates the insight into the phenomenon under study. She believed that the ability to see knowledge is a result of intellectual rigor and readiness (magic). Her ideas support the concept of intuition or, as she labeled it, "abstract knowing" in nursing research.

Sandelowski (1994) took a position on knowing similar to the aesthetic knowing described by Carper (1978): We must accept the art as well as the science of research. Sandelowski believed that the two are not mutually exclusive.

> What differentiates the arts from the sciences is not the search for truth per se, but rather the kinds of truths that are sought. Science typically is concerned with propositional truths, or truth about something. Art is concerned with universal truths, with being true to: even with being more true to life than life itself (Hospers as cited in Sandelowski, 1994, p. 52).

Both May (1994) and Sandelowski (1994) provide us with an expansion of the original positions on truth offered by Carper (1978). These authors provide a validation for knowing other than in the empirical sense. Most important, they offer nurse–researchers a way to discover knowledge that complements the positivist paradigm and gives voice to other ways of knowing. In the case of qualitative research and nursing practice, it is only through examination of the prevailing ideologies that nurses will be able to decide which ideology most reflects their personal patterns of discovery and creation of meaning.

MEANING OF SCIENCE

Science is defined in a number of ways. Kerlinger (1986) described the static view of science as a "way of explaining observed phenomena" (p. 7). Namenwirth (1986) defined it as "a system of gathering, verifying, and systematizing information about reality" (p. 19). Guba (1990), in sharing a view of empirical science, articulated the meaning of science as it is practiced within the premise of value-neutral, logical empirical methods that promise "the growth of rational control over ourselves and our worlds" (p. 317). Parse (2001) offers the term *sciencing* to describe "coming to know and understand the meaning of a phenonmena of concern to a discipline" (p. 1). Each of these definitions or descriptions gives a different perception of what is considered truth.

Much of what individuals know about science in the nursing profession is based on the empirical view of science, which places significant value on rationality, objectivity, prediction, and control. The question arises: Is this view of science consistent with the phenomena of interest to nurses? The empirical view of science permeates many aspects of human activity. In adopting this view, one adopts a value system. Many empiricists believe that if a phenomenon is not observable, the question that should be asked is, Is it real? If a particular phenomenon does not conform to reality as is currently known, empiricists could judge it to be irrational and therefore unimportant. If a phenomenon is studied without controls protecting the objectivity of the study, then it is said to lack rigor or is soft science and therefore results in unusable data. If the findings from an inquiry do not lead to generalization that contributes to the prediction and control of the phenomena under study, some empiricists would argue that this is not science.

An empiricist view of science has permeated society and has structured what is valued. Feminist scholars have suggested that the scientific paradigm that focuses on prediction and control has gained wide acceptance because of its roots in a male paradigm. Historically, women have played only a small role in the creation of knowledge. Therefore, the definitions and values of science have been largely created by male scientists who have valued prediction and control over description and understanding.

An empirical, objective, rational science has significant value when the phenomenon of interest is other than human behavior. However, the goals of this type of science—prediction and control—are less valuable when the subject of the inquiry is unable to be made objective.

As a result of the limitations that result from a positivist view of science, philosophers and social scientists have offered an alternative path to discovery that places value on the study of human experiences. In this model, researchers acknowledge and value subjectivity as part of any scientific inquiry. Human values contribute to scientific knowledge; therefore, neutrality is impossible. Prediction is thought to be limiting and capable of creating a false sense of reality. In a human science framework, the best scientists can hope for in creating new knowledge is to provide understanding and interpretation of phenomena within context. Human science and the methods of inquiry that accompany it offer an opportunity to study and create meaning that will enrich and inform human life. Burnard and Hannigan (2000) state that irregardless of the paradigm, "research is nearly always a searching for patterns, similarities and differences" (p. 5).

Induction Versus Deduction

Knowledge is generated from either an inductive or deductive posture. *Inductive reasoning* is a process that starts with the details of the experience and moves to a more general picture of the phenomenon of interest (Liehr & Smith, 2002, p. 110). For example, a nurse interested in studying the experiences of women in labor would interview women who have undergone labor to discover their experiences of labor. Within context, the nurse could make statements about the labor experience that might be applicable to understanding the labor experience for women not in the study. Hence, qualitative research methods are inductive.

Deductive reasoning "moves from the general to the particular" (Feldman, 1998, p. 137). A researcher interested in conducting research within a deductive framework would develop a hypothesis about a phenomenon and then would seek to prove it. For example, a nurse wanting to know about the labor experience might hypothesize that women in labor experience more pain when they do not use visualization techniques during transition. The researcher's responsibility in such a study would be to identify a pain measure and then collect data on women in the transition phase of labor to determine whether they experience more or less pain based on the use of visualization techniques. Within a deductive framework, the researcher could use the study findings to predict and ultimately control the pain experience of laboring women. Deductive reasoning is the framework for quantitative research studies.

Both frameworks are important in the development of knowledge. Based on the question being asked, the researcher will select either an inductive or deductive stance.

RELATIONSHIP OF THEORY TO RESEARCH

In addition to understanding the framework from which the researcher enters the research enterprise, it is important to be aware of the relationship of theory to research, specifically, qualitative research. Mitchell and Cody (1992) proposed that "all knowledge is theory-laden" (p. 170). What exactly is theory? According to Chinn and Kramer (1999), a theory is "a creative and rigorous structuring of ideas that projects a tentative, purposeful, and systematic view of phenomena" (p.

51). If we think about qualitative research, which advocates the necessity of being atheoretical, the idea of theory appears in opposition to the basic tenets of the qualitative research process. However, this idea may not be true. From a philosophic standpoint, Mitchell and Cody (1992) have suggested that all knowledge is theory laden. The intersection of these two apparently divergent positions occurs in light of the definition of theory and its position in the qualitative research process. Mitchell and Pilkington (1999) see theory in a much larger context, similar to what might be called a philosophy of science. Chinn and Kramer defined *philosophy* as "a form of disciplined inquiry for the purpose of discerning general traits of reality and principles of value" (p. 256). Given Mitchell and Pilkington's dialogue about science, it appears that for the general reader, they are talking about the way one practices science and for them, the way of science should be consistent with the way of practicing nursing. These authors support the work of Parse and as such believe that knowledge generation and practice are based in a philosophy of mutuality.

Chinn and Kramer's (1999) definition of theory *is* contradictory to the basic tenets of qualitative research as a discovery process. However, the discovered information may lead to the development of yet unknown theories. Not all qualitative research studies lead to theory development, but certainly specific approaches used in qualitative research will lead to theory development. Grounded theory is an example of such an approach (see Chapter 7). In grounded theory, the researcher's goal is to develop theory to describe a particular social process.

As an example of how a study or group of studies may lead to theory development, Estabrooks, Field, and Morse (1994) proposed that through an analysis and synthesis of completed qualitative research studies, the aggregation of qualitative research studies can lead to the development of midrange theory. This example clearly demonstrates the potential use of qualitative research for theory development.

If we review the position of Mitchell and Cody (1992) stated earlier, it is necessary to reexamine the definition of theory. According to these authors, qualitative research approaches represent a theoretical position and thus a way in which qualitative research is theory driven. To accept the position of Mitchell and Cody (1992), and many philosophers before them, one must accept the notion that the concepts and constructs represented in qualitative research methodologies represent a form of theory. Morse (1992) also has supported this position: She stated that conceptual frameworks and theories may be used as the theoretical basis for research to fit the research within the paradigmatic perspective of a discipline. As an example, she offered anthropologic use of culture as the underlying theory in ethnography.

The point of offering these descriptions of theory is to place the role of theory development within the context of qualitative research. It is generally accepted that qualitative research findings have the potential to create theory. In the instance of grounded theory, the method is dedicated to the discovery of theory. With regard to theoretical positions attributed to method, the term *theory* represents a particular epistemologic position that many qualitative researchers accept.

Objective Versus Subjective Data Within a Nursing Context

Empirical scientists believe that the study of any phenomena must be devoid of subjectivity (Namenwirth, 1986). Furthermore, they have contended that objectivity is essential in guiding the way to truth. The problem with this position is that no human activity can be performed without subjectivity. Because it is a human quest for knowledge, it is logical to presume that human activity will be necessary to seek knowledge.

Based on his reading and interpretation of Hanson (1958), Phillips (1987) has suggested that objectivity is impossible: "The theory, hypothesis, framework, or background knowledge held by an investigator can strongly influence what he sees" (p. 9). Kerlinger (1979) also proposed that "the procedures of science are objective and not the scientists. Scientists, like all men and women, are opinionated, dogmatic, and ideological" (p. 264). Therefore, the idea of objectivity loses its meaning. On some level, all research endeavors have the subjective influence of the scientist. Procedural objectivity is the goal; however, even it is biased because the scientist will interpret the findings. Even if the findings of a study are statistical (thought to be an objective measure), the scientist interprets the statistical data through a lens of opinions and biases about what the numbers say (MacKenzie, 1981; Taylor, 1985).

Humanistic scientists value the subjective component of the quest for knowledge. They embrace the idea of subjectivity, recognizing that humans are incapable of total objectivity because they have been situated in a reality constructed by subjective experiences. Meaning, and therefore the search for the truth, is possible only through social interaction. The degree to which the scientist is part of the development of scientific knowledge is debated even by the humanistic scientists. Post-empiricists accept the subjective nature of inquiry but still support rigor and objective study through method. The objectivity post-empiricists speak of is one of context. For example, post-empiricist scientists would acknowledge their subjective realities and then, always being aware of them, seek to keep them apart from data collection, but to include them in the analysis and the final report.

Constructivist humanistic scientists believe that "knowledge is the result of a dialogical process between the self-understanding person and that which is encountered—whether a text, a work of art, or the meaningful expression of another person" (Smith, 1990, p. 177). Clearly, subjectivity is acknowledged, but the degree to which it is embraced is based on philosophic beliefs.

Humanistic scientists see objectivity in its empirical definition to be impossible. The degree to which a researcher can be objective, and therefore, unbiased, is determined by the philosophic tradition to which the human scientist ascribes. That subjectivity is included in the discussion of human science conveys an understanding that participation in the world prohibits humans from ever being fully objective.

Nurse–researchers engaged in qualitative research recognize the subjective reality inherent in the research process and embrace it. They are bound by method to acknowledge their subjectivity and to place it in a context that permits full examination of the effect of subjectivity on the research endeavor and description of the phenomenon under study.

GROUNDING RESEARCH IN THE REALITIES OF NURSING

Nurse–scientists have the responsibility of developing new knowledge. Fawcett (1999) offers that nursing needs three types of research: basic, applied, and clinical. The question that needs answering will drive the research type and paradigm selected. If a nurse–scientist is interested in discovering the most effective way to suction a tracheostomy tube, then a quantitative approach will be the appropriate way to study the problem. But, if the nurse–scientist is interested in discovering what the experience of suctioning is for people who are suctioned, qualitative research methods are more appropriate. What the nurse–scientist must do is clearly define the problem and then identify whether it requires an inductive or deductive approach. Only the researcher can determine what the explicit question is and how best to answer it. As Lincoln (1992) pointed out, the area of health research is open to inquiry and the qualitative model is a superior choice over conventional methods.

Emancipation

In recent years, much has been written about "emancipatory research" (Henderson, 1995). Two predominant paradigms permeate what is published: critical theory and feminist theory. *Critical theory*, as described by Habermas (1971), is a way to develop knowledge that is free, undistorted, and unconstrained. According to Habermas, the predominant paradigm in science was not reflective of people's reality. He found that empiricism created cognitive dissonance. The goal of critical theory is to "unfreeze lawlike structures and to encourage self reflections for those whom the laws are about" (Wilson-Thomas, 1995, p. 573). "Critical [theorists] . . . sought to expose oppressive relationships among groups and to enlighten those who are oppressed" (Bent, 1993, p. 296).

Similarly, *feminist theory* takes the idea of emancipation further and speaks specifically to women's lives. Feminist theorists value women and women's experiences (Hall & Stevens, 1991). Feminist scholars believe that the traditional laws of science limit and preclude the discovery of what is uniquely feminist. Seibold (2000) identifies feminist research as being focused first and foremost on women's experiences. Feminist researchers attempt to see the world from the view of the women studied and be critical in examination of the issues and activist in improving the condition of those studied.

In both paradigms, the predominant themes are liberating the study participants and making their voices heard. Sigsworth (1995) identified seven fundamental conditions that are necessary for feminist research that, when editorialized, are appropriate for critical theorist ideas about research as well. These conditions are (1) the research should be focused on the experiences of the population studied, their perceptions, and their truths; (2) "artificial dichotomies and sharp boundaries are suspect in research involving human beings" (Sigsworth, 1995, p. 897); (3) history and concurrent events are always considered when planning, conducting, analyzing, and interpreting findings; (4) the questions asked are as important as the answers discovered; (5) research should not be hierarchical; (6) researchers' assumptions, biases, and presuppositions are part of the research enterprise; and (7) researchers and research participants are partners whose discoveries lead to understanding.

According to Hall and Stevens (1991), qualitative methods are more in line with the feminist perspective as well as with critical theorist ideas. The tenets offered earlier are primary in conducting a study regardless of the methodology used. However, by their stated purposes, the methods of qualitative research are far more accommodating to the ideas supported by critical and feminist theorists. Researchers who wish their work to be emancipating and liberating should consider the methods of qualitative research described in this text.

SUMMARY

This chapter has offered the fundamental ideas supporting qualitative research as a specific research paradigm. In addition, the chapter has shared the relationship of historical, practical, and theoretical ideas. It is hoped that these ideas have piqued the reader's interest and will lead to exploration of the specifics of qualitative research as they are developed in this text.

REFERENCES

Atkinson, P. (1995). Some perils of paradigms. *Qualitative Health Research, 5*(1), 117–124.

Belenky, M. F., Clinchy, B. M., Goldberger, N. R., & Tarule, J. M. (1986). *Women's ways of knowing*. New York: Basic Books.

Benner, P. (1984). *From novice to expert*. Menlo Park, CA: Addison-Wesley.

Bent, K. N. (1993). Perspectives on critical and feminist theory in developing nursing praxis. *Journal of Professional Nursing, 9*(5), 296–303.

Burnard, P., & Hannigan, B. (2000). Qualitative and quantitative approaches in mental health nursing: Moving the debate forward. *Journal of Psychiatric and Mental Health Nursing, 7*, 1–6.

Carper, B. (1978). Fundamental patterns of knowing in nursing. *Advances in Nursing Science, 1*(1), 13–23.

Cheek, J. (1996). Taking a view: Qualitative research as representation. *Qualitative Health Research, 6*(4), 492–505.

Chinn, P. L., & Kramer, M. K. (1999). *Theory and nursing: Integrated knowledge development* (5th ed). St. Louis: Mosby.

Denzin, N. K., & Lincoln, Y. S. (Eds.). (1994). *Handbook of qualitative research*. Thousand Oaks, CA: Sage.

Ermath, M. (1978). *Wilhelm Dilthey:* The critique of historical reason. Chicago: University of Chicago Press.

Estabrooks, C. A., Field, P. A., & Morse, J. M. (1994). Aggregating qualitative findings: An approach to theory development. *Qualitative Health Research, 4*(4), 503–511.

Fawcett, J. (1999). The state of nursing science: Hallmarks of the 20th and 21st centuries. *Nursing Science Quarterly, 12*(4), 311–318.

Feldman, H. (1998). Theoretical framework. In G. LoBiondo-Wood & J. Haber (Eds.), *Nursing research: Methods, critical appraisal, and utilization* (4th ed., pp. 133–154). St. Louis, MO: Mosby.

Guba, E. G. (1990). *The paradigm dialogue.* Newbury Park, CA: Sage.

Habermas, J. (1971). *Knowledge and human interests* (J. J. Strapiro, trans.). Boston: Beacon Press.

Hall, J. M., & Stevens, P. E. (1991). Rigour in feminist research. *Advances in Nursing Science, 22*(3), 16–29.

Hamilton, D. (1994). Traditions, preferences, and postures in applied qualitative research. In N. K. Denzin & Y. S. Lincoln (Eds.), *Handbook of qualitative research* (pp. 60–69). Thousand Oaks, CA: Sage.

Hanson, N. R. (1958). *Patterns of discovery.* Cambridge: Cambridge University Press.

Henderson, D. J. (1995). Consciousness raising in participatory research: Method and methodology for emancipatory inquiry. *Advances in Nursing Science, 17*(3), 58–69.

Kerlinger, F. N. (1979). *Behavioral research: A conceptual approach.* New York: Holt, Rinehart & Winston.

Kerlinger, F. N. (1986). *Foundations of behavioral research* (3rd ed.). New York: Holt, Rinehart & Winston.

Krasner, D.L. (2000). Qualitative research: A different paradigm—part 1. *Journal of Wound, Ostomy and Continence Nursing, 28,* 70–72.

Liehr, P., & Smith, M.J. (2002). Theoretical frameworks. In G. LoBiondo-Wood & J. Haber (Eds.), *Nursing research: Methods, critical appraisal, and utilization* (5th ed., pp. 107–120). St. Louis, MO: Mosby.

Lincoln, Y. S. (1992). Sympathetic connections between qualitative methods and health research. *Qualitative Health Research, 2*(4), 375–391.

MacKenzie, D. (1981). *Statistics in Great Britain: 1885–1930.* Edinburgh, Scotland: Edinburgh University Press.

May, K. A. (1994). Abstract knowing: The case for magic in method. In J. Morse (Ed.), *Critical issues in qualitative research methods* (pp. 10–21). Thousand Oaks, CA: Sage.

Mitchell, G. J. (2001). Prescription, freedom, and participation: Drilling down into theory-based nursing practice. *Nursing Science Quarterly, 14*(3), 205–210.

Mitchell, G. J., & Cody, W. K. (1992). The role of theory in qualitative research. *Nursing Science Quarterly, 6*(4), 170–178.

Mitchell, G. J. & Pilkington, F. B. (1999). A dialogue on the comparability of research paradigms—and other theoretical things. *Nursing Science Quarterly, 12*(4), 283–289.

Morse, J. M. (1992). The power of induction. *Qualitative Health Research, 2*(1), 3–6.

Munhall, P. L. (2001). Epistemology in nursing. In P. L. Munhall (Ed.), *Nursing research: A qualititative perspective* (pp. 37–64). Boston: Jones and Bartlett.

Namenwirth, M. (1986). Science seen through a feminist prism. In R. Bleier (Ed.), *Feminist approaches to science* (pp. 18–41). New York: Pergamon Press.

Parse, R. R. (2001). *Qualitative inquiry: The path of sciencing.* Boston: Jones and Bartlett.

Phillips, D. C. (1987). *Philosophy, science, and social inquiry.* New York: Pergamon Press.

Sandelowski, M. (1994). The proof is in the pottery: Toward a poetic for qualitative inquiry. In J. Morse (Ed.), *Critical issues in qualitative research methods* (pp. 44–62). Thousand Oaks, CA: Sage.

Seibold, C. (2000). Qualitative research from a feminist perspective in the postmodern era: Methodological, ethical and reflexive concerns. *Nursing Inquiry, 7*(3), 147–155.

Sigsworth, J. (1995). Feminist research: Its relevance to nursing. *Journal of Advanced Nursing, 22,* 896–899.

Smith, J. K. (1990). Alternative research paradigms and the problem of criteria. In E. G. Guba (Ed.), *The paradigm dialogue* (pp. 167–187). Newbury Park, CA: Sage.

Taylor, C. (1985). *Human agency and language.* Cambridge, England: Cambridge University Press.

Thorne, S. (1997). Phenomenological positivism and other problematic trends in health science research. *Qualitative Health Research, 7*(2), 287–293.

Wainwright, P. (2000). Towards an aesthetics of nursing. *Journal of Advanced Nursing, 32*(3), 750–756.

Wilson-Thomas, L. (1995). Applying critical social theory in nursing education to bridge the gap between theory, research and practice. *Journal of Advanced Nursing, 21*, 568–575.

The Conduct of Qualitative Research: Common Essential Elements

In the past few years, it has become increasingly more important to examine how and why nurses make the decisions that they do with regard to their research. To fully comprehend the importance of this examination, the following question is offered. Are research foci selected to address research dissertation advisors' agendas, class objectives, employers' agendas, funding agency priorities, and promotion and tenure criteria or to meet the needs of those persons nurses serve? This question is not meant to suggest that conducting research for "practical" reasons is not legitimate and ultimately will not serve the needs of those nurses care for. However, it remains primary that nurses focus on development of nursing knowledge. And, since the time and energy required to conduct research are significant, it should be work that nurse–researchers are deeply invested in.

One of the differences in nursing research presently that may have not been as true in the past is that nurse–researchers spend more time developing their research questions and clarifying what it is they are planning to study. It becomes increasingly more important that research studies be based on sound rationale and a clear understanding of the research question. Denzin (2000) suggests that in addition to carefully developing the research question, researchers must also examine the political nature of their work. All research represents a political enterprise that carries significant implications. The more nurses understand the motivating factors involved in their work, the more explicit they can be about its benefits.

Once the research question is clearly articulated and the researcher has an understanding of the problem and what impact the research activity will have on those studied, the discipline, and those to whom the results may be meaningful, the researcher will need to decide which research paradigm will most appropriately answer the question. This chapter offers the reasons for choosing a qualitative approach to inquiry, describes the common elements of the qualitative research process, and shares with the reader very practical information regarding how to enter the field. Based on this overview of the important aspects of qualitative research, readers will be able to assess whether qualitative inquiry offers an opportunity to explore the questions that arise from their practice.

Without doubt, to fully engage in one of the methods discussed in this book, the reader will need a solid understanding of the method and its assumptions. In addition, it is essential to engage a research mentor (Morse, 1997). As Morse has offered, one cannot learn to drive a car by reading the manual; hence, the researcher should not assume that one could conduct a qualitative study by reading this or any other qualitative research text. A mentor will make "shifting gears" a more effective process.

INITIATING THE STUDY: CHOOSING A QUALITATIVE APPROACH

Exploring the Common Characteristics of Qualitative Research

In the conduct of research, certain attributes are common to the discovery process. This is true of both qualitative and quantitative designs. This section explores those common characteristics of qualitative research. Table 2.1 offers a comparison of qualitative and quantitative methods.

Qualitative researchers emphasize six significant characteristics in their research: (1) a belief in multiple realities, (2) a commitment to identifying an approach to understanding that supports the phenomenon studied, (3) a commitment to the participant's viewpoint, (4) the conduct of inquiry in a way that limits disruption of the natural context of the phenomena of interest, (5) acknowledged participation of the researcher in the research process, and (6) the reporting of the data in a literary style rich with participant commentaries.

TABLE 2.1	COMPARISON OF QUANTITATIVE AND QUALITATIVE RESEARCH METHODS
Quantitative	**Qualitative**
Objective	Subjectivity valued
One reality	Multiple realities
Reduction, control, prediction	Discovery, description, understanding
Measurable	Interpretative
Mechanistic	Organismic
Parts equal the whole	Whole is greater than the parts
Report statistical analyses	Report rich narrative
Researcher separate	Researcher part of research process
Subjects	Participants
Context free	Context dependent

The idea that multiple realities exist and create meaning for the individuals studied is a fundamental belief of qualitative researchers. "Qualitative researchers direct their attention to human realities rather than to the concrete realities of objects" (Boyd, 2001, p. 76). Instead of searching for one reality—one truth—researchers committed to qualitative research believe that individuals actively participate in social actions, and through these interactions that occur based on previous experiences, individuals come to know and understand phenomena in different ways. Because people do understand and live experiences differently, qualitative researchers do not subscribe to one truth but, rather, to many truths. Qualitative researchers believe that there are always multiple realities (perspectives) to consider when trying to fully understand a situation (Boyd, 2001).

Qualitative researchers are committed to discovery through the use of multiple ways of understanding. These researchers address questions about particular phenomena by finding an appropriate method or approach to answer the research question. The discovery leads the choice of method rather than the method leading the discovery. In some cases, more than one qualitative approach or more than one data collection strategy may be necessary to fully understand a phenomenon. For example, in her work on substance-dependent African American women's feelings about maternal role, Ehrmin (2001) used both participant observation and focused individual interviews to discover the nursing care needs of these women. The interviews provided the researcher with each individual's perceptions of her unique situation. The observations offered the opportunity to view the women as they "lived" their experiences. In this instance and in other qualitative research studies, researchers are committed to *discovery*. Therefore, the discovery process in qualitative research provides the opportunity for variation in the use of data collection strategies. Method and data collection strategies may change as needed, rather than being prescribed before the inquiry begins. As Maggs-Rapport (2000) suggests, "there are benefits to be derived from an approach which combines...methods and methodologies, provided that methodological rigor is applied without compromising the underlying value of any one methodology" (p. 224). This process differs from the way traditional or positivist science is developed.

Commitment to participants' viewpoints is another characteristic of qualitative research. Use of unstructured interview, observation, and artifacts grounds researchers in the real life of study participants. Researchers are co-participants in the discovery and understanding of the realities of the phenomena studied. Qualitative researchers will conduct extensive interviews and observations, searching documents and artifacts of importance to fully understand the context of what is researched. The purpose of the extensive investigation is to provide a view of reality that is important to the study participants, rather than to the researchers. For example, in research focused on African American women's experiences of breast cancer screening, Phillips, Cohen and Tarzian (2001) provided the framework for the African American women to share their experience by using a hermeneutic phenomenological approach. Instead of using an instrument to examine the women's perceptions, which would include preestablished ideas about what the women's experiences were, Phillips et al. used open-ended questions to collect their experiences. An open-ended question allowed the participants to share *their* experiences, in *their own* words, rather than being forced into preestablished lines of thinking developed by researchers.

Another characteristic of qualitative research is conduct of the inquiry in a way that does not disturb the natural context of the phenomena studied. Researchers are obligated to conduct a study so that it alters the environment of the phenomena as little as possible. Using ethnographic research to illustrate this characteristic, the ethnographer would study a particular culture with as little intrusion as possible. Living among study participants is one way to minimize the intrusion and maintain the natural context of the setting. It is unrealistic to believe that the introduction of an unknown individual will not change the nature of the relationships and activities observed; however, the researcher's prolonged presence should minimize the effect of the intrusion.

All research affects the study participants in some way. The addition of any new person or experience changes the way people think or act. The important factor in qualitative research that makes the difference is the serious attention to discovering the *emic view*, that is, the insider's perspective. What is it like for the participant? Qualitative researchers explore the insider's view with utmost respect for the individual's perspective and his or her space. As stated earlier, prolonged engagement by the researcher has the effect of reducing overt changes in behavior of those studied.

Researcher as instrument is another characteristic of qualitative research. The use of the researcher as instrument requires an acceptance that the researcher is part of the study. Because the researcher is the observer, interviewer, or the interpreter of various aspects of the inquiry, objectivity serves no purpose. Qualitative investigators accept that all research is conducted with a subjective bias. They further believe that researcher participation in the inquiry has the potential to add to the richness of data collection and analysis. Objectivity is a principle in quantitative research that documents the rigor of the science. In qualitative research, rigor is most often determined by the study participants. Do they recognize what the researcher has reported to be their culture or experience? The acknowledgment of the subjective nature of qualitative research and the understanding that researchers affect what is studied is fundamental to the conduct of qualitative inquiry.

Whether the approach is phenomenological, ethnographic, action research, grounded theory, or historical, qualitative researchers will report the study findings in a rich literary style. Participants' experiences are the findings of qualitative research. Therefore, it is essential these experiences be reported from the perspective of the people who have lived them. Inclusion of quotations, commentaries, and stories adds to the richness of the report and to the understanding of the experience and context in which they occur. Table 2.1 describes the contrasts between quantitative and qualitative research.

All six characteristics guide qualitative researchers on a journey of discovery and participation. Doing qualitative research is similar to reading a good novel. When conducted in the spirit of the philosophy that supports it, qualitative research is rich and rewarding, leaving researchers and consumers with a desire to understand more about the phenomena of interest.

Selecting the Method Based on Phenomenon of Interest

An acceptance of the basic tenets of qualitative research is the first step in deciding whether to initiate a qualitative research study. Once researchers understand that these essential elements will guide all that is done, they can begin to explore various qualitative methods. It is important to note that all qualitative approaches "share a similar goal in that they seek to arrive at an understanding of a particular phenomenon from the perspective of those experiencing the phenomenon" (Woodgate, 2000, p. 194). What the researcher will need to determine is which approach will answer the research question. The choice of method depends on the question being asked.

Because each method is explained in depth in the following chapters, the examples that follow serve only as an introduction to method selection based on the phenomena of interest. While reading the examples, keep in mind that the qualitative nurse–researcher is more concerned with values, beliefs, and meaning attached to health and illness than to aggregates of conditions (Hayes, 2001).

For example, while working in a nursing home a nurse observes individuals who seem to be very happy in their setting while others are not. The nurse is interested in discovering what the experience of living in the nursing home is for those who seem to be well adjusted. In this case, the nurse would use phenomenology to learn more about the experience of living in a nursing home from those who seem to enjoy being there. The purpose of phenomenology is to explore the lived experience of individuals. Phenomenology provides researchers with the framework for discovering what it is like to live an experience.

If the nurse–researcher is interested in the nursing home as an institution that cares for the elderly in a particular community as well as its political antecedents, a historical inquiry is the research approach of choice. Clearly, review of institutional documents such as meeting minutes, policy manuals in addition to community meeting minutes, personal documents, diaries, research papers and proceedings, newspaper articles, and commentaries will provide the information for this type of study.

Another question that might be important to answer is, What is it like to make the decision to become a nursing home resident? Based on the preceding comments, phenomenology may be the method of choice; however, assume that it is not the experience of being a resident that the researcher is interested in but, rather, the process that the individual goes through to arrive at the decision that the nursing home is the right place to be. In this case, the research method selected would be grounded theory. The researcher is more interested in understanding the process of choosing to leave one's home and enter a nursing home rather than the actual experience of being a nursing home resident. The outcome is what determines the method. More specifically, the grounded theory researcher interested in the process of choosing to leave one's residence to be cared for in a nursing home is committed to developing a theory about the process an individual goes through to arrive at that decision.

In a related situation, a nurse might be interested in studying the culture of family support groups for those with loved ones in a nursing home. The nurse–researcher would want to observe and collect information about group members, their activities, values, and life ways, as well as participate in group sessions. In doing so, a full understanding of the culture of the support group studied would become available. Ethnography would be the method of choice.

If a nurse–researcher is interested in social change as it relates to nursing home residents and their ability to participate in the setting, an action research study might be the appropriate choice. By studying those who have been active in maintaining an independent environment, the researcher has the potential to learn from the experiences of those residents who have been most involved, how they participate in maintaining their independence, and how they ultimately participated in effecting a change. In this case, the action researcher would be serving two masters: theory and practice (Jenks, 1995). Because of the action/change orientation, participatory action research would be the method of choice.

Clearly, this limited description suggests researchers may use a number of research methods to address specific practice questions. Researchers need to clearly identify the focus of the inquiry and then choose the method that will most effectively answer the question.

Understanding the Philosophic Position

After researchers have identified the research question and have made explicit the approach to studying the question, a thorough understanding of the philosophic assumptions that are the foundation of the method is essential. Too frequently, novice qualitative researchers develop and implement research studies without having a solid understanding of the philosophic underpinnings of the chosen method. This lack of understanding has the potential of leading to sloppy science, resulting in misunderstood findings. For instance, phenomenology is an approach that can be used to study lived experience. Based on the philosophic position supported by the researcher, different interpretations might occur. To further illustrate this point, phenomenologists who support Edmund Husserl—a prominent leader of the phenomenological movement—and his followers believe that the purpose of phenomenology is to provide pure understanding. Supporters of the philosophic positions of Martin Heidegger and his colleagues believe that phenomenology is interpretive. Neither group is incorrect; rather, each approaches the study of lived experience with different sets of goals and expectations.

The comments offered here should help the reader develop an appreciation for the importance of understanding the method chosen and its philosophic underpinnings. Making explicit the school of thought that guides an inquiry will help researchers to conduct a credible study and help those people who use the findings apply the results within the appropriate context.

Using the Literature Review

In the development of a quantitative research study, an interested researcher would begin with an extensive literature search on the topic of interest. This review documents the necessity for the study and provides a discussion of the area of interest and related topics. It helps the researcher determine whether the planned study has been conducted, and if so, whether significant results were discovered. Furthermore, it helps the researcher refine the research question and build a case for why the topic of interest should be studied and how the researcher will approach the topic.

Qualitative researchers do not generally begin with an *extensive* literature review. Some qualitative researchers would suggest that no literature review should be conducted before the inquiry begins. Others accept that a cursory review of the literature may help focus the study. The reason for not conducting the literature review initially is to reduce the likelihood that the investigator will develop suppositions or biases about the topic under consideration. Further, by not developing preconceived ideas about the topic, it is assumed that the researcher will be protected from leading the participants during the interviewing process in the direction of what the researcher knows or believes. For instance, if a researcher is interested in developing a theory about the process a client goes through in accepting the necessity of an amputation, the review of the literature before the study might lead to the development of preconceived notions about amputees. The researcher may not have held these beliefs before the review, but, following it, now has information that could affect how he or she collects and analyzes data. Pinch (1993) suggested that researchers learn more about phenomena when conducting qualitative studies if they are "strangers." One way to remain a stranger is to limit the acquisition of information about the focus of the study prior to conducting it.

It is, however, essential to conduct the literature review after analyzing the data. The purpose of reviewing the literature in a qualitative study is to place the findings of the study in the context of what is already known. Unlike a quantitative study, qualitative researchers do not use the literature review to establish grounds for the study or to suggest a theoretical or conceptual framework. The purpose of the literature review in a qualitative study is to tell the reader how the findings fit into what is already known about the phenomena. In addition, the literature review is not meant to confirm or argue existing findings.

Explicating the Researcher's Beliefs

Before starting a qualitative study, it is in the researcher's best interest to explicate his or her thoughts, ideas, suppositions, or presuppositions about the topic as well as personal biases. The purpose of this activity is to bring to consciousness and reveal what is believed about a topic. By bringing to consciousness the researcher's beliefs, he or she should be in a better position to approach the topic honestly and openly. Explication of personal beliefs makes the investigator more aware of the potential judgments that may occur during data collection and analysis based on the researcher's belief system rather than on the actual data collected from participants. One of the best ways to make one's beliefs known is to write them down. Writing out what one believes before actually conducting the study gives the author a frame of reference. Journaling during the time that one is engaged in the research also helps to keep an open mind and differentiate what the researcher's thoughts are versus the ideas, comments, and activities of the participants. As qualitative researchers conduct their studies, they can use their journal to "reality test" what is being observed or heard against what they have chronicled (the researcher's ideas or presuppositions).

As an example, let's say that the topic of interest is quality of life for individuals diagnosed with multiple sclerosis (MS). The researcher has an interest in the topic based on a long history of working with individuals with end-stage disease. Based on the researcher's experience, his or her perception is that people with MS live sad, limited existences. If researchers do not explicate these perceptions, they may lead informants to describe their experiences in the direction of the researchers' own beliefs about what is real or important. This can occur as a result of the questions asked. In asking questions, the researcher might try to validate his or her ideas about MS without really discovering the meaning of MS for those who live it. Remember, the way the questions are worded can affect the outcome of the interview and sometimes impose answers on respondents (McDougall, 2000). The act of expressing one's ideas should help remind the researcher to listen and see what is real for the informants rather than what is real for the researcher. Schutz (1970) recommended that researchers follow this process of describing personal beliefs about their assumptions to help them refrain from making judgments about phenomena based on personal experiences.

Once the researcher has explicated his or her thoughts, feelings, and perceptions about phenomena, it is recommended that the researcher bracket those thoughts, feelings, and perceptions. *Bracketing* is the cognitive process of putting aside one's own beliefs, not making judgments about what one has observed or heard, and remaining open to data as they are revealed. Specifically, in descriptive phenomenology, this activity is carried out before the beginning of the study and is repeated throughout data collection and analysis. In ethnographic work, keeping a diary of personal thoughts and feelings is an excellent way to explicate the researcher's ideas. Once revealed, the researcher can set them aside. *Setting them aside* means to be constantly aware of what the researcher believes and trying to keep it separate from what is being shared by the informant. By conducting this self-disclosure, researchers are more likely to be able to keep their eyes open and to remain cognizant of when data collection and analysis reflect their own personal beliefs rather than informants' beliefs.

Ahern (1999) states that the process of bracketing is iterative and part of a reflexive journey. She states that it is important to process your thoughts about the phenomenon of interest. As suggested earlier, writing down one's thoughts is one of the best ways to be aware of what you believe. Once they have been written down, you should reflect on what you have written and try to understand why you have written what you did, what are the values inherent in your statements, and how do they affect the study? It is essential that the researcher be aware of the potential impact that imposing personal agendas can have on the process of data collection and analysis. Bracketing is essential if the researcher is to share the informants' views of the studied phenomena.

Choosing the Setting for Data Collection

The setting for qualitative research is the field. The *field* is the place where individuals of interest live—where they experience life. The inquiry will be conducted in the homes, neighborhoods, classrooms, or sites selected by the study participants. The reason for conducting data collection in the field is to maintain the natural settings where phenomena occur. For instance, if an investigator is interested in studying the culture of an intensive care unit (ICU), he or she would visit an ICU. If a researcher is interested in studying the clinical decision-making skills of nurses, he or she would go to nurses who carry out this skill and ask them where they want to be interviewed or observed.

Being in the field requires reciprocity in decision making. The researcher is not in control of the study setting or those who inform the inquiry. Participants will decide what information they give the researcher access to. For instance, if the researcher was interested in studying the experiences of people who have received a cancer diagnosis, he or she would need access to people who have had this life situation. The researcher may make the decision to enter the setting and may select appropriate individuals to interview. However, participants may not wish to share their thoughts or feelings in one sitting or at all. Negotiation may be possible to obtain information that the participants are reluctant to share. It is essential to remember that using qualitative research methods requires good interpersonal skills and a willingness to relinquish control. The mutual trust that develops based on the reciprocal nature of decision making will enhance the discovery process by allowing access to personal information and private spaces usually reserved for significant persons in the lives of informants. The conduct of qualitative research with its requirement of close social interaction may create situations that can either limit or enhance access to information. The close social interaction also has the potential to create ethical dilemmas that need careful attention. Only by being aware of the distinctive nature of the interactions and being in the field will the researcher be truly aware of the strengths and potential weaknesses of this form of research.

Selecting Participants

Qualitative researchers generally do not label the individuals who inform their inquiries as *subjects*. The use of the terms *participants* or *informants* illustrates the position those studied play in the research process. That is, individuals who take part in the research are not acted on but, rather, are active participants in the study

(Morse, 1991). The participants' active involvement in the inquiry helps those who are interested in their experiences or cultures to better understand their lives and social interactions.

Individuals are selected to participate in qualitative research based on their first-hand experience with a culture, social process, or phenomenon of interest. For instance, if an ethnographer is interested in studying the culture of a first-year nursing class, then the informants for the study must be those students who have experienced and participated in the culture. The participants are selected for the purpose of describing an experience that they have been part of. Unlike quantitative research, there is no need to randomly select individuals, because manipulation, control, and generalization of findings are not the intent of the inquiry. The outcome of a qualitative study should be greater understanding of the phenomena (Krasner, 2001). Therefore, the researcher interested in a first-year nursing class culture should interview as many first-year nursing students as possible to obtain a clear understanding of the culture. Lincoln and Guba (1985) and Patton (1990) labeled this type of sampling *purposeful sampling*. It has also been called purposive sampling (Field & Morse, 1985). A similar type of sampling is *theoretical sampling* (Glaser & Strauss, 1967; Patton, 1980). Theoretical sampling, used primarily in grounded theory, is one particular type of purposeful sampling (Coyne, 1997). Theoretical sampling is a complex form of sampling based on concepts that have proven theoretical relevance to the evolving theory (Coyne, 1997; Strauss & Corbin, 1990). More specifically, Glaser (1978) states:

> Theoretical sampling is the process of data collection for generating theory whereby the analyst jointly collects, codes, and analyses his data and decides what data to collect next and where to find them in order to develop his theory as it emerges (p. 36).

Theoretical sampling "is a valuable way of encouraging studies to develop and build on theory at an early stage" (Thompson, 1999, p. 816).

What both purposeful and theoretical sampling represent is a commitment to observing and interviewing people who have had experience with or are part of the culture or phenomenon of interest. The goal for researchers is to develop a rich or dense description of the culture or phenomenon, rather than using sampling techniques that support generalizability of the findings.

Cohen, Phillips, and Palos (2001) discuss the value of including cultural minorities in qualitative research studies. They share that not only is it valuable to include minorities, but that it has been mandated by the National Institutes of Health. Therefore when studying a particular culture or phenomenon, the qualitative nurse–researcher should be aware of the importance and overall benefits of including minorities in the study when appropriate. Cohen et al. discuss the potential skepticism that may be encountered when nurses of different cultural backgrounds try to enlist members of other cultures. They suggest that nurse–researchers engage diverse populations by using some of the following strategies: (1) seek endorsement and support from community leaders, (2) commit to giving back something to the group you wish to study, (3) develop an ongoing relationship of trust and respect, (4) develop cultural competence and sensitivity, (5) become well acquainted with the group before you approach them, (6) recognize the heterogeneous nature of a group, and (7) use anthropologic strategies when conducting the research (p. 194).

Choosing the setting and participants appropriately will assist in developing a successful research study. Knowing how to access the site, knowing what to expect from those who are part of a particular group, and knowing how to most effectively develop a trusting relationship with those from whom you intend to learn will support achievement of the research goals.

Achieving Saturation

A feature that is closely related to the topic of sampling is saturation. *Saturation* refers to the repetition of discovered information and confirmation of previously collected data (Morse, 1994). This means that rather than sampling a specific number of individuals to gain significance based on statistical manipulation, the qualitative researcher is looking for repetition and confirmation of previously collected data. For example, Beck (2000) was interested in studying the experience of choosing nursing as a career. Her sample consisted of nursing students from a large university in New England. Beck continued interviewing this group until she achieved repetition of the salient points (themes). She was able to recognize the repetition and determined that the addition of new informants confirmed her findings rather than added new information. The repetitive nature of data is the point at which the researcher declares that saturation has been achieved.

Morse (1989), however, has warned that saturation may be a myth. She believes that if another group of individuals were observed or interviewed at another time, new data might be revealed. The best that a qualitative researcher can hope for in terms of saturation is to saturate the specific culture or phenomenon at a particular time.

SUMMARY

This chapter has described the common elements of qualitative research. It also offers an introduction to how a nurse–researcher makes the decision to use a qualitative approach. Based on knowledge of the expectations related to the approach and the things to consider when entering the field, this chapter lays the foundation for conducting the qualitative research study. The actual conduct of a qualitative study will be described in Chapter 3.

REFERENCES

Ahern, K. J. (1999). Ten tips for reflexive bracketing. *Qualitative Health Research*, 9(3), 407–412.
Beck, C. T. (2000). The experience of choosing nursing as a career. *Journal of Nursing Education*, 39(7), 320–322.

Boyd, C. O. (2001). Philosophical foundations of qualitative research. In P. L. Munhall (Ed.), *Nursing research: A qualitative perspective* (pp. 65–89). Sunbury, MA: Jones and Bartlett.

Cohen, M. Z., Phillips, J. M., & Palos, G. (2001). Qualitative research with diverse populations. *Seminars in Oncology Nursing, 17*(3), 190–196.

Coyne, I. T. (1997). Sampling in qualitative research. Purposeful and theoretical sampling: Merging or clear boundaries? *Journal of Advanced Nursing, 26,* 623–630.

Denzin, N. K. (2000). Aesthetics and the practice of qualitative inquiry. *Qualitative Inquiry, 6*(2), 253–265.

Ehrmin, J. T. (2001). Unresolved feelings of guilt and shame in the maternal role with substance-dependent African American women. *Journal of Nursing Scholarship, 33*(1), 47–52.

Field, P. A., & Morse, J. M. (1985). *Nursing research: The application of qualitative approaches.* Rockville, MD: Aspen.

Glaser, B. G., & Strauss, A. (1967). *The discovery of grounded theory.* Chicago: Aldine.

Glaser, B. G. (1978). *Theoretical sensitivity: Advances in the methodology of grounded theory.* Mill Valley, CA: The Sociology Press.

Hayes, P. (2001). Diversity in a global society. *Clinical Nursing Research, 10*(2), 99–101.

Jenks, J. M. (1995). New generation research approaches. In H. J. Streubert & D. R. Carpenter (Eds.), *Qualitative research in nursing* (pp. 242–268). Philadelphia: J. B. Lippincott.

Krasner, D. L. (2001). Qualitative research: A different paradigm-Part 1. *Journal of Wound, Ostomy and Continence Nurses Society, 28*(2), 70–72.

Lincoln, Y. S., & Guba, E. G. (1985). *Naturalistic inquiry.* Beverly Hills, CA: Sage.

Maggs-Rapport, F. (2000). Combining methodological approaches in research: Ethnography and interpretive phenomenology. *Journal of Advanced Nursing, 31*(1), 219–225.

McDougall, P. (2000). In-depth interviewing: The key issues of reliability and validity. *Community Practitioner, 73*(8), 722–724.

Morse, J. M. (1989). Strategies for sampling. In J. M. Morse (Ed.), *Qualitative nursing research: A contemporary dialogue* (pp. 117–131). Rockville, MD: Aspen.

Morse, J. M. (1991). Subjects, respondents, informants and participants? *Qualitative Health Research, 1*(4), 403–406.

Morse, J. M. (1994). Designing funded qualitative research. In N. K. Denzin & Y. S. Lincoln (Eds.), *Handbook of qualitative research* (pp. 220–235). Thousand Oaks, CA: Sage.

Morse, J. M. (1997). Learning to drive from a manual? *Qualitative Health Research, 7*(2), 181–183.

Patton, M.Q. (1980). *Qualitative evaluation methods.* Beverly Hills, CA: Sage.

Patton, M. Q. (1990). *Qualitative evaluation and research methods.* Newbury Park, CA: Sage.

Phillips, J. M., Cohen, M. Z., & Tarzian, A. J. (2001). African American women's experiences with breast cancer screening. *Journal of Nursing Scholarship, 33*(2), 135–140.

Pinch, W. J. (1993). Investigator as stranger. *Qualitative Health Research, 3*(4), 493–498.

Schutz, A. (1970). *On phenomenology and social relations.* Chicago: University of Chicago Press.

Strauss, A., & Corbin, J. (1990). *Basics of qualitative research: Grounded theory procedures and techniques.* Newbury Park, CA: Sage.

Thompson, C. (1999). Qualitative research into nurse decision making: Factors for consideration in theoretical sampling. *Qualitative Health Research, 9*(6), 815–828.

Woodgate, R. (2000). Part 1: An introduction to conducting qualitative research in children with cancer. *Journal of Pediatric Oncology Nursing, 17*(4), 192–206.

Designing Data Generation and Management Strategies

To implement a good qualitative research study, a researcher must make sure that the research question is clear, that the method selected to answer the question is appropriate, and that the people and data needed are available. The researcher will then set out to collect data. Once data are collected, they must be analyzed, conclusions will need to be drawn, and practice implications stated. This chapter will explore the strategies for collecting data and managing it. General concepts of qualitative research will be offered. The specifics of data generation and management to be used for particular qualitative approaches are offered in the chapter that follows.

GENERATING DATA

A variety of strategies can be used to generate qualitative research data: interviews, observations, narrative, and focus groups. "The reconstruction of social phenomena can come in a number of forms: video, photography, film and text" (Maggs-Rapport, 2000, p. 221). The strategies offered in this chapter are not meant to be exhaustive but rather descriptive of the more common data collection techniques. Each researcher will need to determine, based on the question asked, the research approach selected, the sensitivity of the subject matter, and available resources, which methods of data generation are most appropriate. For example, if the researcher is interested in investigating the experiences of comfort for clients living in a nursing home, those who agree to be interviewed may be more willing to speak in a focus group rather than face to face. As the researcher, you will need to carefully assess the research goals and then match those with the best data collection strategy.

Conducting Interviews

One of the most frequently used data collection strategies is the open-ended interview. According to Robinson (2000), it is the mainstay of qualitative nursing research. Formally defined, "the formal qualitative interview is an unstructured conversation with a purpose that usually features audiotaped and verbatim transcription of data, and use of an interview guide rather than a rigid schedule of questions" (Robinson, 2000, p. 18).

Prior to entering the field to conduct an interview, it is important for the researcher to consider the social and cultural context in which data will be collected (McDougall, 2000). The interviewer comes with a history and cultural value system and when he or she engages in an interview, on many levels the cultural and social expectations of both individuals—interviewer and interviewee—will affect what is said and what is heard. At the extreme, "differences in age, social class, race and ethnicity between the interviewer and interviewee may inhibit rapport" (p. 722). To facilitate dialogue during data collection, the researcher needs to be aware of cultural differences and work to reduce their impact as much as possible. One of the ways suggested earlier in this text is to use the researcher's journal as a place to chronicle feelings, attitudes, and values relative to the interview process and those who will be interviewed. Another suggestion is to take the time to build rapport with those from whom you will be soliciting information. In the process of building a relationship, the researcher can assure the informants that their confidentiality will be protected. McDougall (2000) also suggests that there is an important value in building trust and possessing a calm and reassuring manner.

Open-ended interviews provide participants with the opportunity to fully explain the experience of the phenomena of interest. Interviews generally are conducted face to face. To facilitate sharing by the research participants, it is a good practice to conduct the interview in a place and at a time that is most comfortable for the participants. The more comfortable each participant is, the more likely he or she will reveal the information sought.

The actual interviews can be brief with a specific objective, such as verifying previously reported information. Or interviewing can cover a longer period, either in one sitting or over a prolonged time. A life history is an example of data collection that may continue for a long time at each sitting and also over weeks, months, or years.

"The *structured interview* [italics added] refers to a situation in which an interviewer asks each respondent a series of pre-established questions with a limited set of response categories" (Fontana & Frey, 1994, p. 363). Structured interviews are more likely to occur in quantitative rather than qualitative research studies. An *unstructured interview* provides the opportunity for greater latitude in the answers provided. In the unstructured interview, the researcher asks open-ended questions, such as, "Tell me, what is the experience of nursing an abusive client?" In this example, there is no defined response. Using this question, the respondent is able to move about freely in his or her description of caring for an abusive client. The unstructured interview is a common technique in a qualitative study.

In addition to the considerations presented, there are special population-specific concerns. One in particular that has gained significant attention is age. Robinson (2000) and Docherty and Sandelowski (1999) have addressed interviewing the aged and children. Robinson found in her work with institutionalized elderly that the interview had six distinct phases. These included (1) introducing, (2) personalizing, (3) reminiscing, (4) contextualizing, (5) closing, and (6) reciprocating. In describing these phases, Robinson clearly states the relevance and importance of allowing the aged individual to lead the conversation. Although interviews may take longer with the elderly, the time for sharing is well worth the richness of the data collected.

Docherty and Sandelowski (1999) offer advice on interviewing children based on an extensive review of the literature. Based on their review, researchers should be aware that "developmental age, the target event under investigation, interview structure, multiple interviewers, and research design" are all factors requiring the interviewer's attention. In addition, Docherty and Sandelowski raise the issue of attention span and recall, both of which may not be directly linked to developmental age.

Another interview technique gaining support across disciplines is narrative picturing. The definition of this technique has been debated, according to Stuhlmiller and Thorsen (1997). Generally speaking, *narrative picturing* is a strategy that grew out of therapeutic work with survivors of trauma called Traumatic Incident Reduction (Stuhlmiller & Thorsen, 1997). In this technique, interviewers ask participants to imagine or picture an event or sequence of events as a method of describing an experience. It is a medium for conveying understanding and creating meaning of experiences (Brody, 1987; Stuhlmiller & Thorsen, 1997).

Regardless of the data collection strategies used, researchers need to gain access to participants. Access is an extremely important consideration when designing data collection strategies. When interviewing is the major way the researcher will collect data, it is important to determine how he or she will accomplish access. The way in which researchers present themselves to prospective study participants will affect the level and type of participation provided.

After the researcher gains access, it is important to establish rapport by conveying a sense of interest and concern for the research informant. The research participant must trust the researcher before he or she will feel comfortable revealing information.

Using Focus Groups

Focus groups are another strategy for collecting qualitative research data. A *focus group* is "a semi-structured group session, moderated by a group leader, held in an informal setting, with the purpose of collecting information on a designated topic" (Carey, 1994, p. 226). Although focus groups as a method of data collection did not arise from a qualitative tradition, they have been found to be most useful in a number of settings, but most importantly when dealing with sensitive topics. Focus groups are particularly suited to the collection of qualitative data because they have the advantages of being inexpensive, flexible, stimulating, cumulative, elaborative, assistive in information recall, and capable of producing rich data (Fontana & Frey, 1994; MacDougall & Baum, 1997). The major disadvantage of focus groups is *group think*, a process that occurs when stronger members of a group or segments of the group have major control or influence over the verbalizations of other group members (Carey & Smith, 1994). Generally, a good group leader can overcome the tendency of group think if he or she is mindful of its potential throughout data collection. The advantages of focus groups as a data collection strategy outweigh the disadvantage.

Focus groups have been used to collect information on a variety of topics. They are thought to be most useful when the topic of inquiry is considered sensitive. In situations in which the topic may be extremely sensitive, White and Thomson (1995) recommended using telephone focus groups. Through these groups, participants are able to maintain their anonymity as they participate in group conversations about an issue. Murray (1997) suggested using virtual focus groups, which use computer-mediated communications such as e-mail. Murray pointed out that asynchronous computer communication requires the least amount of specialized software, therefore permitting more individuals to participate. Researchers should exercise caution when using e-mail as an information exchange medium because anonymity can be compromised.

It is important to point out that the focus group is not a data collection strategy that should be engaged in without serious attention to its elements. A good focus group session has the potential to learn about both the *focus* and the *group* (Kidd & Parshall, 2000). In order to do so, the group facilitator must have a solid understanding of group process (Joseph, Griffin, & Sullivan, 2000) and should collect data with at least one other researcher/facilitator (Kidd & Parshall).

In addition, when deciding who should attend a focus group, the researcher must be certain that the people invited to participate "have a shared trait or experience on which the discussion can build on" (Lucasey, 2000). Murray (1997) advocates for group size to be between six to eight participants. Others have advocated group size of not larger than eight to 10 (Kennedy, Kools, & Krueger, 2001; Lucasey, 2000).

Recording of focus group data can be problematic and is another area that should be seriously considered before the decision is made to use this strategy for data collection. A number of authors address the complexity of transcribing recorded data when the data are being generated during a focus group. Location of the microphone, intonation, participants talking at the same time, and mechanical difficulties can all preclude complete and accurate data transcription. Joseph et al. (2000) advocate the use of videotaping as a method of data documentation during focus group activity. Videotaping has proven successful particularly with children's focus groups (Kennedy et al., 2001). Videotaping has the advantage of providing a complete recording of individual's statement, group interaction, and individual behavior; however, it also can be viewed as intrusive and a violation of privacy. Researchers interested in using videotaping will need to consider the positives and negatives in its use.

More recently, attention has been directed at the reliability and validity of focus group data. Kidd and Parshall (2000) state that there are three criteria of reliability. These are stability, equivalence, and internal consistency. Stability refers to the consistency of issues over time. Stability becomes an important issue when group membership changes from one meeting of the group to the next.

Equivalence is a term used to describe the consistency of the moderators or coders of the focus group (Kidd & Parshall, 2000). It is essential that to the extent possible, the same moderator lead the discussion with one group and across groups and that one researcher play a predominant role in analysis.

Internal consistency relates to the importance of having one team member assume the major responsibility for "conducting the analysis, participate in as many groups and debriefings as possible, and communicate regularly with other team members as the analysis proceeds" (Kidd & Parshall, 2000, p. 302).

Validity is used by Kidd and Parshall (2000) to describe a form of content validity. In other words, how convinced is the researcher that what the participants have shared is valid information? Paying careful attention to the composition of the group and interviews across groups with similar experiences are two ways to attend to validity of the data when using focus groups.

"The history of focus groups suggests that they were not originally conceived as a stand-alone method" (Kidd & Parshall, 2000). Therefore, to enhance the findings of a study that uses focus groups, the researcher should be prepared to use data triangulation. For a full description of data triangulation, the reader is referred to Chapter 15.

Narratives

Written responses by qualitative research participants are not new as a data collection strategy. Many researchers prefer written narratives to the spoken word because such narratives permit participants to think about what they wish to share. In addition, written narratives reduce costs by eliminating transcription requirements for audiotape interviews. The disadvantage of written narratives is the lack of spontaneity in responses that may occur. The popularity of the written narrative suggests it has proven itself to be an effective means of collecting qualitative research data.

In using written narratives, it becomes extremely important to be clear about what it is researchers wish the participants to write about. Because the researcher often is not present during the actual writing, it is essential that directions be focused to obtain the desired information. Researchers may need to establish mechanisms to request clarification in the event that the written document provided is unclear.

More recently, the nursing literature includes the term *narrative analysis*. Narrative analysis has been addressed primarily as a research method. Bailey (1996) defines narrative analysis as "the systematic study of stories commonly found in ethnographic interviews" (p. 187). Eaves and Kahn (2000) further share that the "terms narrative and story are used interchangeably and refer to any spoken or written presentation that includes a recounting of events that follow each other in time" (p. 29). "Narrative explains by clarifying the importance of events that have taken place based on the outcome that has resulted" (p. 29).

Narrative analysis and narrative, used here as a data collection strategy, are **not** interchangeable concepts. Researchers interested in narrative analysis should read the works of Polkinghorne (1988) and Riessman (1993) to gain a clear understanding of this valuable research methodology. Narrative as referenced here is a data collection strategy used to collect information on the focus of a qualitative research study. It is generally used *in place of* an interview.

Using Chat Rooms

With the increasing use of computer-mediated communications, the opportunities to collect data on-line grow daily. Chat rooms on the World Wide Web allow interested parties to log on and communicate synchronously. The transmissions and responses occur in real time as opposed to being delayed. A number of chat rooms are available on the Internet. Although their use as a data collection strategy has not been fully developed or completely explored, the opportunities abound. As Waskul and Douglas (1996) pointed out, computer-mediated communications present "conceptual, theoretical and methodological challenges—the resolution of which represents the seeds of academic advancement" (p. 130). It is interesting to note that despite the potential for chat rooms as a data collection strategy, little has been written about use of them. The use of chat rooms is most appropriate for data collection in situations where focus groups would serve as the most effective way to approach the research topic. Interestingly, Kirk (2000), in a study of preservice teachers and the use of chat rooms, reported that the use of chat rooms did not increase students' abilities to participate in reflective thought. However, the students offered that providing them with the opportunity to engage in the chat room did give them a forum for response that allowed them to confront issues in an anonymous way. Although the study is limited, it does offer the qualitative researcher interested in using chat rooms something to think about. Does the anonymity provided by the chat room balance the possible lack of engagement on the part of those who participate? There is not a decisive answer to this question; however, it is a question that needs to be examined before one chooses to engage a group in a chat room as a way to collect research data.

Using Participant Observation

Participant observation is a method of data collection that comes from the anthropologic tradition. Therefore, it is the method of choice in ethnography. Generally, four types of participant observation are discussed in the literature. The first is complete observer, in which the researcher is a full observer of participants' activities. There is no interaction between the researcher and participants.

Observer as participant is the second type of participant observation. In this situation, the predominant activity of the researcher is to observe and potentially to interview. The majority of the researcher's time is spent in observation, rather than participation. To "fit" into the setting, the researcher may engage in some activities with the participants.

Participant as observer is the third type of participant observation. In this situation, the researcher acknowledges interest in studying the group; however, the researcher is most interested in doing so by becoming part of the group. A great deal has been written about "going native." This phrase was coined to demonstrate the inherent problem in getting too involved. That is, the researcher becomes so engrossed in group activities, he or she loses sight of the real reason for being with the group.

The fourth type of participant observation is called *complete participant.* Complete participation requires that the researcher conceal his or her purpose. The individual becomes a member of the group. The ethical standard accepted by all disciplines makes concealment unacceptable. It is difficult, if not impossible, to justify this method. Because of a real concern for the ethics involved in data collection, individuals should not become complete participants.

Researchers should explore fully the reasons for selecting the various approaches to participant observation before initiating a study, realizing that, based on the circumstances, they may move among the approaches. There is no requirement to use only one approach. More importantly, the possibility of using only one approach is almost impossible given the nature of fieldwork (Atkinson & Hammersley, 1998). However, it is important for researchers to think carefully about which approach they are interested in using in a given situation.

Using Field Notes

Field notes are the notations ethnographers generally make to document observations. These notes become part of data analysis. When recording field notes, it is important that researchers document what they have heard, seen, thought, or experienced. Chapter 9 offers examples of types of field notes, with detailed descriptions of how to write them.

Qualitative researchers using approaches other than ethnography for their research can use field notes. The field notes or notations made by the researcher may describe observations, assumptions about what is being heard or observed, or personal narrative about what is felt by the researcher during a particular encounter. These notes can be very important during data collection and analysis. For example, in a phenomenological study conducted by the author, during the interviews, notes were used to describe the participants' expressions, changes in position, and other observations that would not be captured by voice recordings. These notes were important additions during data analysis because they provided validation for important points made by the participants and facilitated appropriate emphasis on emerging themes during data analysis.

MANAGING DATA

How researchers manage data will greatly affect the ease with which they analyze the data. As addressed earlier, researchers may collect data in a number of ways. Storage and retrieval are other important considerations. A large amount of qualitative data has the capacity to be stored on computers using a variety of available computer applications. It is beyond the scope of this book to fully share all the qualitative data collection packages available and their uses. It is important for qualitative researchers interested in using computer software to acquire and preview qualitative data analysis software and work with various software packages to determine which will be the most useful. Working with individuals who have used particular packages offers a significant opportunity to learn about the application without hours of reading and "trial and error." However, it is important to remember that what an "expert" in the program knows and what the program can do may not be the same. Therefore, gaining as much knowledge as possible about computer programs is important. Also, it is important to remember that your purpose and needs relative to data analysis may be different from the "expert" you utilize. In conclusion, the time to review data analysis packages is *before* you begin data collection. It can be very distracting and frustrating to try to develop an understanding of the software during the data collection and analysis phases of your research.

Morison and Moir (1998) report that there five classifications of qualitative data analysis packages. These are:

1. Text retrievers—such as Metamorph, Orbis, Sonar Professional, The Text Collector
2. Text base managers—such as askSam, Folio VIEWS, MAX, Tabletop
3. Code and retrievers—such as HyperQual 2, QUALPRO, the Ethnograph
4. Code-based theory builders—such as AQUAD, ATLAS/ti, HyperRE-SEARCH, NUD*IST
5. Conceptual network builders—such as Inspiration, MECA, MetaDesign, SemNet

Each class of programs has the ability to offer its user different types of information. The researcher must carefully match the programs capabilities with the goals of data analysis.

Richards and Richards (1994) offered that if data are in text format and are part of a word processing document, computer analysis offers several features. Seven of these features are as follows:

1. The ability to handle multiple documents on-screen in separate windows, which will facilitate viewing text that is similar throughout the document and will allow "cut and paste" editing
2. The ability to format files
3. The ability to include pictures, graphs, or charts to illustrate ideas
4. The ability to add video or audio data
5. Good text-searching abilities

6. Publish and subscribe facility, which allows for text to be changed in one document and automatically updated in a linked document
7. The ability to link documents using hypertext, which permits readers to easily move from document to document and creates a unique ability to annotate text using hypertext links; these links facilitate memo writing about identified information. These features are available in computer applications that would not be accessible in the more traditional storage formats such as handwritten files.

Table 3.1 offers an overview of commonly used computer packages. "The CAQDAS (Computer Assisted Qualitative Data Analysis) World Wide Web Page (http://www.soc.surrey.ac.uk/caqdas/) makes available to the research community a selection of demonstration versions of qualitative data analysis packages for download" (Lewins, 1996, p. 300) and preview.

CAQDAS Networking Project also offers "Internet resources, a support line, training courses and academic seminars" (Morison & Moir, 1998, p. 116). The

TABLE 3.1 COMPUTERIZED QUALITATIVE DATA MANAGEMENT PROGRAMS	
Computer Programs	**Source**
ATLAS/ti	SCOLARI, Sage Publications, Inc. 6 Bonhill Street London, EC2A 4PU, UK +44(0) 20-7330-1222 info@scolari.co.uk http://www.scolari.co.uk
Ethnograph (Version 5)	Qualis Research Associates P.O. Box 3356 Salt Lake City, UT 84110 (801) 532-3090 Qualis@Qualisresearch.com http://www.Qualisresearch.com
Hyper Research 2.0	Research Ware, Inc. P.O. Box 1258 Randolph, MA 02368-1258 (781) 961-3909 researchwr@aol.com http://www.researchware.com/
QRS N5 (NUD*IST)	SCOLARI, Sage Publications, Inc. 6 Bonhill Street London, EC2A 4PU, UK +44(0) 20-7330-1222 info@scolari.co.uk http://www.scolari.co.uk

Network's goal is to encourage debate and discussion in addition to training and support for social and behavioral scientists interested in use of data analysis packages (Morison & Moir, 1998).

Qualitative researchers will need to practice working with these packages and, in some cases, use computer consultants to navigate all the various program features. However, ultimately, the rewards of using a qualitative data analysis package will outweigh the time spent in learning about the various packages.

PERFORMING DATA ANALYSIS

When researchers have collected all data, it is then necessary to begin analysis. The amount of data collected and the style in which researchers have stored the data will either facilitate or impede data analysis. Analysis of qualitative research is a hands-on process. Thorne (2000) states, "unquestionably, data analysis is the most complex and mysterious of all of the phases of a qualitative project" (p. 68). Researchers must become deeply immersed in the data (sometimes referred to as "dwelling" with the data). This process requires researchers to commit fully to a structured analytic process to gain an understanding of what the data convey. It requires a significant degree of dedication to reading, intuiting, analyzing, synthesizing, and reporting the discoveries.

Data analysis in qualitative research actually begins when data collection begins. As researchers conduct interviews or observations, they maintain and constantly review records to discover additional questions they need to ask or to offer descriptions of their findings. Usually these questions or descriptions are embedded in observations and interviews. Qualitative researchers must "listen" carefully to what they have seen, heard, and experienced to discover the meanings. The cyclic nature of questioning and verifying is an important aspect of data collection and analysis. In addition to the analysis that occurs throughout the study, a protracted period of immersion occurs at the conclusion of data collection. During this period of dwelling, investigators question all prior conclusions in light of what they have discovered in the context of the whole. Generally, this period of data analysis consumes a considerable amount of time. Researchers will spend weeks or months with data based on the amount of data available for analysis.

The actual process of data analysis usually takes the form of clustering similar data. In many qualitative approaches, these clustered ideas are labeled *themes*. Themes are structural meaning units of data. DeSantis and Ugarriza (2000) tell us that themes emerge from the data; they are not superimposed on it. Further they share that "a theme is an abstract entity that brings meaning identity to a recurrent experience and its variant manifestations. As such, a theme captures and unifies the nature or basis of the experience into a meaningful whole" (p. 400). For example, in a study about clinical experience, conducted by the author, male nursing students used sports language when describing their feelings about clinical experience. For instance, two students offered the following, "I need to be part of the team. Nobody wants to be the bat boy when they can be a part of the team"

(Streubert, 1994, p. 30); and "Health care is a team-oriented profession, PT, OT, nurses, physicians. You have to interact. They all have a mutual goal and they have to interact to reach that goal. That's how I see it—as a team"(p. 30). Comments such as these lead Streubert to identify team as an essential theme in describing what clinical experience is for male nursing students.

Once researchers have explicated all themes relevant to a study, they report them in a way that is meaningful to the intended audience. In a phenomenological study, the researcher will relate the themes to one another to develop an *exhaustive description* of the experience being investigated.

Thorne (2000) shares that in each approach to qualitative data analysis, there is a different purpose for and different process used to draw conclusions. In grounded theory, the process for analyzing data is labeled *constant comparative method*. Using this process, the researcher compares each new piece of data with data previously analyzed. Questions are asked each time relative to the similarities or differences between each compared piece of data. The ultimate goal is the development of a theory about why a particular phenomenon exists as it does. What is the basic social-psychological process that is occurring? For a full description of the process, the reader is directed to Glaser and Strauss (1967).

In phenomenology, the process of interpretation may vary based on the philosophical tradition used. However, both traditions support "immersing oneself in data, engaging with data reflectively, and generating a rich description that will enlighten a reader as to the deeper essential structures underlying the human experience" (Thorne, 2000, p. 69).

For ethnographers, the focus of data analysis is to offer a description of a culture based on participant observation, interviews, and artifacts. "Ethnographic analysis uses an iterative process in which cultural ideas that arise during active involvement 'in the field' are transformed, translated or represented in written document" (Thorne, 2000, p. 69). The researcher asks questions, analyzes the answers, develops more questions, and analyzes the answers in a repeating pattern until a full picture of the culture emerges.

Regardless of the methodological approach used, the goal of data analysis is to illuminate the experiences of those who have lived them by sharing the richness of lived experiences and cultures. The researcher has the responsibility of describing and analyzing what is presented in the raw data to bring to life particular phenomena. It is only through rich description that we will come to know the experiences of others. As Krasner (2001) states, "Stories illuminate meaning, meaning stimulates interpretation, and interpretation can change outcome" (p. 72).

DEMONSTRATING TRUSTWORTHINESS

Much debate is ongoing regarding rigor or goodness in qualitative research. The debate has mostly moved beyond the positivist convention of reliability and validity. This section of the chapter takes a conservative position regarding the ongoing debate and offers a set of criteria that have been meaningful to qualitative researchers for the last 10 to 15 years. However, taking the conservative position for the sake of sharing the *fundamentals* of qualitative research does not negate the need for or the importance of the debate surrounding rigor. It is the authors' position that rigor in qualitative research is most important in demonstrating to the respective publics who read qualitative research that it is a respectable approach to science. On the other hand, there is an important need to constantly question the predominant paradigm's structure and function. Dualist thinking does not advance nursing knowledge nor does it add substantially to what we know about the people we care for or the lives they lead. Advocacy for being open to alternative ways of knowing is essential. Emden and Sandelowski (1999) offer as an important criterion for addressing rigor in qualitative research a "criterion of uncertainty" (p. 5). This criterion provides for "an open acknowledgement that claims about research outcomes are at best tentative and that there may indeed be no way of showing otherwise" (p. 5).

At the outset, it is important to state that "no one set of criteria can be expected to 'fit the bill' for every research study" (Emden & Sandelowski, 1999, p. 6). Further, it is important to recognize that ultimately, our decisions regarding the rigor in a research study amount to a judgment call (p. 6). With these two assumptions in mind, rigor in qualitative research is demonstrated through researchers' attention to and confirmation of information discovery. The goal of rigor in qualitative research is to accurately represent study participants' experiences. There are different terms to describe the processes that contribute to rigor in qualitative research. Guba (1981) and Guba and Lincoln (1994) have identified the following terms that describe operational techniques supporting the rigor of the work: credibility, dependability, confirmability, and transferability.

Credibility includes activities that increase the probability that credible findings will be produced (Lincoln & Guba, 1985). One of the best ways to establish credibility is through prolonged engagement with the subject matter. Another way to confirm the credibility of findings is to see whether the participants recognize the findings of the study to be true to their experiences (Yonge & Stewin, 1988). Lincoln and Guba (1985) call this activity "member checks" (p. 314). The purpose of this procedure is to have those people who have lived the described experiences validate that the reported findings represent their experiences.

Dependability is a criterion met once researchers have demonstrated the credibility of the findings. The question to ask is, How dependable are these results? Similar to validity in quantitative research, in which there can be no validity without reliability, the same holds true for dependability: There can be no dependability without credibility (Lincoln & Guba, 1985).

Confirmability is a process criterion. The way researchers document the confirmability of the findings is to leave an *audit trail*, which is a recording of activities over time that another individual can follow. This process can be compared to a fiscal audit (Lincoln & Guba, 1985). The objective is to illustrate as clearly as possible the evidence and thought processes that led to the conclusions. This particular criterion can be problematic, however, if you subscribe to Morse's (1989) ideas regarding the related matter of saturation. It is the position of this author that another researcher may not agree with the conclusions developed by the original researcher. Sandelowski (1998a) argues that only the researcher who has collected the data and been immersed in them can confirm the findings.

Transferability refers to the probability that the study findings have meaning to others in similar situations. Transferability has also been labeled "fittingness." The expectation for determining whether the findings fit or are transferable rests with potential users of the findings and not with the researchers (Greene, 1990; Lincoln & Guba, 1985; Sandelowski, 1986). As Lincoln and Guba (1985) have stated,

> It is...not the naturalist's task to provide an *index of transferability*; it is his or her responsibility to provide the *data base* that makes transferability judgment possible on the part of potential appliers (p. 316).

These four criteria for judging the rigor of qualitative research are important. They define for external audiences the attention qualitative researchers render to their work.

PRESENTING THE DATA

"There is no one style for reporting the findings of a qualitative research study" (Sandelowski, 1998b, p. 376). Researchers interested in sharing their results must take several things into consideration. First, who is the audience? Second, what is the purpose of the report? Third, for whom am I writing the report? Although presented linearly, the questions offered do not need to be answered linearly. The most important question, which is overarching, is, How do I most effectively communicate the findings of my study to make them useful for others?

Sandelowski (1998b) offers some important parameters in developing the research report. These include determining focus of the narrative; balancing description, analysis, and interpretation; emphasizing character, scene, or plot; deciding whose voice will be heard; and learning how to effectively use metaphor.

Determining the focus of the study is essential. The researcher must consider carefully what needs to be told. All qualitative research studies create voluminous amounts of data. The researcher needs to decide based on the purpose of his or her study what will be told. For instance, if the purpose of the study is to discover the meaning of health to those who lived in lower Manhattan in the months following the destruction of the World Trade Center, then the purpose is to tell the story of those who experienced living there. The research report should include a rich description of what the meaning of health was for those individuals given the living conditions following the collapse of the Towers.

The way in which one tells the story is guided by the purpose of the study. If the researcher is conducting a phenomenological study, then the focus is on the description with much less attention to analysis and interpretation. This is not to suggest that the raw data are presented without analysis. Rather, the researcher will have the responsibility of digesting the narrative and distilling it into a meaningful representation of a phenomenon based on those whose experiences are shared.

If, however, the purpose of the research study is to develop a theory about recovery in the aftermath of a major crisis, then the narrative will give rise to analysis and interpretation leading ultimately to the new theory. The descriptions of individuals' recovery will not be what are highlighted in the report. The descriptions will be the groundwork from which the theory will be derived. What will be highlighted is the analysis and interpretation, the reformulations of the data, that lead to the creation of the theory.

Sandelowski (1998b) suggests that qualitative researchers also might want to consider "whether the stories they want to tell are best told by emphasizing, and consciously using devices to showcase, character, scene or plot" (p. 37). For example, if the researcher has studied the history of a college of nursing over 25 years, the researcher can approach the study report in a number of ways. One way is to look at an individual. Let's say the same dean presided over the college for that period of time. The researcher can look at the institution through the eyes of the dean or can analyze the findings within the context of the dean's influence over the college's growth and development. The researcher might also look at the institution in terms of its politics. For instance, if the institution was a publicly funded entity in a state with representation whose primary agenda in the state was improving the health of the populace, then the college can be described based on the effect the politics had in its growth and development. There is no one way to tell the story. The researcher should consider carefully the emphasis of the report.

Deciding whose voice will be heard is a decision that needs careful consideration. Power structures frequently overshadow choice of research topic, data collection, sampling, and analysis. Often, researchers do not even consider how what they share is cloaked in power relationships. Although the researcher needs to stay attuned to the issues of power constantly, it is enormously important when telling the story. Whose voice will be heard and how it will be shared is extremely important. For example, if the researcher has studied the culture of a trauma unit in a major city for the purpose of sharing what life is like for the health professionals and clients who use the unit, the question should be asked whose voice will be predominate and why? If the researcher tells the story primarily from the health professionals' points of view, is there a slant on the research report that is different than if it is told from the clients' perspectives? Power is an important factor in research. It is a particularly important factor to consider in qualitative research which has as one of its underlying principles the commitment to convey the experiences of those studied.

Finally, Sandelowski (1998b) offers the importance of metaphor and its use in reporting qualitative research. She shares that frequently when metaphor is used in research reports, it is used incorrectly or incompletely. Metaphor is a powerful tool in helping the reader to fully grasp what the researcher is trying to convey. Therefore, it needs to be selected carefully. Those who choose to use it must realize that it is only a tool or device to help the reader understand the data. It is a directional tool and not an outcome.

SUMMARY

The focus of this chapter has been on data collection, management, and analysis. The reader has been offered a variety of strategies to collect data. The focus of the data management section was on the use of computer packages to handle interview data. Specific data analysis techniques were offered in general and specifically for phenomenology, grounded theory, and ethnography. Finally, important facets of trustworthiness and reporting were shared.

REFERENCES

Atkinson, P., & Hammersley, M. (1998). Ethnography and participant observation. In N. K. Denzin & Y. S. Lincoln (Eds.), *Strategies of qualitative inquiry* (pp. 110–136). Thousand Oaks, CA: Sage.

Bailey, P. H. (1996). Assuring quality in narrative analysis. *Western Journal of Nursing Research, 18*(2), 186–195.

Brody, H. (1987). *Stories of sickness.* New Haven, CT: Yale University Press.

Carey, M. A. (1994). The group effect in focus groups: Planning, implementing, and interpreting focus group research. In J. M. Morse (Ed.), *Critical issues in qualitative research methods* (pp. 225–241). Thousand Oaks, CA: Sage.

Carey, M. A., & Smith, M. W. (1994). Capturing the group effect in focus groups: A special concern for analysis. *Qualitative Health Research, 4*(1), 123–127.

DeSantis, L., & Ugarriza, D. N. (2000). The concept of theme as used in qualitative research. *Western Journal of Nursing Research, 22*(3), 351–377.

Docherty, S., & Sandelowski, M. (1999). Focus on qualitative methods: Interviewing children. *Research in Nursing and Health Care, 22,* 177–185.

Eaves, Y. D., & Kahn, D. L. (2000). Coming to terms with perceived danger. *Journal of Holistic Nursing, 18*(1), 27–45.

Emden, C., & Sandelowski, M. (1999). The good, the bad and relative, part two: Goodness and the criterion problem in qualitative research. *International Journal of Professional Nursing Practice, 5*(1), 2–7.

Fontana, A., & Frey, J. H. (1994). Interviewing: The art and science. In N. K. Denzin & Y. S. Lincoln (Eds.), *Handbook of qualitative research* (pp. 361–376). Thousand Oaks, CA: Sage.

Glaser, B. G., & Strauss, A. (1967). *The discovery of grounded theory.* Chicago: Aldine.

Greene, J. C. (1990). Three views on nature and role of knowledge in social science. In E. Guba (Ed.), *The paradigm dialogue* (pp. 227–245). Newbury Park, CA: Sage.

Guba, E. G. (1981). Criteria for assessing the trustworthiness of naturalistic inquiries. *Educational Communication and Technology Journal, 29,* 75–92.

Guba, E. G., & Lincoln Y. S. (1994). Competing paradigms in qualitative research. In N. K. Denzin & Y. S. Lincoln (Eds.), *Handbook of qualitative research* (pp. 105–117). Thousand Oaks, CA: Sage.

Joseph, D. H., Griffin, M., & Sullivan, E. D. (2000). Videotaped focus groups: Transforming a therapeutic strategy into a research tool. *Nursing Forum, 35*(1), 15–20.

Kennedy, C., Kools, S., & Krueger, R. (2001). Methodological considerations in children's focus groups. *Nursing Research, 50*(3), 184–187.

Kidd, P. S., & Parshall, M. B. (2000). Getting the focus and the group: Enhancing analytical rigor in focus group research. *Qualitative Health Research, 10*(3), 293–309.

Kirk, R. (2000). A study of the use of a private chat room to increase reflective thinking in preservice teachers. *College Student Journal, 34*(1), 115–123.

Krasner, D. L. (2001). Qualitative research: A different paradigm—Part 1. *Journal of Wound, Ostomy and Continence Nurses Society, 28*(2), 70–72.

Lewins, A. (1996). The CAQDAS Networking Project: Multilevel support for the qualitative research community. *Qualitative Health Research, 6(2)*, 298–303.

Lincoln, Y. S., & Guba, E. (1985). *Naturalistic inquiry*. Beverly Hills, CA: Sage.

Lucasey, B. (2000). Qualitative research and focus group methodology. *Orthopedic Nursing, 19(1)*, 53–55.

MacDougall, C., & Baum, F. (1997). The devil's advocate: A strategy to avoid group think and stimulate discussion in focus groups. *Qualitative Health Research, 7(4)*, 532–541.

Maggs-Rapport, F. (2000). Combining methodological approaches in research: Ethnography and interpretive phenomenology. *Journal of Advanced Nursing, 31(1)*, 219–225.

McDougall, P. (2000). In-depth interviewing: The key issues of reliability and validity. *Community Practitioner, 73(8)*, 722–724.

Morison, M., & Moir, J. (1998). The role of computer software in the analysis of qualitative data: efficient clerk, research assistant or Trojan horse? *Journal of Advanced Nursing, 28(1)*, 106–116.

Morse, J. M. (1989). Strategies for sampling. In J. M. Morse (Ed.), *Qualitative nursing research: A contemporary dialogue* (pp. 117–131). Rockville, MD: Aspen.

Murray, P. J. (1997). Using virtual focus groups in qualitative research. *Qualitative Health Research, 7(4)*, 542–549.

Patton, M. Q. (1980). *Qualitative evaluation methods*. Beverly Hills, CA: Sage.

Polkinghorne, D. E. (1988). *Narrative knowing and the human sciences*. Albany: State University of New York Press.

Richards, T. J., & Richards, L. (1994). Using computers in qualitative research. In N. K. Denzin & Y. S. Lincoln (Eds.), *Handbook of qualitative research* (pp. 445–462). Thousand Oaks, CA: Sage.

Riessman, C. K. (1993). *Narrative analysis*. Newbury Park, CA: Sage.

Robinson, J. P. (2000). Phases of the qualitative research interview with institutionalized elderly individuals. *Journal of Gerontological Nursing, 26(11)*, 17–23.

Sandelowski, M. (1986). The problem of rigor in qualitative research. *Advances in Nursing Science, 8(3)*, 27–37.

Sandelowksi, M. (1998a). The call to experts in qualitative research. *Research in Nursing & Health, 21*, 467–471.

Sandelowski, M. (1998b). Writing a good read: Strategies for re-presenting qualitative data. *Research in Nursing and Health, 21*, 375–382.

Streubert, H. J. (1994). Male nursing students' perceptions of clinical experience. *Nurse Educator, 19(5)*, 28–32.

Stuhlmiller, C. M., & Thorsen, R. (1997). Narrative picturing: A new strategy for qualitative data collection. *Qualitative Health Research, 7(1)*, 140–149.

Thorne, S. (2000). Data analysis in qualitative research. *Evidence-Based Nursing, 3(3)*, 68–70.

Waskul, D., & Douglas, M. (1996). Considering the electronic participant: Some polemical observations on the ethics of on-line research. *Information Society, 12*, 129–139.

White, G. E., & Thomson, A. N. (1995). Anonymized focus groups as a research tool for health professionals. *Qualitative Health Research, 5(2)*, 256–261.

Yonge, O., & Stewin, L. (1988). Reliability and validity: Misnomers for qualitative research. *The Canadian Journal of Nursing, 20(2)*, 61–67.

Writing a Qualitative Research Proposal

The implementation of any research study requires clear articulation of the question and appropriate application of the method. Once these components are developed a proposal must be presented to the designated review boards. The research proposal is essentially a formal request to conduct a study. The proposal generally includes the problem and purpose statements, a review of relevant literature, and a detailed description of the planned study methodology. The proposal must communicate, in a formal manner, the critical material necessary for a review board to grasp the scope and significance of the investigation. Additionally, the proposal is essential for the conduct and possible funding of any research project. This chapter will explore issues related to the development of a qualitative research proposal, elements of the research report, and challenges facing qualitative researchers. A discussion of the essential elements and philosophical underpinnings relevant to a qualitative research proposal is important given the increased interest in these methodological approaches to the development of a research agenda. The reader is also referred to Chapter 17 for an example of a funded qualitative proposal.

SELECTING AN AREA OF RESEARCH

Beck (1997) emphasized that "A productive research program for nurse scientists in both academic and clinical settings is critical to career advancement" (p. 265). Given the significance one's scholarly work can potentially have on a professional career, selecting an area of research must be guided by several factors. First and foremost the researcher must be immersed enough in the nursing research literature to know what areas of research have been developed and where research is still needed. Since research in nursing is still evolving, myriads of opportunities exist to select an area of interest and develop a research agenda that is relevant and that will make a meaningful contribution to nursing's substantive body of knowledge. Secondly, it is critical to select an area of research that is not only meaningful to the discipline but also to the researcher. One's research agenda should essentially merge with one's professional career in nursing practice, education, or administration. The effort needed and the significant amount of time required to develop a research agenda requires that the researcher become immersed in and feel connected to what they are doing. Boyd and Munhall (2001) articulate this position skillfully:

> On some level, most researchers settle on a research topic because of some personal reason. Even for the opportunistic researcher with an eye on funding priorities, personal interest is usually aroused with ties to the researcher as person. For the qualitative researcher, personal interest is a strategic tool in the research project; it provides the energy and the motivation to persevere with the challenges and tedium inherent in any scholarly work. More importantly, however, personal interest can position the researcher to attend to the phenomenon under study in a certain way; it establishes figure and ground for the research endeavor in what can be highly personalized ways that make the research a passion, a preoccupation, an intimate companion (p. 615).

Additionally, establishing an area of research requires that the investigator confirm the significance of the problem and articulate not only why the study needs to be done, but also why the study requires a qualitative format. This stage is complex, and requires diligence and clarity of thought. The process is one that takes time and requires an ongoing process of evaluation. Reading, sharing ideas with colleagues, writing, and rewriting are all necessary aspects of the refinement of one's research agenda. When conducting a qualitative study for the first time, investigators inexperienced in this methodology should consider enlisting the help of a seasoned qualitative researcher to serve as a mentor during the development of a new project. For a detailed discussion of specific methodologies and a selected review of qualitative research topics, the reader should refer to the chapters that follow.

GENERAL CONSIDERATIONS

Identifying a research agenda requires that the researcher make clear the problem or phenomenon of interest to be studied. Articulating the need for a particular study and clarifying one's purpose will provide the appropriate direction needed to proceed with proposal development. Ideas must be logically developed and clearly articulated.

Determining scientific merit and quality of the proposal are guided by the researcher's ability to articulate the research paradigm and method. The conduct of any research study requires precision and rigor. The proposal must be clear, concise, and complete (Dexter, 2000). Knowledge of qualitative methodology, prior experience with the methodology and availability of appropriate resources to successfully complete the study are important considerations. The depth required of a research proposal is essentially determined by its ultimate purpose. Variation exists depending on whether you are preparing a proposal for a dissertation, a grant, or an individual research project. For academics, guidelines can generally be obtained from the office of research services. If you are writing a grant proposal, then the granting agency's requirements determine how you prepare your materials. The content of the proposal must address all the stipulations set forth in enough depth to be meaningful, clear, and educational.

Brink and Woods (2001) differentiate between the development of a research plan and a research proposal.

> The research plan is the basic outline of your entire research idea, with your bibliography cards, your working definitions, and so on. Your research proposal is your essay that fills in all the gaps of the outline, makes all the logical transitions for the reader, and shows the consistent development of the idea from question to answer (pp. 241–242).

Therefore, once a general plan has been devised for a qualitative research project, the proposal must follow with enough detail to clarify and ensure rigor of method for all those who must review it.

Very often, members of institutional review boards are grounded in quantitative research approaches. Therefore, the composition of the board may result in qualitative research proposals that face unnecessary obstacles. Qualitative research cannot be evaluated from a quantitative paradigm. This should be clear at this point in the textbook. The abstract nature of many qualitative approaches is so different from a qualitative worldview that the proposal will require excellent rationale and explanation of qualitative method applications. The proposal should be written in such a way as to provide enough theoretical support for the research paradigm so as to answer the questions of individuals reviewing the project that may not be familiar with qualitative approaches. The content of any proposal must always be written with the interest and expertise of the reviewers in mind. According to Boyd and Munhall (2001), when the *"guardians of the dominant paradigm"* (p. 614) are reviewing your qualitative research proposal, the readers should be provided with:

- Education about and description of the method from its aim to its outcome. Such detail also enhances confirmability by leaving a decision trail.
- Justification for using the method through a logically developed explanation of why the researcher has chosen to use it.
- Translation of language unique to the method in terms that are likely to be understood by readers (p. 614).

The overall appearance of the proposal is an additional consideration. It is expected that the work is done professionally; therefore, in addition to articulate and accurate content, the writer must also ensure that there are no spelling, punctuation, or grammatical errors. The document must be aesthetically appealing in addition to being described clearly (Dexter, 2000). The reader will now be provided with an overview of the essential components of the research proposal. The detail needed to complete a written account of each aspect of the proposal can be found in method-specific chapters.

ELEMENTS OF THE RESEARCH PROPOSAL

The purpose of the research proposal is similar for both quantitative and qualitative research paradigms. The document must communicate to the reviewers the essential elements of the study in such a way that the study's purpose, method, data generation, and treatment strategies are clear and methodologically precise. Further, the document must communicate to the reader that the participants of the project will be protected from harm. An overview of each component of the proposal follows. Box 4.1 lists the elements that should be included in a complete proposal. Once again, the reader is referred to Chapter 17 for a reprint of a research proposal that received funding for the conduct of a phenomenological investigation. As with any document, the writer should begin with an introduction and overview of the project.

Introduction and Overview of the Project

Any research study must begin with a judgment regarding the importance of the project to the development of knowledge in the discipline. Introducing the study requires identification of the phenomenon of interest, the problem statement, and purpose. The researcher must clearly describe the background and significance of the project. Linking the proposed investigation to the current body of nursing knowledge adds to the development of the significance of the research for the discipline of nursing and verifies that what is currently known about the topic is insufficient, requiring additional investigation. The literature review refines the questions and builds the case for the conduct of the study.

Chapter 2 addresses issues related to the conduct of the literature review in a qualitative investigation. The discussion addresses the fact that often qualitative researchers do not begin with an extensive literature review to reduce the likelihood that researchers might bias their data collection or analysis through development of preconceived notions about the topic under investigation. Should the qualitative researcher choose to maintain this standard, then rationale should be provided for the reviewers. In any case, the researcher should include a cursory review of the literature.

Marshall and Rossman (1999) suggest the following questions when addressing the significance of a particular study: (1) Who has interest in this area of inquiry?; (2) What is already known about the topic?; (3) What has not been answered adequately in previous research and practice?; and (4) How will this research add to knowledge, practice and policy in this area? Answering these questions in relationship to a particular research study will add clarity to the proposal.

Research Approach

Following the study's introduction, it is important to discuss the rationale for selecting a qualitative format, and the philosophical underpinnings that support the approach. Qualitative research approaches vary, and consequently the conceptual foundations that support the approaches vary as well. The underlying

Box 4.1

ELEMENTS OF THE RESEARCH PROPOSAL

The Introduction

1. Identify the phenomenon or problem of interest
2. Statement of purpose
3. Rationale for research approach
4. Significance of the phenomenon to nursing

The Literature Review

1. Review of relevant theoretical and research literature
2. Discussion of literature review and how it will be used in the qualitative investigation

The Research Design

1. Introduce the research design (phenomenology, grounded theory, ethnography, action research, historical research)
2. Describe the philosophical correlates
3. List the procedural steps
4. Describe strengths and potential limitations of the design

Methodology

1. Researcher's role and credentials
2. Participant selection/sample
3. Gaining access, entering the setting for data generation
4. Protection of participants and ethical considerations relevant to qualitative inquiry
5. Data generation and treatment (process, data collector's training, data management, data analysis)

Discussion of Communication of the Findings

1. Within the proposal briefly address how the findings will be addressed within the context of the literature review
2. Address rigor in relationship to the method
3. Discuss implications for nursing practice, education, and administration
4. What are the implications for future research?

References

Appendices

1. Consent forms
2. Any other relevant supporting documents

assumptions relevant to the qualitative methodology selected must be described in detail. See Chapter 2 for a detailed discussion of how different qualitative approaches may be used to study particular phenomena.

Method

Once the phenomenon of interest has been fully described and the research approach is selected, the investigator must then proceed with a detailed discussion of the actual application of the design. This is a critical component of the proposal. Discussion of the research protocol will ensure consistent application of the method. Decisions made related to method application are essential to the overall cohesiveness of the project. They culminate in a road map of how the study will be conducted. The method also has implications related to resources needed to conduct the study such as time, money, and personnel.

Within the section addressing method, the strengths and weaknesses of the research design must also be addressed. A level of expertise in the application of qualitative methods is expected from the researcher and should be evident in a description of the researcher's credentials. If the individual is not a skilled qualitative researcher, then the mentor's credentials should be included. The emerging nature of a qualitative investigation should also be addressed. Explicit description of the philosophical correlates guiding method application will enhance the credibility of the proposal. The researcher should also address the possibility that the study may need to be modified at any point during implementation. The rationale for potential modifications must be provided (Sandelowski, Davis, & Harris, 1989).

In addition to the researcher's credentials, the proposal must include how participants will be selected, how the researcher will gain entry into the setting where data will be collected, and once there how the rights of participants will be protected. For a detailed discussion of protection of human subjects and the ethical issues facing qualitative researchers, the reader is referred to Chapter 16.

Data generation and treatment in a qualitative investigation generally consists of in-depth interviewing. Often the interviews are tape-recorded and can range from very open-ended to very structured interviews. Data analysis techniques should be discussed along with issues related to how the researcher will ensure authenticity and trustworthiness of the data (see Chapter 3).

Protection of Human Subjects

Protection of human subjects is without question a critical component of any research study and must be addressed articulately in the proposal. "The government's system for regulating research involving human subjects was born out of fear that researchers might, whether wittingly or not, physically or mentally injure the human beings that they study" (American Association of University Professors, 2001, p. 55). This report further notes that "IRB's, in carrying out their responsibilities, too often mistakenly apply standards of clinical and biomedical research to social science research, to the detriment of the latter" (p. 56). Clearly, informed consent takes on a new and different meaning when applied to qualitative studies as opposed to clinical or biomedical research. For this reason Boyd and Munhall (2001) have suggested that qualitative researchers address the idea of *process consent* as opposed to *informed consent*. This essentially involves renegotiating informed consent throughout the study as data emerge and the research evolves. If the proposal author plans to use process consent, then this type of consent should be explained fully in terms of its definition and application.

Qualitative Research Findings

The proposal is prepared in an effort to gain permission to conduct a formal study. Although the results cannot be addressed in the proposal, a brief discussion of why the findings will be important and how they will be used may be helpful in adding a sense of completeness to the proposal. Again, the writer must be sure to address the specific guidelines provided as they relate to the type of proposal being written.

Appendices and References

Appendices and references of the proposal should include an example of the consent form to be used as well as any other supplemental material to be included in the research. For example, if participants will be asked to write detailed responses to open-ended questions, the format and items to be included should be placed in the appendix. The reference list provided will verify the need for the study and will substantiate the researcher's expertise in the research area as well as the methodology planned.

SUMMARY

This chapter has addressed issues related to the development of a qualitative research proposal. The fundamental elements necessary for proposal development are highlighted along with some suggestions for avoiding roadblocks with institutional review boards. Detailed discussions of all elements of the proposal are included within individual chapters of this book. Further, application is addressed in the sample grant in Chapter 17.

REFERENCES

American Association of University Professors. (2001). Protecting human beings: Institutional review boards and social science research. *ACADEME* (May-June), 55–67.

Beck, C. T. (1997). Developing a research program using qualitative and quantitative approaches. *Nursing Outlook, 45,* 265–269.

Boyd, C. O., & Munhall, P. L. (2001). Qualitative research proposals and reports. In P. L. Munhall (Ed.), *Nursing research: A qualitative perspective* (3rd ed., pp. 613–638). Boston: Jones and Bartlett.

Brink, P. J., & Woods, M. J. (2001). *Basic steps in planning nursing research: From question to proposal.* Boston: Jones and Bartlett.

Dexter, P. (2000). Tips for scholarly writing in nursing. *Journal of Professional Nursing, 16*(1), 6–12.

Marshall, C., & Rossman, G. B. (1999). *Designing qualitative research* (3rd ed.). New York: Altamira Press.

Sandelowski, M., Davis, D. H., & Harris, B. G. (1989). Artful design: Writing the proposal for research in the naturalist paradigm. *Research in Nursing and Health, 12*(2), 77–84.

Phenomenology as Method

Phenomenology has been and continues to be an integral field of inquiry that cuts across philosophical, sociologic, and psychologic disciplines. This rigorous, critical, systematic method of investigation is a recognized qualitative research approach applicable to the study of phenomena important to the discipline of nursing. Phenomenological inquiry brings to language perceptions of human experience with all types of phenomena. Because professional nursing practice is enmeshed in people's life experiences, phenomenology as a research approach is well suited to the investigation of phenomena important to nursing.

As several authors have noted, phenomenology, both as philosophy and research approach, allows nursing to explore and describe phenomena important to the discipline (Beck, 1994; Caelli, 2000; Todres & Wheeler, 2001; Van der Zalm & Bergum, 2000).

Phenomenological inquiry as a philosophy and developing science continues to undergo interpretation and explication in terms of its pragmatic use as a nursing research method. This chapter addresses the variety of methodological interpretations detailed within the discipline of phenomenological inquiry. Phenomenology as philosophy and as method is discussed along with fundamental differences between descriptive and interpretive phenomenology. Highlights of specific elements and interpretations of phenomenology as a research approach provide readers with a beginning understanding of common phenomenological language and themes. Chapter 5 also addresses methodological concerns specific to conducting a phenomenological investigation.

Introductory concepts for researchers interested in conducting a phenomenological investigation are presented in the content that follows. The reader should keep in mind that there is no quick step-by-step method to phenomenological inquiry. The methodology is philosophically complex and the analytic processes required to participate in the method require scientific discipline. Researchers interested in following through with a qualitative investigation must read original philosophically based work and identify a mentor with expertise in the discipline to acquire an in-depth understanding of phenomenology both as a philosophy and as a research approach.

PHENOMENOLOGY DEFINED

Phenomenology is a science whose purpose is to describe particular phenomena, or the appearance of things, as lived experience. Cohen (1987) has pointed out that phenomenology was first described as the study of phenomena or things by Immanuel Kant in 1764. Merleau-Ponty (1962) asked the question, What is phenomenology?, in the preface to his text *Phenomenology of Perception*. His description reflects the flow of phenomenological thinking, but Merleau-Ponty never offered a definitive answer as to what phenomenology actually entailed. Essentially, not much has changed in the past 40 years. Merleau-Ponty offered the following description:

> Phenomenology is the study of essences; and according to it, all problems amount to finding definitions of essences: the essence of perception, or the essence of consciousness, for example. But phenomenology is also a philosophy, which puts essences back into existence, and does not expect to arrive at an understanding of man and the world from any starting point other than that of their "facticity." It is a transcendental philosophy which places in abeyance the assertions arising out of the natural attitude, the better to understand them: but it is also a philosophy for which the world is always "already there" before reflection begins—as an inalienable presence; and all its efforts are concentrated upon re-achieving a direct and primitive contact with the world, and endowing that contact with a philosophical status. It is the search for a philosophy which shall be a "rigorous science," but it also offers an account of space, time and the world as we "live" them. It tries to give a direct description of our experience as it is, without taking account of its psychological origin and the causal explanations which the scientist, the historian or the sociologist may be able to provide (p. vii).

The historian Herbert Spiegelberg (1975) explained phenomenology as a movement, rather than a uniform method or set of doctrines. The account provided by Spiegelberg emphasizes the fluid nature of phenomenology and the fact that a list of steps to the approach would not reflect the philosophical depth of the discipline. Spiegelberg defined phenomenology as "the name for a philosophical movement whose primary objective is the direct investigation and description of phenomena as consciously experienced, without theories about their causal explanation and as free as possible from unexamined preconceptions and presuppositions" (p. 3).

Spiegelberg (1975) and Merleau-Ponty (1962) described phenomenology as both a philosophy and a method. Phenomenology was further explained by Wagner (1983) as a way of viewing ourselves, others, and everything else whom or with which we come in contact in life. "Phenomenology is a system of interpretation that helps us perceive and conceive ourselves, our contacts and interchanges with others, and everything else in the realm of our experiences in a variety of ways, including to describe a method as well as a philosophy or way of thinking" (Wagner, 1983, p. 8).

Omery (1983) addressed the question, What is the phenomenological method? Although researchers have interpreted this question in a variety of ways, the approach is inductive and descriptive in its design. Phenomenological method is "the trick of making things whose meanings seem clear, meaningless, and then, discovering what they mean" (Blumensteil, 1973, p. 189).

Lived experience of the world of everyday life is the central focus of phenomenological inquiry. Schutz (1970) described the world of everyday life as the "total sphere of experiences of an individual which is circumscribed by the objects, persons, and events encountered in the pursuit of the pragmatic objectives of living" (p. 320). In other words, it is the lived experience that presents to the individual what is true or real in his or her life. Furthermore, it is this lived experience that gives meaning to each individual's perception of a particular phenomenon and is influenced by everything internal and external to the individual. Perception is important in phenomenological philosophy and method, as explained by Merleau-Ponty (1956):

> Perception is not a science of the world, nor even an act, a deliberate taking up of a position. It is the basis from which every act issues and it is presupposed by them. The world is not an object the law of whose constitution I possess. It is the natural milieu and the field of all my thoughts and of all my explicit perceptions. Truth does not "dwell" only in the "interior man" for there is no interior man. Man is before himself in the world and it is in the world that he knows himself. When I turn upon myself from the dogmatism of common sense or the dogmatism of science, I find, not the dwelling place of intrinsic truth, but a subject committed to the world (p. 62).

Phenomenology is as much a way of thinking or perceiving as it is a method. The goal of phenomenology is to describe lived experience. To further clarify both the philosophy and method of phenomenology, it is helpful to gain a sense of how the movement developed historically. An overview of the roots of phenomenology as a philosophy and science follows.

PHENOMENOLOGICAL ROOTS

The phenomenological movement began around the first decade of the twentieth century. This philosophical movement consisted of three phases: (1) Preparatory, (2) German, and (3) French. The following describes common themes of phenomenology within the context of these three phases.

Preparatory Phase

The Preparatory phase was dominated by Franz Brentano (1838–1917) and Carl Stumpf (1848–1936). Stumpf was Brentano's first prominent student, and through his work demonstrated the scientific rigor of phenomenology. Clarification of the concept of intentionality was the primary focus during this time (Spiegelberg, 1965). *Intentionality* means that consciousness is always consciousness of something. Merleau-Ponty (1956) explained "interior perception is impossible without exterior perception, that the world as the connection of phenomena is anticipated in the consciousness of my unity and is the way for me to realize myself in consciousness" (p. 67). Therefore, one does not hear without hearing something or believe without believing something (Cohen, 1987).

German Phase

Edmund Husserl (1857–1938) and Martin Heidegger (1889–1976) were the prominent leaders during the German or second phase of the phenomenological movement. Husserl (1931, 1965) believed that philosophy should become a rigorous science that would restore contact with deeper human concerns and that phenomenology should become the foundation for all philosophy and science. According to Spiegelberg (1965), Heidegger followed so closely in the steps of Husserl that his work is probably a direct outcome of Husserl's. The concepts of essences, intuiting, and phenomenological reduction were developed during the German phase (Spiegelberg, 1965).

Essences are elements related to the ideal or true meaning of something, that is, those concepts that give common understanding to the phenomenon under investigation. Essences emerge in both isolation and in relationship to one another. According to Natanson (1973), "Essences are unities of meaning intended by different individuals in the same acts or by the same individuals in different acts" (p. 14). Essences, therefore, represent the basic units of common understanding of any phenomenon. For example, in a study on experiences of elder women living off of the coast of Maine, Roberts & Cleveland (2001) describe the essences (or basic units of common understanding) related to the experiences of elder women living alone. The essences described included: "no one is an island, no one lives alone; securely anchored in safe harbor; and weathering the storms" (p. 45). In another study by Tarzian (2000) entitled "Caring for Dying Patients Who Have Air Hunger," the major themes or essences described were "(a) the patient's look—panic beckons, (b) surrendering and sharing control, and (c) fine-tuning dying indicated ways nurses responded to relieve a patient's air hunger, including being prepared before air hunger occurs, calming patients and families, medicating patients, improvising care, attending to family members' needs, and drawing a distinction between palliating and killing" (p. 137). Neil and Munjas (2000) describe the experience of living with a chronic wound as "Contending with the wound and staying home" and "Staying back." Themes of oozing and smelling, losing sleep, being in pain, and noticing are described in the article (p. 28).

Intuiting is an eidetic comprehension or accurate interpretation of what is meant in the description of the phenomenon under investigation. The intuitive process in phenomenological research results in a common understanding about the phenomenon under investigation. Intuiting in the phenomenological sense requires that researchers imaginatively vary the data until a common understanding about the phenomenon emerges. Through imaginative variation, researchers begin to wonder about the phenomenon under investigation in relationship to the various descriptions generated. To further illustrate, in a study on commitment to nursing (Rinaldi, 1989), the essences of commitment gleaned from the data were varied in as many ways as possible and compared with participants' descriptions.

From this imaginative variation, a relationship between the essences of commitment and to whom or what the nurse was committed emerged. For example, the nurse may be committed to clients, colleagues, the employing institution, the profession, or self. To whom or what the nurse is committed is then examined in relationship to the essences of commitment. Researchers might vary the essences of commitment with each example of the person to whom or thing to which the nurse is committed. Some essences may apply when the issue is commitment to clients and other essences if the issue is commitment to the institution.

Phenomenological reduction is a return to original awareness regarding the phenomenon under investigation. Husserl specified how to describe, with scientific exactness, the life of consciousness in its original encounter with the world through phenomenological reduction. Husserl (1931, 1965) challenged individuals to go "back to the things themselves" to recover this original awareness. Husserl's reference "to the things" meant "a fresh approach to concretely experienced phenomena, as free as possible from conceptual presuppositions and an attempt to describe them as faithfully as possible" (Spiegelberg, 1975, p. 10).

Phenomenological reduction begins with a suspension of beliefs, assumptions, and biases about the phenomenon under investigation. Isolation of pure phenomenon, versus what is already known about a particular phenomenon, is the goal of the reductive procedure. The only way to really see the world clearly is to remain as free as possible from preconceived ideas or notions. Complete reduction may never be possible because of the intimate relationship individuals have with the world (Merleau-Ponty, 1956).

As part of the reductive process, phenomenological researchers must first identify any preconceived notions or ideas about the phenomenon under investigation. Having identified these ideas, the researchers must bracket or separate out of consciousness what they know or believe about the topic under investigation. *Bracketing* requires researchers to remain neutral with respect to belief or disbelief in the existence of the phenomenon. Bracketing begins the reductive process and, like that process, must continue throughout the investigation. Essentially, researchers set aside previous knowledge or personal beliefs about the phenomenon under investigation to prevent this information from interfering with the recovery of a pure description of the phenomenon. Bracketing must be constant and ongoing if descriptions are to achieve their purest form. Haggman-Laitila (1999) holds the position that the researcher cannot detach from his or her own view and offers practical aspects to help in overcoming the researcher's views during data gathering and analysis. Chapter 16 offers an overview of strategies to address this very issue within the context of ethical standards.

French Phase

Gabriel Marcel (1889–1973), Jean Paul Sartre (1905–1980), and Maurice Merleau-Ponty (1905–1980) were the predominant leaders of the French or third phase of the phenomenological movement. The primary concepts developed during this phase were embodiment and being-in-the-world. These concepts refer to the belief that all acts are constructed on foundations of perception or original awareness of some phenomenon. Lived experience, given in the perceived world, must be described (Merleau-Ponty, 1956). Munhall (1989) explained these key concepts, originally described by Merleau-Ponty, as follows:

> Embodiment explains that through consciousness one is aware of being-in-the-world and it is through the body that one gains access to this world. One feels, thinks, tastes, touches, hears, and is conscious through the opportunities the body offers. There is talk sometimes about expanding the mind or expanding waistlines. The expansion is within the body, within the consciousness. It is important to understand that at any point in time and for each individual a particular perspective and/or consciousness exists. It is based on the individual's history, knowledge of the world, and perhaps openness to the world. Nursing's focus on the individual and the "meaning" events may have for an individual, is this recognition that experience is individually interpreted (p. 24).

The philosophical underpinnings of phenomenology are complex. Given this understanding one can appreciate why the methodological applications remain dynamic and evolving. Different philosophers may have different interpretations of phenomenology as both a philosophy and method. The dynamic nature and evolving interpretations provide phenomenological researchers with a variety of options from which to choose when embarking on an investigation of this nature. The content that follows presents these options, in a very pragmatic format, along with other issues related to actually conducting a phenomenological investigation.

At this particular juncture the following words of caution are offered: Imperative to gaining an in-depth understanding of the method and philosophy of phenomenology is a return to the original works. Readers should take the time to read the works of Husserl, Heidegger, Merleau-Ponty, Spiegelberg, Ricoeur, Gadamer, and others to ensure a solid foundation and understanding of the philosophy behind the method. It is also advised that beginning researchers connect with a mentor who can guide their development in the area of phenomenology. Paley (1997) suggested that "a problematic feature of the way in which phenomenology has been imported into nursing is that sources tend to be second-hand and several 'tiers' in the literature are apparent" (p. 187). Paley's work addresses how original concepts can become distorted when interpreted secondhand and emphasizes the point made earlier; researchers who are embarking on a phenomenological investigation must return to the original works, secure a mentor with expertise in the discipline, and recognize that there is no simplistic step-by-step approach to phenomenological inquiry.

FUNDAMENTAL CHARACTERISTICS OF THE PHENOMENOLOGICAL METHOD

Phenomenology as a research method is a rigorous, critical, systematic investigation of phenomena. "The purpose of phenomenological inquiry is to explicate the structure or essence of the lived experience of a phenomenon in the search for the unity of meaning which is the identification of the essence of a phenomenon, and its accurate description through the everyday lived experience" (Rose, Beeby, & Parker, 1995, p. 1124).

Several procedural interpretations of phenomenological method are available as guidelines to this research approach (Colaizzi, 1978; Giorgi, 1985; Paterson & Zderad, 1976; Spiegelberg, 1965, 1975; Streubert, 1991; van Kaam, 1959; van Manen, 1984). Because there is more than one legitimate way to proceed with a phenomenological investigation, the researcher must be familiar with the philosophical underpinnings and ground the study in the approach that would offer the most rigorous and accurate interpretations of the phenomenon under investigation. Appropriateness of the method to the phenomenon of interest should guide the method choice. Clearly, phenomenology is grounded in a variety of philosophical positions and procedural interpretations. The philosophical underpinnings of phenomenology are critical to the discipline. The guidelines in Table 5.1 provide meaningful direction for method application and highlight various procedural interpretations. Once again the reader is encouraged to return to the original works to ensure a comprehensive understanding of the philosophical positions associated with the method. Chapter 6 provides a critical discussion of method application along with selected examples of research that apply the approaches described in Table 5.1.

TABLE 5.1	METHODOLOGICAL INTERPRETATIONS
Author	**Procedural Steps**
van Kaam (1959)	1. Obtain a core of common experiences.
	2. List and prepare a rough preliminary grouping of every expression presented by participants.
	3. Reduce and eliminate.
	Test each expression for two requirements:
	(a) Does it contain a moment of the experience that might eventually be a necessary and sufficient constituent of the experience?
	(b) If so, is it possible to abstract this moment and to label it, without violating the formulation presented by the participant?
	Expressions not meeting these two requirements are eliminated. Concrete, vague, and overlapping expressions are reduced to more exactly descriptive terms. Example: "I feel like I could pull my hair out by the roots" could be reduced to "feelings of frustration."
	4. Tentatively identify the descriptive constituents; bring together all common relevant constituents in a cluster labeled with the more abstract formula expressing the common theme.

(continued)

TABLE 5.1   METHODOLOGICAL INTERPRETATIONS (CONTINUED)

Author	Procedural Steps
	5. Finally, identify the descriptive constituents by application; this operation consists of checking the tentatively identified constituents against random cases of the sample to see whether they fulfill the following conditions: Each constituent must: (a) be expressed explicitly in the description. (b) be expressed explicitly or implicitly in some or the large majority of descriptions. (c) be compatible with the description in which it is not expressed. If a description is found incompatible with a constituent, the description must be proven not to be an expression of the experience under study, but of some other experience that intrudes on it.
Giorgi (1985)	1. Read the entire description of the experience to get a sense of the whole. 2. Reread the description. 3. Identify the transition units of the experience. 4. Clarify and elaborate the meaning by relating constituents to each other and to the whole. 5. Reflect on the constituents in the concrete language of the participant. 6. Transform concrete language into the language or concepts of science. 7. Integrate and synthesize the insight into a descriptive structure of the meaning of the experience.
Paterson & Zderad (1976)	1. Compare and study instances of the phenomenon wherever descriptions of it may be found (putting descriptions in a logbook). 2. Imaginatively vary the phenomenon. 3. Explain through negation. 4. Explain through analogy and metaphor. 5. Classify the phenomenon.
Colaizzi (1978)	1. Describe the phenomenon of interest. 2. Collect participants' descriptions of phenomenon. 3. Read all participants' descriptions of the phenomenon. 4. Return the original transcripts and extract significant statements.

(continued)

TABLE 5.1	METHODOLOGICAL INTERPRETATIONS (CONTINUED)
	5. Try to spell out the meaning of each significant statement.
	6. Organize the aggregate formalized meanings into clusters of themes.
	7. Write an exhaustive description.
	8. Return to the participants for validation of the description.
	9. If new data are revealed during the validation, incorporate them into an exhaustive description.
van Manen (1984)	1. Turn to the nature of lived experience by orienting to the phenomenon, formulating the phenomenologic question, and explicating assumptions and pre-understandings.
	2. Engage in existential investigation, which involves exploring the phenomenon: generating data, using personal experience as a starting point, tracing etymologic sources, searching idiomatic phrases, obtaining experiential descriptions from participants, locating experiential descriptions in the literature, and consulting phenomenologic literature, art, and so forth.
	3. Engage in phenomenologic reflection, which involves conducting thematic analysis, uncovering thematic aspects in life-world descriptions, isolating thematic statements, composing linguistic transformations, and gleaning thematic descriptions from artistic sources.
	4. Engage in phenomenologic writing, which includes attending to the speaking of language, varying the examples, writing, and rewriting.
Streubert (1991)	1. Explicate a personal description of the phenomenon of interest.
	2. Bracket the researcher's presuppositions.
	3. Interview participants in unfamiliar settings.
	4. Carefully read the interview transcripts to obtain a general sense of the experience.
	5. Review the transcripts to uncover essences.
	6. Apprehend essential relationships.
	7. Develop formalized descriptions of the phenomenon.
	8. Return to participants to validate descriptions.
	9. Review the relevant literature.
	10. Distribute the findings to the nursing community.

Six Core Steps

Spiegelberg (1965, 1975) identified a core of steps or elements central to phenomenological investigations. These six steps are (1) descriptive phenomenology, (2) phenomenology of essences, (3) phenomenology of appearances, (4) constitutive phenomenology, (5) reductive phenomenology, and (6) hermeneutic phenomenology (Spiegelberg, 1975). A discussion of each of the six elements follows. As Spiegelberg (1965) has explained, the purpose of this discussion is to "present this method as a series of steps, of which the later will usually presuppose the earlier ones, yet not be necessarily entailed by them" (p. 655). As such, phenomenology as a movement is described. A combination of one or more of the elements identified as central to the movement can be found in the plethora of published qualitative investigations.

Descriptive Phenomenology

Descriptive phenomenology involves "direct exploration, analysis, and description of particular phenomena, as free as possible from unexamined presuppositions, aiming at maximum intuitive presentation" (Spiegelberg, 1975, p. 57). Descriptive phenomenology stimulates our perception of lived experience while emphasizing the richness, breadth, and depth of those experiences (Spiegelberg, 1975, p. 70). Spiegelberg (1965, 1975) identified a three-step process for descriptive phenomenology: (1) intuiting, (2) analyzing, and (3) describing.

Intuiting

The first step, *intuiting*, requires the researcher to become totally immersed in the phenomenon under investigation and is the process whereby the researcher begins to know about the phenomenon as described by the participants. The researcher avoids all criticism, evaluation, or opinion and pays strict attention to the phenomenon under investigation as it is being described (Spiegelberg, 1965, 1975).

The step of intuiting the phenomenon in a study of quality of life would involve the "researcher as instrument" in the interview process. The researcher becomes the tool for data collection and listens to individual descriptions of quality of life through the interview process. The researcher then studies the data as they are transcribed and reviews repeatedly what the participants have described as the meaning of quality of life.

Analyzing

The second step is *phenomenological analyzing*, which involves identifying the essence of the phenomenon under investigation based on data obtained and how the data are presented. As the researcher distinguishes the phenomenon with regard to elements or constituents, he or she explores the relationships and connections with adjacent phenomena (Spiegelberg, 1965, 1975).

As the researcher listens to descriptions of quality of life and dwells with the data, common themes or essences will begin to emerge. Dwelling with the data essentially involves complete immersion in the generated data to fully engage in this analytic process. The researcher must dwell with the data for as long as necessary to ensure a pure and accurate description.

Describing

The third step is *phenomenological describing*. The aim of the describing operation is to communicate and bring to written and verbal description distinct, critical elements of the phenomenon. The description is based on a classification or grouping of the phenomenon. The researcher must avoid attempting to describe a phenomenon prematurely. Premature description is a common methodological error associated with this type of research (Spiegelberg, 1965, 1975). Description is an integral part of intuiting and analyzing. Although addressed separately, intuiting and analyzing are often occurring simultaneously.

In a study on quality of life, phenomenological describing would involve classifying all critical elements or essences that are common to the lived experience of quality of life and describing these essences in detail. Critical elements or essences are described singularly and then within the context of their relationship to one another. A discussion of this relationship follows.

Phenomenology of Essences

Phenomenology of essences involves probing through the data to search for common themes or essences and establishing patterns of relationships shared by particular phenomena. *Free imaginative variation,* used to apprehend essential relationships between essences, involves careful study of concrete examples supplied by the participants' experiences and systematic variation of these examples in the imagination. In this way, it becomes possible to gain insights into the essential structures and relationships among phenomena. Probing for essences provides a sense for what is essential and what is accidental in the phenomenological description (Spiegelberg, 1975). The researcher follows through with the steps of intuiting, analyzing, and describing in this second core step (Spiegelberg, 1965, 1975). According to Spiegelberg (1975), "Phenomenology in its descriptive stage can stimulate our perceptiveness for the richness of our experience in breadth and in depth" (p. 70).

Phenomenology of Appearances

Phenomenology of appearances involves giving attention to the ways in which phenomena appear. In watching the ways in which phenomena appear, the researcher pays particular attention to the different ways in which an object presents itself. Phenomenology of appearances focuses attention on the phenomenon as it unfolds through dwelling with the data. Phenomenology of appearances "can heighten the sense for the inexhaustibility of the perspectives through which our world is given" (Spiegelberg, 1975, p. 70).

Constitutive Phenomenology

Constitutive phenomenology is studying phenomena as they become established or "constituted" in our consciousness. Constitutive phenomenology "means the process in which the phenomena 'take shape' in our consciousness, as we advance from first impressions to a full 'picture' of their structure" (Spiegelberg, 1975, p. 66). According to Spiegelberg (1975), constitutive phenomenology "can develop the sense for the dynamic adventure in our relationship with the world" (p. 70).

Reductive Phenomenology

Reductive phenomenology, although addressed as a separate process, occurs concurrently throughout a phenomenological investigation. The researcher continually addresses personal biases, assumptions, and presuppositions or sets aside these beliefs to obtain the purest description of the phenomenon under investigation. Suspending judgment can make us more aware of the precariousness of all our claims to knowledge, "a ground for epistemological humility" (Spiegelberg, 1975, p. 70).

This step is critical for the preservation of objectivity in the phenomenological method. For example, in a study investigating the meaning of quality of life for individuals with type I (insulin-dependent) diabetes mellitus, the investigator begins the study with the reductive process. The researcher identifies all presuppositions, biases, or assumptions he or she holds about what quality of life means or what it is like to have diabetes. This process involves a critical self-examination of personal beliefs and an acknowledgment of understandings that the researcher has gained from experience. The researcher takes all he or she knows about the phenomenon and brackets it or sets it aside in an effort to keep what is already known separate from the lived experience as described by the participants.

Phenomenological reduction is critical if the researcher is to achieve pure description. The reductive process is also the basis for postponing any review of the literature until the researcher has analyzed the data. The researcher must always keep separate from the participants' descriptions what he or she knows or believes about the phenomenon under investigation. Therefore, postponing the literature review until data analysis is complete facilitates phenomenological reduction.

INTERPRETIVE NURSING RESEARCH AND HERMENEUTIC PHILOSOPHY

Interpretive frameworks within phenomenology are used to search out the relationships and meanings that knowledge and context have for each other (Lincoln & Guba, 1985). Increasingly, published nursing research is grounded in the philosophical theory of hermeneutics (see Table 6.1) and several authors have discussed the philosophical underpinnings of this particular research approach, offering clarity and direction for others (Geanellos, 1999; Todres & Wheeler, 2001; Van der Zalm & Bergum, 2000). A phenomenological-hermeneutic approach is essentially a philosophy of the nature of understanding a particular phenomenon and the scientific interpretation of phenomena appearing in text or written word. Hermeneutics as an interpretive approach is based on the work of Ricoeur (1976), Heidegger (1927/1962), and Gadamer (1976). Allen and Jenson (1990) emphasized that:

> The value of knowledge in nursing is, in part, determined by its relevance to and significance for an understanding of the human experience. In order to obtain that understanding, nursing requires modes of inquiry that offer the freedom to explore the richness of this experience. Hermeneutics offers such a mode of inquiry. With this interpretive strategy, a means is provided for arriving at a deeper understanding of human existence through attention to the nature of language and meaning. (p. 241)

Hermeneutic phenomenology is a "special kind of phenomenological interpretation, designed to unveil otherwise concealed meanings in the phenomena" (Spiegelberg, 1975, p. 57). Gadamer (1976) elaborated by noting that hermeneutics bridges the gap between what is familiar in our worlds and what is unfamiliar: "Its field of application is comprised of all those situations in which we encounter meanings that are not immediately understandable but require interpretive effort" (p. xii). As in all research, congruence between the philosophical foundations of the study and the methodological processes of the research are critical. The basic elements of hermeneutic philosophy and interpretive inquiry are addressed in the following narrative within the context of the work of Ricoeur (1976), Heidegger (1927/1962), and Gadamer (1976).

Paul Ricoeur's interpretive approach is one way in which nurse researches can apply hermeneutic philosophy to a qualitative investigation. Ricoeur (1976) described the interpretive process as a series of analytic steps and acknowledged the "interrelationship between epistemology (interpretation) and ontology (interpreter)" (Geanellos, 2000, p. 112). Analysis is essentially the hermeneutic circle, which proceeds from a naïve understanding to an explicit understanding that emerges from explanation of data interpretation. There are three main steps:

1. First, during the *naïve reading*, the researcher reads the text as a whole to become familiar with the text and begins to formulate thoughts about its meaning for further analysis. Lindholm, Uden, and Rastem (1999) in a study on nursing management note that during this particular component of data analysis they "read all the interviews individually to gain a sense of the whole text. Their impressions of the text were then documented and discussed. The naïve reading directed attention to the phenomenon of power" (p. 103).

2. *Structural analysis* follows as the second step and involves identifying patterns of meaningful connection. This step is often referred to as an *interpretive reading*. To illustrate, Lindholm et al. (1999) noted that the researchers met to compare and discuss the texts. They describe this step in the follow-

ing manner: "The text was divided into meaning units, which were transformed with the contents intact. Arising from every transformed meaning unit a number of labels were created, to discover common themes. During the analysis there was continuous movement between the whole and the parts of the text" (p. 103).

3. Thirdly, *interpretation of the whole* follows and involves reflecting on the initial reading along with the interpretive reading to ensure a comprehensive understanding of the findings. Several readings are usually required. Lindholm et al. (1999) performed a separate interpretation of their data during this step and described themes and subthemes within the data.

Ricoeur (1981) has addressed the difference between text and discourse, referring to these differences as distancing. The four principles of distancing are (1) the transcription itself and the meaning of the written word, (2) the relationship between what has been written and the intent of the person who wrote the text, (3) the meaning of the text beyond its original intent as well as the author's original intent, and (4) the new interpreted meaning of the written word and the audience.

As described by Allen and Jenson (1990):

The hermeneutical circle of interpretation moves forward and backward, starting at the present. It is never closed or final. Through rigorous interaction and understanding, the phenomenon is uncovered. The interpretive process that underlies meaning arises out of interactions, working outward and back from self to event and event to self (p. 245).

Allen and Jenson (1990) illustrated the application of hermeneutic inquiry in their exploration of what it means to have eye problems and to be visually impaired. Their example emphasizes the applicability of hermeneutics in the description and explanation of human phenomena. According to Allen and Jenson (1990):

The task...of modern hermeneutics is to describe and explain human phenomena (such as health and illness). The purpose of hermeneutical description and explanation is to achieve understanding through interpretation of the phenomena under study. It is the written description of the phenomena (text) that is the object of interpretation (p. 242).

Interpretive phenomenology is a valuable method for the study of phenomena relevant to nursing education, research, and practice. Several investigations have used interpretive phenomenology in areas such as educational innovation (Diekelmann, 2001), caring for dying patients with air hunger (Tarzian, 2000), and examining the experience of isolation in blood and marrow transplantation (Cohen, Ley, & Tarzian, 2001).

Examples of the different interpretations describing phenomenology are outlined in Table 5.1. Applying any of these interpretations to a particular investigation will require a careful examination of the researcher's role, generation and treatment of data, and ethical issues connected with a phenomenological investigation. A discussion of these topics as they relate to the selection of phenomenology as a research method follows.

SELECTION OF PHENOMENOLOGY AS METHOD

How do researchers decide to use the phenomenological method for the investigation of phenomena important to nursing? This is a complex decision that should be grounded in the understanding that the approach selected must be the best one to answer the questions relevant to the study. Nursing's philosophical beliefs about humans and the holistic nature of professional nursing will provide direction and guidance as well.

Nursing encourages detailed attention to the care of people as humans and grounds its practice in a holistic belief system that nurses care for mind, body, and spirit. Holistic care and avoidance of reductionism are at the center of professional nursing practice. The holistic approach to nursing is rooted in the nursing experience and is not imposed artificially from without. Just as caring for only part of the client is inconsistent with nursing practice, so, too, is the study of humans by breaking them down into parts. The following example illustrates the nature of holistic nursing practice. When caring for a client who has had a mastectomy, the nurse addresses not only body image but also the effect the surgery may have on family, work, and psychological well-being. The nurse might ask, "How are you feeling about your surgery?" or "What kinds of changes in your life do you anticipate as a result of your mastectomy?" These questions elicit more about the client as a person, with a life and feelings, as opposed to a question such as, "Do you want to look at the scar?" An approach that deals only with the body part removed narrows the understanding of the overall impact of this life-altering event and can potentially result in misdirected care.

Because phenomenological inquiry requires that the integrated whole be explored, it is a suitable method for the investigation of phenomena important to nursing practice, education, and administration. Spiegelberg (1965) remarked that phenomenological method investigates subjective phenomena in the belief that essential truths about reality are grounded in lived experience. What is important is the experience as it is presented, not what anyone thinks or says about it. Therefore, investigation of phenomena important to nursing requires that researchers study lived experience as it is presented in the everyday world of nursing practice, education, and administration.

A holistic perspective and the study of experience as lived serve as the foundation for phenomenological inquiry. A positive response to the following questions will help researchers clarify if phenomenological method is the most appropriate approach for the investigation. First, researchers should ask, Is there a need for further clarity on the chosen phenomenon? Evidence leading researchers to conclude that they need further clarity may be that there is little if anything published on a subject, or perhaps what is published needs to be described in more depth. Second, researchers should consider the question, Will the shared lived experience be the best data source for the phenomenon under investigation? Because the primary method of data collection is the voice of the people experiencing a particular phenomenon, researchers must determine that this approach will provide the richest and most descriptive data. Third, as in all research, investigators should ask, What are the available resources, the time frame for the completion of the research, the audience to which the research will be presented, and my own personal style and ability to engage in the method in a rigorous manner while accepting the inherent ambiguity?

Topics appropriate to phenomenological research method include those central to humans' life experiences. Examples include happiness, fear, being there, commitment, being a chairperson, being a head nurse, or the meaning of stress for nursing students in the clinical setting. Health-related topics suitable for phenomenological investigation might include a myriad of topics including the meaning of pain, living with chronic illness, and end of life issues. Chapter 6 offers readers a selective sample of published research using phenomenological research methodology in the areas of practice, education, and administration.

ELEMENTS AND INTERPRETATIONS OF THE METHOD

Researcher's Role

As lived experience becomes the description of a particular phenomenon, the investigator takes on specific responsibilities in transforming the information. Reinharz (1983) articulated five steps that occur in phenomenological transformation as the investigator makes public what essentially was private knowledge. The first transformation occurs as people's experiences are transformed into language. During this step, the researcher, through verbal interaction, creates an opportunity for the lived experience to be shared (Reinharz, 1983). In the example of research on quality of life for individuals with type I diabetes mellitus, the researcher would create an opportunity for individuals living with this chronic illness to share their experiences related to the meaning of quality of life.

The second transformation occurs as the researcher transforms what is seen and heard into an understanding of the original experience. Because one person can never experience what another person has experienced in exactly the same manner, researchers must rely on the data participants have shared about a particular experience and from those develop their own transformation (Reinharz, 1983). In this instance, the researcher studying quality of life takes what participants have said and produces a description that lends understanding to the participants' original experiences.

Third, the researcher transforms what is understood about the phenomenon under investigation into conceptual categories that are the essences of the original experience (Reinharz, 1983). Data analysis of interviews addressing the meaning of quality of life would involve clarifying the essences of the phenomenon. For example, the data may reveal that quality of life for an individual with type I diabetes mellitus may center around freedom from restrictions in daily activities, independence, and prevention of long-term complications.

Fourth, the researcher transforms those essences into a written document that captures what the researcher has thought about the experience and reflects the participants' descriptions or actions. In all transformations, information may be lost or gained; therefore, it is important to have participants review the final description to ensure the material is correctly stated and nothing has been added or deleted (Reinharz, 1983).

Fifth, the researcher transforms the written document into an understanding that can function to clarify all preceding steps (Reinharz, 1983). The intent of this written document, often referred to as the exhaustive description, is to synthesize and capture the meaning of the experience into written form without distorting or losing the richness of the data. In other words, the exhaustive description of quality of life would reveal the richness of the experience identified from the very beginning of the investigation as perceived by individuals with type I diabetes mellitus.

In addition to the five transformational steps outlined by Reinharz (1983), the investigator must possess certain qualities that will permit access to data participants possess. The abilities to communicate clearly and to help participants feel comfortable expressing their experiences are essential qualities in a phenomenological researcher. The researcher is the instrument for data collection and must function effectively to facilitate data collection. The researcher must recognize that personal characteristics such as manner of speaking, gender, age, and other personality traits may interfere with data retrieval. For this reason, researchers must ask whether they are the appropriate people to access a given person's or group's experiences (Reinharz, 1983).

Data Generation

Purposeful sampling is used most commonly in phenomenological inquiry. This method of sampling selects individuals for study participation based on their particular knowledge of a phenomenon for the purpose of sharing that knowledge. "The logic and power of purposeful sampling lies in selecting information-rich cases for study in depth. Information-rich cases are those from which one can learn a great deal about issues of central importance to the purpose of the research, thus the term purposeful sampling" (Patton, 1990, p. 169).

Sample selection provides the participants for the investigation. Researchers should contact participants, once they have agreed to participate, before the interview to prepare them for the actual meeting and to answer any preliminary questions. At the time of the first interview, the researcher may obtain informed consent and permission to tape-record if using this data-gathering instrument. Piloting interview skills and having a more experienced phenomenological researcher listen to the tape of an interview can assist in the development of interviewing skills. According to Benoliel (1988), an "effective observer-interviewer needs to bring knowledge, sensitivity, and flexibility into a situation. Interviewing is not an interpersonal exchange controlled by the interviewer but rather a transaction that is reciprocal in nature and involves an exchange of social rewards" (p. 211).

Researchers should help participants describe lived experience without leading the discussion. Open-ended, clarifying questions such as the following facilitate this process: What comes to mind when you hear the word *commitment*? What comes to mind when you think about quality of life? Open-ended interviewing allows researchers to follow participants' lead, to ask clarifying questions, and to facilitate the expression of the participants' lived experience. Interviews usually end when participants believe they have exhausted their descriptions. If interviews are not feasible, researchers may ask participants to write an extensive description of some phenomenon by responding to a preestablished question or questions. The concern with written responses versus tape-recorded interviews is that saturation may not be achieved. During the interview, researchers can help participants explain things in more detail by asking questions. This valuable opportunity is eliminated when participants write their descriptions.

The interview allows entrance into another person's world and is an excellent source of data. Complete concentration and rigorous participation in the interview process improve the accuracy, trustworthiness, and authenticity of the data. However, researchers must remember to remain centered on the data, listen attentively, avoid interrogating participants, and treat participants with respect and sincere interest in the shared experience.

Data generation or collection continues until the researcher believes saturation has been achieved, that is, when no new themes or essences have emerged from the participants and the data are repeating. Therefore, predetermination of the number of participants for a given study is impossible. Data collection must continue until the researcher is assured saturation has been achieved.

Morse (1989) stated that saturation is a myth. She proposed that, given another group of informants on the same subject at another time, new data may be revealed. Therefore, investigators will be able to reach saturation only with a particular group of informants and only during specific times. "The long term challenge for the phenomenologist interested in generating theory is to interview several samples from a variety of backgrounds, age ranges and cultural environments to maximize the likelihood of discovering the essences of phenomena across groups" (Streubert, 1991, p. 121).

Ethical Considerations

The personal nature of phenomenological research results in several ethical considerations for researchers. Informed consent differs in a qualitative study as opposed to a quantitative investigation. There is no way to know exactly what might transpire during an interview. Researchers must consider issues of privacy. When preparing a final manuscript, researchers must determine how to present the data so that they are accurate yet do not reveal participants' identities. For an in-depth discussion of ethical issues in qualitative research, see Chapter 16.

Data Treatment

Researchers may handle treatment of the data in a variety of ways. Use of open-ended interviewing techniques, tape recordings, and verbatim transcriptions will increase the accuracy of data collection. High-quality tape-recording equipment is essential. Researchers will also make handwritten notes. Adding handwritten notes to verbally transcribed accounts helps to achieve the most comprehensive and accurate description. A second interview may be needed, giving researchers an opportunity to expand, verify, and add descriptions of the phenomenon under investigation and assist participants in clarifying and expounding on inadequate descriptions. In addition, often participants will have additional thoughts about the phenomenon under study after the initial interview. Following an interview, researchers should immediately listen to the tape, checking that the interview made sense and verifying the need for a follow-up interview. Also, researchers should make extensive, detailed notes immediately following the interview in case the tape recording has failed.

When data collection begins, so, too, does data analysis. From the moment researchers begin listening to descriptions of a particular phenomenon, analysis is occurring. These processes are inseparable. Therefore, the importance of the reductive process cannot be overemphasized. Separating one's beliefs and assumptions from the raw data occurs throughout the investigation. Journaling helps in continuing the reductive process. Researchers' use of a journal can facilitate phenomenological reduction. Writing down any ideas, feelings, or responses that emerge during data collection supports reductive phenomenology. Drew (1989) has offered the added perspective that journaling that addresses a researcher's own experience can be "considered data and examined within the context of the study for the part it has played in the study's results" (p. 431).

Following data collection and verbatim transcription, researchers should listen to the tapes while reading the transcriptions for accuracy. This step will help to familiarize them with the data and begin immersing them in the phenomenon under investigation.

Data Analysis

Data analysis requires that researchers dwell with or become immersed in the data. The purpose of data analysis, according to Banonis (1989), is to preserve the uniqueness of each participant's lived experience while permitting an understanding of the phenomenon under investigation. This begins with listening to participants' verbal descriptions and is followed by reading and rereading the verbatim transcriptions or written responses. As researchers become immersed in the data, they may identify and extract significant statements. They can then transcribe these statements onto index cards or record them in a data management file for ease of ordering later in the process. Apprehending or capturing the essential relationships among the statements and preparing an exhaustive description of the phenomenon constitutes the final phase. Through free imaginative variation, researchers make connections between statements obtained in the interview process. It is critical to identify how statements or central themes emerged and are connected to one another if the final description is to be comprehensive and exhaustive.

Microcomputers and word processing software can make data storage and retrieval more efficient. Examining available software packages for qualitative data analysis may be an appropriate option, depending on researchers' personal preferences. See Chapter 3 for an in-depth discussion of data generation and management strategies including available software for data storage, retrieval, and analysis.

Review of the Literature

The review of literature generally follows data analysis. The rationale for postponing the literature review is related to the goal of achieving a pure description of the phenomenon under investigation. The fewer ideas or preconceived notions researchers have about the phenomenon under investigation, the less likely their biases will influence the research. A cursory review of the literature may be done to ensure the necessity of the study and the appropriateness of method selection. Once data analysis is complete, researchers review the literature to place the findings within the context of what is already known about the topic.

Trustworthiness and Authenticity of Data

The issue of trustworthiness in qualitative research has been a concern for researchers engaging in these methods and is discussed at length in the literature (Beck, 1993; Krefting, 1991; Yonge & Stewin, 1988). The issue of rigor in qualitative research is important to the practice of good science.

The trustworthiness of the questions put to study participants depends on the extent to which they tap the participants' experiences apart from the participants' theoretical knowledge of the topic (Colaizzi, 1978). Consistent use of the method and bracketing prior knowledge helps to ensure pure description of data. To ensure trustworthiness of data analysis, researchers return to each participant and ask if the exhaustive description reflects the participant's experiences. Researchers should incorporate content added or deleted by participants into a revised description.

Requesting negative descriptions of the phenomenon under investigation is helpful in establishing authenticity and trustworthiness of the data. For example, in the study investigating the meaning of quality of life in individuals with type I diabetes mellitus, the researcher may ask, "Can you describe a situation in which you would feel that you did not have quality of life?" This question gives an opportunity to compare and contrast data. For additional discussion of issues surrounding reliability and validity in qualitative research, see Chapter 2.

SUMMARY

Phenomenology is an integral field of inquiry to nursing, as well as philosophy, sociology, and psychology. As a research method, phenomenology is a rigorous science whose purpose is to bring to language human experiences. The phenomenological movement has been influenced by the works of Husserl, Brentano, Stumpf, Merleau-Ponty, and others. Concepts central to the method include intentionality, essences, intuiting, reduction, bracketing, embodiment, and being-in-the-world.

Phenomenology as a method of research offers nursing an opportunity to describe and clarify phenomena important to practice, education, and research. Researchers selecting this approach for the investigation of phenomena should base their decision on suitability and a need for further clarification of selected phenomenon. Specific consideration must be given to the issues of researcher as instrument, data generation, data treatment and authenticity, and trustworthiness of data. Investigations that use this approach contribute to nursing's knowledge base and can provide direction for future investigations.

The relevance of phenomenology as a research method for nursing is clear. Within the qualitative paradigm, this method supports "new initiatives for nursing care where the subject matter is often not amenable to other investigative and experimental methods" (Jasper, 1994, p. 313). Nursing maintains a unique appreciation for caring, commitment, and holism. Phenomena related to nursing can be explored and analyzed by phenomenological methods that have as their goal the description of lived experience.

REFERENCES

Allen, M. N., & Jenson, L. (1990). Hermeneutical inquiry, meaning and scope. *Western Journal of Nursing Research, 12*(2), 241–253.

Banonis, B. C. (1989). The lived experience of recovering from addiction: A phenomenological investigation. *Nursing Science Quarterly, 2*(1), 37–42.

Beck, C. T. (1993). Qualitative research: The evaluation of its credibility, fittingness, and auditability. *Western Journal of Nursing Research, 15*(2), 263–265.

Beck, C. T. (1994). Phenomenology: Its use in nursing research. *International Journal of Nursing Studies, 31*(6), 499–510.

Benoliel, J. Q. (1988). Commentaries on special issue. *Western Journal of Nursing Research, 10*(2), 210–213.

Blumensteil, A. (1973). A sociology of good times. In G. Psathas (Ed.), *Phenomenological sociology: Issues and applications.* New York: Wiley.

Caelli, K. (2000). The changing face of phenomenological research: Traditional and American phenomenology in nursing. *Qualitative Health Research, 10*(3), 366–377.

Cohen, M. Z. (1987). A historical overview of the phenomenological movement. *Image, 19*(1), 31–34.

Cohen, M. Z., Ley, C., & Tarzian, A. J. (2001). Isolation in blood and marrow transplantation, *Journal of Nursing Scholarship, 23*(6), 592–609.

Colaizzi, P. F. (1978). Psychological research as the phenomenologist views it. In R. Valle & M. King (Eds.), *Existential phenomenological alternative for psychology* (pp. 48–71). New York: Oxford University Press.

Diekelmann, N. (2001). Narrative pedagogy: Heideggerian hemeneutical analysis of lived experiences of students, teachers, and clinicians. *Advances in Nursing Science, 23*(3), 53–71.

Drew, N. (1989). The interviewer's experience as data in phenomenological research. *Western Journal of Nursing Research, 11*(4), 431–439.

Gadamer, H. G. (1976). *Philosophical hermeneutics* (D. E. Linge, Trans. & Ed.). Los Angeles: University of California Press.

Geanellos, R. (2000). Exploring Ricoeur's hermeneutic theory of interpretation as a method of analyzing research texts. *Nursing Inquiry, 7*(2), 112–119.

Giorgi, A. (1985). *Phenomenology and psychological research.* Pittsburgh, PA: Duquesne University Press.

Haggman-Laitila, A. (1999). The authenticity and ethics of phenomenological research: How to overcome the researcher's own views. *Nursing Ethics, 6*(1), 12–22.

Heidegger, M. (1962). *Being and time.* New York: Harper & Row. (Original work published 1927.)

Husserl, E. (1931). *Ideas: General introduction to pure phenomenology* (W. R. Boyce Gibson, Trans.). New York: Collier.

Husserl, E. (1965). *Phenomenology and the crisis of philosophy* (Q. Laver, Trans.). New York: Harper & Row.

Jasper, M. A. (1994). Issues in phenomenology for researchers of nursing. *Journal of Advanced Nursing, 19*, 309–314.

Krefting, L. (1991). Rigor in qualitative research: The assessment of trustworthiness. *American Journal of Occupational Therapy, 45*(3), 214–222.

Lincoln, Y. S., & Guba, E. G. (1985). *Naturalistic inquiry.* Beverly Hills, CA: Sage.

Lindholm, M., Uden, G., and Rastam, R. (1999). Management from four different perspectives. *Journal of Nursing Management, 7*, 101–111.

Merleau-Ponty, M. (1956). What is phenomenology? *Cross Currents, 6*, 59–70.

Merleau-Ponty, M. (1962). *Phenomenology of perception* (C. Smith, Trans.). New York: Humanities Press.

Morse, J. M. (1989). *Qualitative nursing research: A contemporary dialogue.* Rockville, MD: Aspen.

Munhall, P. (1989). Philosophical ponderings on qualitative research. *Nursing Science Quarterly, 2*(1), 20–28.

Natanson, M. (1973). *Edmund Husserl: Philosopher of infinite tasks.* Evanston, IL: Northwestern University Press.

Neil, J. A., & Munjas, B.A. (2000). Living with a chronic wound: The voices of sufferers. *Ostomy/Wound Management, 46*(5), 28–38.

Omery, A. (1983). Phenomenology: A method for nursing research. *Advances in Nursing Science, 5*(2), 49–63.

Paley, J. (1997). Husserl, phenomenology and nursing. *Journal of Advanced Nursing, 26*, 187–193.

Paterson, G. J., & Zderad, L. T. (1976). *Humanistic nursing.* New York: Wiley.

Patton, M. Q. (1990). *Qualitative evaluation and research methods* (2nd ed.). Newbury Park, CA: Sage.

Reinharz, S. (1983). Phenomenology as a dynamic process. *Phenomenology and Pedagogy, 1*(1), 77–79.

Ricoeur, P. (1976). *Interpretation theory: Discourse and the surplus of meaning.* Fort Worth, TX: Texas Christian University Press.

Ricoeur, P. (1981). *Hermeneutics and the social sciences* (J. Thompson, Trans. & Ed.). New York: Cambridge University Press.

Rinaldi, D. M. (1989). The lived experience of commitment to nursing. *Dissertation Abstracts International* (University Microfilms No. 1707).

Roberts, D. C., & Cleveland, L. A. (2001). Surrounded by ocean, a world apart...The experience of elder women living alone. *Holistic Nursing Practice, 15*(3), 45–55.

Rose, P., Beeby, J., & Parker, D. (1995). Academic rigour in the lived experience of researchers using phenomenological methods in nursing. *Journal of Advanced Nursing, 21*, 1123–1129.

Schutz, A. (1970). *On phenomenology and social relations.* Chicago: University of Chicago Press.

Spiegelberg, H. (1965). *The phenomenological movement: A historical introduction* (2nd ed., Vol. 1–2). Dordrecht, The Netherlands: Martinus Nijhoff.

Spiegelberg, H. (1975). *Doing phenomenology.* Dordrecht, The Netherlands: Martinus Nijhoff.

Streubert, H. J. (1991). Phenomenological research as a theoretic initiative in community health nursing. *Public Health Nursing, 8*(2), 119–123.

Tarzian, A. J. (2000). Caring for dying patients who have air hunger. *Journal of Nursing Scholarship, 32*(2), 137–143.

Todres, L., & Wheeler, S. (2001). The complexity of phenomenology, hermenutics and existentialism as a philosophical perspective for nursing research. *International Journal of Nursing Studies, 38,* 1–8.

Van der Zalm, J. E., & Bergum, V. (2000). Hermeneutic phenomenology: Providing living knowledge for nursing practice. *Journal of Advanced Nursing, 31*(1), 211–218.

van Kaam, A. (1959). A phenomenological analysis exemplified by the feeling of being really understood. *Individual Psychology, 15,* 66–72.

van Manen, M. (1984). Practicing phenomenological writing. *Phenomenology and Pedagogy, 2*(1), 36–69.

Wagner, H. R. (1983). *Phenomenology of consciousness and sociology of the life and world: An introductory study.* Edmonton, Alberta: University of Alberta Press.

Yonge, O., & Stewin, L. (1988). Reliability and validity: Misnomers for qualitative research. *Canadian Journal of Nursing Research, 20*(2), 61–67.

Phenomenology in Practice, Education, and Administration

The acceptance of qualitative methods as legitimate approaches to the discovery of knowledge continues to grow as an increasing number of nurse–researchers apply qualitative methods to investigations that have as their phenomena of interest people's life experiences. Very often in nursing we are faced with practice, education, and administrative experiences that seem to present patterns that are familiar to us. In order to validate our perceptions, research must be conducted to explore and describe phenomenon fully and accurately. This process, in turn, leads to improved understanding and ultimately better outcomes in all domains of nursing. Hudacek's (2000) work, *Making A Difference: Stories from the Point of Care,* which is published in book form, uses phenomenological principles to analyze nurse stories. Her work has implications for nursing practice, education, and administration. As evidenced by published works, phenomenology as one approach to qualitative investigations has made a significant contribution to the substantive body of nursing knowledge. Qualitative methods allow exploration of humans by humans in ways that acknowledge the value of all evidence, the inevitability and worth of subjectivity, the value of a holistic view, and the integration of all patterns of knowing (Chinn, 1985).

This chapter provides an overview and critique of three phenomenological investigations, published as journal articles, in the areas of nursing practice, education, and administration. A reprint of Butcher, Holkup, and Buckwalter's (2001) article addressing a nursing practice problem is reprinted at the end of the chapter to provide readers with a sample of a phenomenological investigation while they use the critiquing guidelines. The practice, education, and administrative studies presented in this chapter were reviewed according to the qualitative critique criteria in Box 6.1. These guidelines offer readers of qualitative investigations a guide to recognizing the essential methodological points of a published report. The guidelines also allow readers to examine how the research has contributed to the scientific base of nursing knowledge. This chapter also provides readers with selected examples of published research using the phenomenological method. These examples are presented in Table 6.1.

Box 6.1

QUALITATIVE CRITIQUE CRITERIA

Focus/Topic

1. What is the focus or the topic of the study? What is it that the researcher is studying? Is the topic researchable? Is it focused enough to be meaningful but not too limited so as to be trivial?
2. Why is the researcher using a qualitative design? Would the study be more appropriately conducted in the quantitative paradigm?
3. What is the philosophical tradition or qualitative paradigm upon which the study is based?

Purpose

1. What is the purpose of the study? Is it clear?

Significance

1. What is the relevance of the study to what is already known about the topic?
2. How will the results be useful to nursing and/or health care?

Method

1. Given the topic of the study and the researcher's stated purpose, how does the selected research method help to achieve the stated purpose?
2. What methodological components/strategies (?) has the researcher identified to conduct the study?
3. Based on the material presented, how does the researcher demonstrate that he or she has followed the method?
4. If the researcher used any form of triangulation, explain how he or she maintained the integrity of the study.

Sampling

1. How were participants selected?
2. Explain how the selection process supports a qualitative sampling paradigm.

(continued)

APPLICATION TO PRACTICE

Many nursing interventions performed in clinical settings lend themselves to quantitative measurement. Examples include measurement of blood pressure, central venous pressure, or urine-specific gravity. However, nurses enmeshed in practice settings are well aware that much of what is done for clients is subjective and based on how nurses come to know their clients and the clients' life experiences. For example, caring, reassurance, and quality of life are phenomena central to nursing practice, but they do not necessarily lend themselves to quantitative measurement. Even areas

Box 6.1

QUALITATIVE CRITIQUE CRITERIA (CONTINUED)

3. Are the participants in the study the appropriate people to inform the research? Explain.

Data Collection

1. How does the data collection method reported support discovery, description, or understanding?
2. What data collection strategies does the researcher use?
3. Does the researcher clearly state how human subjects were protected?
4. How was data saturation achieved?
5. Are the data collection strategies appropriate to achieve the purpose of the study? Explain.

Data Analysis

1. How were data analyzed?
2. Based on the analysis reported, can the reader follow the researcher's stated processes?

Findings/Trustworthiness

1. How do the reported findings demonstrate the participants' realities?
2. How does the researcher relate the findings of the study to what is already known?
3. How does the researcher demonstrate that the findings are meaningful to the participants?

Conclusions/Implications/Recommendations

1. How does the researcher provide a context for use of the findings?
2. Are the conclusions drawn from the study appropriate? Explain.
3. What are the recommendations for future research?
4. Are the recommendations, conclusions, and implications clearly related to the findings? Explain.

of practice that are studied primarily from a quantitative perspective can be enriched when examined from a qualitative lens. Therefore, subjective phenomena unique to the practice of professional nursing need investigative approaches suitable to their unique nature. Phenomenology as a qualitative research method has been used to explore a variety of practice-related experiences and facilitates understanding of subjective interactive experiences (Beck, 1990; Caelli, 2000; Omery, 1987; Pallikkathayil & Morgan, 1991; Paterson, 1971; Taylor, 1993; Todres & Wheeler, 2001; Van der Zalm & Bergum, 2000). Examples of published research related to the practice domain can be found in Table 6.1.

text continued on page 82

TABLE 6.1   SELECTIVE SAMPLING OF PHENOMENOLOGICAL RESEARCH STUDIES

Author	Date	Domain	Phenomenon of Interest	Method
Cohen, Ley, & Tarzian	2001	Practice	To describe the experience of isolation in patients who had undergone autologous bone marrow transplantation	Hermeneutics
Daley	2001	Education	How does clinical nursing practice facilitate learning?	Qualitative Interpretivist Perspective
Diekelmann	2001	Education	To describe common experiences of students, teachers, and clinicians in nursing with the goal of reforming nursing education	Hermeneutics
Heinrich	2001	Education	To describe the experiences of self-described passionate dissertations scholars	Hermeneutics
Roberts & Cleveland	2001	Practice	To discover, describe, and understand the lived experience of isolated elder women loving alone on islands off the coast of Maine	Phenomenology
Berggren & Severinsson	2000	Education/ Practice	To investigate the influence of clinical supervision on nurses' moral decision making	Hermeneutics
Rasmussen, Jansson, & Norberg	2000	Practice	To describe the effects of nursing care on patients in a hospice setting in Sweden	Phenomenological-hermeneutic approach of Ricoeur

Sample	Data Generation	Findings
20 patients who had undergone autologous bone marrow transplantations	Tape-recorded interviews, transcribed verbatim	Three themes emerged: Physical Isolation (Protecting Self and Others). Emotional Isolation (Protecting Self and Others), and Physical and Emotional Isolation (Supporting Self and Others).
40 nurses in acute care, long-term care, and home care	Tape-recorded interviews, transcribed verbatim	Clinical nursing practice was found to facilitate personal and professional development of nurses through examination of self-respect, hope, control, vulnerability, acceptance, loss, and persistence.
200 students, teachers, and clinicians	Tape-recorded interviews, transcribed verbatim	Longitudinal study describing "Narrative Pedagogy" uses conventional, phenomenological, critical, and feminist pedagogies, with postmodern discourse to revision nursing education.
6 doctoral candidates	Focus group	Passionate scholarship was described as exciting and risky, personally meaningful, and socially relevant life's work.
9 women age 80 and older	Tape-recorded interviews transcribed verbatim	Themes essential to rural island life were described as: No one is an island, no one lives alone; securely anchored in safe harbor, and weathering storms. Women remained actively engaged in life, feeling valued and connected, safe and secure. They were also resilient and determined.
15 registered nurses	Tape-recorded interviews, transcribed verbatim	Four themes were identified: Increased self-assurance, an increased ability to support the patient, an increased ability to be in a relationship with the patient, and an increased ability to take responsibility.
12 patients in a hospice in Sweden	Tape-recorded interviews, transcribed verbatim	The findings revealed that the effects of and reactions to nursing care by hospice patients were inseparable from the setting. Themes of becoming homeless and isolated emerged.

(continued)

TABLE 6.1		SELECTIVE SAMPLING OF PHENOMENOLOGICAL RESEARCH STUDIES (CONTINUE[]		
Author	**Date**	**Domain**	**Phenomenon of Interest**	**Method**
Vydelingum	2000	Practice	The lived experience of acute hospital care from the perspectives of South Asian patients and their family caregivers	Heideggerian Hermeneutics
Tarzian	2000	Practice	To understand nurses' experiences caring for dying patients who have "air hunger"	Phenomenology
Tongprateep	2000	Practice	How do rural Thai elders experience and describe spirituality in their daily lives?	Hermeneutic Phenomenological Inquiry
Zerwekh	2000	Practice	To describe the unique nature of caring for disenfranchised and outcast patients	Phenomenology

Sample	Data Generation	Findings
10 patients and 6 caregivers	Tape-recorded interview and field notes	Five themes were identified and included feelings of satisfaction with care, unhappy about the service, fitting-in strategies and post-discharge coping mechanisms. Implications for South Asian patients requiring hospitalization and caring for minority patients are discussed.
10 hospice, long-term care, oncology, or emergency medicine nurses	Tape-recorded interviews, transcribed verbatim	Themes identified included "The patient's look-panic beckons," "Surrendering and sharing control," and "Fine-tuning dying" indicated ways nurses responded to relieve a patient's air hunger.
12 rural Thai elders	Tape-recorded interviews, transcribed verbatim	Three categories and nine themes emerged that provide a knowledge base for Thai nurses to explore and explain spirituality among rural Thai elders. The category of Spiritual Beliefs included the themes of The Law of Karma and Life After Death; the category of Religious Practices included the themes of Merit Making, Observance of Moral Precepts, Gratitude and Caring and Meditation, and the third category, that of Consequences of Spirituality, included Coping With the Vicissitudes of Life, Being Hopeful, and Having a Peaceful Mind.
7 nurses who work with clients estranged from mainstream society	Tape-recorded interviews, transcribed verbatim	Ten themes were identified as describing "Caring on the Edge." The themes are organized as three meta-themes, which included the Human Connection, the Community Connection, and Making Self-Care Possible.

Nurses are in a special position to influence patient care. They not only are responsible for the patient as an individual in the health care setting but they also frequently make observations about the effects of illness on family members and other related aspects of the illness experience. They are in a prime position to identify issues related to nursing practice that need to be understood and described more fully. One example of a phenomenological research study as applied to the practice setting is "The Experience of Caring for a Family Member With Alzheimer's Disease" by Butcher et al. (2001). In this study, the authors share how they used qualitative data to provide a fuller understanding of the health care experience for caregivers of family members with Alzheimer's. This article was reviewed using the criteria presented in Box 6.1.

The purpose of the study by Butcher et al. (2001) was "to describe the experience of caring for a family member with Alzheimer's disease or related disorder (ADRD) living at home" (p. 33). The purpose was clearly articulated in the abstract and early in the article. Further, extensive evidence is provided regarding the focus of the study and the importance of the research to nursing and health care. Butcher et al. provide an extensive review of the literature supporting the rationale and need for their study noting the devastation and challenges experienced when one is caring for a family member with ADRD. They emphasize the severe physical and behavioral problems associated with the illness and the increased incidence of the disease with an aging population. They have made explicit the importance of the research at the outset of this comprehensive and well articulated phenomenological investigation. It is clear to the reader that a problem exists that lends itself to a qualitative approach.

Butcher et al. (2001) emphasize the need for a qualitative research design, noting that "the bulk of ADRD family caregiving research has been conducted by means of surveys, and closed-ended interview methods that rely heavily on standardized psychometric instruments including various depression and anxiety scales, caregiver burden scales, symptom checklists, and structural diagnostic assessment tools"(p. 35). Through narrative review of published research and detailed discussion of the need to understand lived experience from the caregiver perspective, the authors have supplied the reader with sound rationale for the research approach as well as the study's significance. Clearly research has been conducted from a quantitative perspective. The researchers further note, "There are relatively few phenomenological studies or naturalistic studies of any type on family ADRD caregiving" (Butcher et al., p. 35). The qualitative approach applied by this team of researchers provides an added and important dimension to understanding the lived experience of caring for a family member with Alzheimer's disease.

Butcher et al. (2001) describe in detail the methodological strategies used to conduct their study. The author's detailed description clearly demonstrates how the method was followed throughout the study. For purposes of this investigation, the researchers used van Kaam's four-stage, 12-step phenomenological method. Although the philosophical underpinnings of phenomenological method were not specifically addressed, the authors did discuss in detail the method used for this investigation and supported the discussion with other research using van Kaam's methodology. This approach was selected for its rigorous methods, and usefulness in analyzing large narrative data samples. The authors note that "(o)ne of the unique features of van Kaam's phenomenological method is the reporting of frequencies and percentages of participants for each of the preliminary structural elements and essential structural elements. The reporting of frequencies provides easier comparison and summary of the categorization of all data"(p. 37).

This particular phenomenological study is unique in that it involved secondary analysis of in-depth transcribed interview data. Butcher et al. (2001) note:

> The secondary analysis of this data allowed for expansion of the original data through an in-depth and rigorous analysis of the baseline transcribed interviews. The baseline transcribed interviews came from a larger 4-year, longitudinal study designed to evaluate the efficacy of a 12-month, community-based psychoeducational nursing intervention (p. 38).

The methodology was appropriate for this phenomenological study, and the method application was clearly articulated by the researchers. The authors have applied triangulation strategies in their research with clear rationale. This study used data, method, and researcher triangulation. This approach adds richness to the study as well as increasing the overall complexity of the work. Chapter 15 discusses these research strategies in detail.

Sampling is clearly addressed by Butcher et al. (2001). Participants volunteered to participate and were solicited through radio and newspaper notices and word-of-mouth referrals. All caregivers participating in the study met specific selection criteria and were caregivers for a family member or friend with Alzheimer's. Interviews and participant selection underwent rigorous testing and evaluation to prevent bias and ensure completeness and quality of the data collected. This particular study has an unusually large sample for a qualitative investigation. This is related to the fact that the data are part of a larger quantitative study. The concept of saturation is not addressed but this may be related to the unusually large sample.

The authors note that the study was reviewed and approved by an Institutional Review Board. Based on this statement the reader can make the assumption that protection of human subjects was addressed. Baseline open-ended interviews were conducted. The researchers noted:

> Consistent with a phenomenological interviewing approach, the interviewer asked each caregiver to describe what caregiving was like for her or him in the context of caring for a family member with Alzheimer's disease living at home. The interviews were unstructured and open-ended, with the interviewer providing neutral probes when appropriate. The interviewers avoided introducing topics or discussion relating to the assessment of the care recipient or the intervention until after the interview was concluded. The in-depth interviews averaged 45 to 60 minutes in length. They were conducted and audio taped in the caregivers' home setting and transcribed using a word-processing program (Butcher et al., 2001, p. 39).

Data analysis was described in detail and followed the rigorous research methodology described by van Kaam. The reader can easily follow the processes stated by the researchers for data analysis. The steps of van Kaam's methodology also are used to clarify how essential and preliminary structural elements were developed and percentages calculated. This adds to the authenticity and trustworthiness of the findings.

The findings demonstrate the participants' realities as they relate to the caregiving experience for family members with Alzheimer's. Eight essential structural elements were presented with supporting verbatim descriptive expressions from participants. Two tables are included in the article that illustrate further the application of van Kaam's methodology. The author's research resulted in the following findings:

> In this study of 103 ADRD family caregivers, caring for a family member living at home with ADRD was experienced as being immersed in caregiving/enduring stress and frustration/suffering through the losses/integrating ADRD into our lives/preserving integrity/gathering support/moving with continuous change/and finding meaning and joy (Butcher et al., 2001, p. 43).

The findings of the study are discussed within the context of what is already known about the topic, followed by detailed recommendations for future research. As the authors note, "The methodological innovativeness of this study expands and deepens understanding of the experience of caring for a family member with ADRD" (Butcher et al., 2001, p. 51). Butcher et al. provide an excellent example of phenomenological research using van Kaam's approach to data analysis. This study also offers and excellent example of some of the benefits to be achieved through triangulation.

APPLICATION TO EDUCATION

Nursing education also lends itself to objective and subjective research interests. Test construction and critical thinking are education-related examples that are appropriate for quantitative investigation, although not exclusively. The educational domain of nursing also lends itself to qualitative investigation in areas such as educational experiences, caring and the curriculum, or the effect of evaluation on student performance in the clinical setting.

Several authors have used qualitative methods to investigate phenomena unique to nursing education. For example, Heinrich (2001) described scholarship from the view of doctoral students; Dickerson, Neary, and Hyche-Johnson (2000) identified learning needs of Native American graduate nursing students; and Daley (2001) studied the impact of clinical practice on learning. Nursing education is an important area of research that can be studied using qualitative approaches. An overview and critique of the study "Technological Competence as a Fundamental Structure of Learning in Critical Care Nursing: A Phenomenological Study" by Little (2000) is provided for this example of the phenomenological method applied to the educational domain of nursing.

The phenomenon of interest for this study is relevant to nursing education and had as its purpose to understand "the extent to which a prescribed curriculum in critical care nursing met students' most immediate learning needs" (Little, 2000, p. 392). Little provides rationale for her study through a literature review of topics related to critical care and learning. She emphasized the importance of her study in the following statement: "Also concerned with learning and practice development in critical care, this phenomenological study attempts to provide further insight into the most fundamental concepts that characterize the nature of the critical care learners' world" (Little, 2000, p. 392).

Little's (2000) work is consistent with Heidegger's hermeneutic phenomenology. Rationale for the method and philosophical underpinnings are clearly articulated. Little makes this clear to the reader in the following:

> The philosophical assumptions that underpin the study are consistent with those of Heidegger's hermeneutic phenomenology. Essential notions of Heideggerian philosophy offer a perspective on learning in critical care that differs from the traditional view. As self-interpreting beings who co-constitute their world, learners are seen to define themselves and their learning needs in terms of being able to participate within their own, unique environment—their "world." Furthermore, participation in the world is fundamentally dependent on embodiment of common activities that are symbolic of shared practices and shared understanding (p. 392).

Little (2000) described her participant selection in detail. Her selection process supported a qualitative framework in that it was purposeful, and subjects had experience with the phenomenon under investigation. The author notes:

> Participants comprised 10 qualified nurses who were practising in the specialty either of intensive care or intensive care combined with coronary care and who were employed in one of three District General Hospitals located in the South of England. Participants represented two consecutive cohorts that had recently completed and English National Board post-registration education programme in Intensive and Coronary Care Nursing (Little, 2000, p. 392).

Little (2000) also addresses the protection of human subjects and she notes that ethical principles were honored. Although the specific details were not described, the researcher noted that issues related to informed consent, privacy and confidentiality were addressed.

The data collection strategies used by Little (2000) support phenomenological approaches to discovery, description, and understanding. The strategies used by the researcher are detailed and appropriate to achieve the purposes of the study. "Data were collected and audio recorded during individual or collective interviews. The first cohort provided six individual interviews whilst the second cohort provided one collective interview. Interviews took the form of reflective dialogue that recognized the value of both participant and researcher in the generation of research data and was considered to be consistent with hermeneutic techniques (Little, 2000, p. 392).

Data analysis follows the interpretive approach described by Little (2000). In addition to her narrative analysis, Little diagrams for the reader her analysis process and the relationship of her findings, thereby facilitating a clearer understanding of her line of thinking in the data analysis process. Saturation is not addressed.

Discussion of the findings demonstrates how the data reflected participants' realities and how the researcher related findings of the study to what is already known. Little describes in detail for the reader the three relational themes that resulted. They included "learning as focusing, learning as questioning and learning as technological mastery" (p. 393). Examples of raw data related to each relational theme are provided, allowing the reader to follow the line of thinking of the researcher and adding credibility to the study.

The conclusions drawn from the study are appropriate, and recommendations for future research are made. Additional qualitative research related to the impact of technology and critical care nursing are needed. The recommendations, conclusion, and implications discussed by the author are clearly related to the findings.

APPLICATION TO ADMINISTRATION

There is limited literature on studies related to nursing administration that use qualitative approaches. This is a domain of nursing that is in need of further qualitative investigation. The development of qualitative research that describes phenomena important to nursing administration might include research that examines professional nurse behavior and work satisfaction, successful leadership strategies, and perspectives on nurse empowerment

An overview of the study "Management from Four Different Perspectives" by Lindholm, Uden, and Rastam (1999) is presented as an example of the application of qualitative research in the area of nursing administration. The phenomenon of interest, clearly identified in the study, focused on gaining an understanding of the process of nursing management in a developing organization. The specific rationale for using a qualitative format, as well as the philosophic underpinnings of the approach, was clearly described. Despite the fact that the Swedish health care system has a variety of management positions to which nurses have legal access, nurses have traditionally held middle management positions. Ongoing decentralization has moved nurses into senior management positions. Therefore, "Elucidating the significance of nursing management increases the possibility of developing the management area of the nursing profession and of using recently acquired knowledge to influence the development of the nursing profession" (Lindholm et al., 1999, p. 102).

The purpose of the study was to "illuminate nursing management in a developing organization from the perspectives of nurse managers, chief physicians, hospital directors and politicians, respectively" (Lindholm et al., 1999, p. 102). The authors make explicit their purpose and support it with a review of the literature.

The sample included 15 nurse managers, 11 chief physicians, and three politicians who were chairmen of the local health boards. "The nurse managers were all women, except for one. In the other groups all the participants were men"(Lindholm et al., 1999, p. 102).

The method used to collect data was compatible with the research purpose and adequately addressed the phenomenon of interest. Lindholm et al. (1999) interviewed their participants individually. All interviews were tape recorded and transcribed verbatim. The authors used Ricoeur's process of phenomenological hermeneutics. Detailed examples of the steps of the hermeneutic circle are provided, demonstrating for the reader how the researchers followed the stated method. Although the researchers do not make an explicit statement regarding data saturation, they do comment that the interviews were comprehensive and "provided good coverage of the issues leaving no need to increase the number of informants" (Lindholm et al., 1999, p. 102).

Data analysis followed the phenomenological hermeneutic approach inspired by Ricoeur. The author provides clear examples of the data analysis process in relationship to each step of the hermeneutic circle.

> The first step was the naïve reading of each interview to acquire a sense of the whole of the text, to gain an impression and to formulate ideas for further analysis. The second step was a structural analysis to identify meaning units, to explain, through revealing the structure and the internal dependent relations, what constitutes the static state of the text. The third step was the understanding of the interpreted whole, from reflection on the naïve reading and the structural analysis (Lindholm et al., 1999, p. 103).

The findings demonstrate the participants' realities and the researchers relate the findings of the study to what is already known. Through the discussion of the findings the researchers provide a context for their use and conclusions are drawn. Recommendations for future research are made and the conclusions and implications are clearly related to the findings. This work makes an important contribution to the nursing administration knowledge base.

SUMMARY

The body of published phenomenological research has grown considerably since the first publication of this textbook. Clearly, the body of practice related research is expanding with considerable development of research in the area of education and administration. Examples of phenomenological research applied to the areas of nursing practice, education, and administration emphasize the important contribution that phenomenological research has made to nursing's substantive body of knowledge. The critiquing guidelines provide the reader with a guide to evaluating phenomenological research. Examples of phenomenological research using the method interpretations described in Chapter 5 have been highlighted to facilitate method comprehension and application.

Phenomenology as a research approach provides an avenue for investigation that allows description of lived experiences. The voice of professional nurses in practice, education, and administration can be a tremendous source of data that have yet to be fully explored. Identifying subjective phenomena unique to the domains of nursing education, practice, and administration is important to the ever-expanding body of nursing knowledge.

REFERENCES

Beck, C. T. (1990). Qualitative research: Methodologies and use in pediatric nursing. *Issues in Comprehensive Pediatric Nursing, 13*, 193–201.

Butcher, H. K., Holkup, P. A., & Buckwalter, K. C. (2001). The experience of caring for a family member with Alzheimer's disease. *Western Journal of Nursing Research, 23*(1), 33–55.

Caelli, K. (2000). The changing face of phenomenological research: Traditional and American phenomenology in nursing. *Qualitative Health Research, 10*(3), 366–377.

Chinn, P. (1985). Debunking myths in nursing theory and research. *Image, 17*(2), 171–179.

Cohen, M. Z., Ley, C., & Tarzian, A. J. (2001). Isolation in blood and marrow transplantation. *Western Journal of Nursing Research, 23*(6), 592–609.

Daley, B. J. (2001). Learning in clinical practice. *Holistic Nursing Practice, 16*(1), 43–54.

Dickerson, S. S., Neary, M. A., & Hyche-Johnson, M. (2000). Native American graduate nursing students' learning experiences. *Journal of Nursing Scholarship, 32*(2), 189–196.

Diekelmann, N. (2001). Narrative pedagogy: Heideggerian hermeneutic analyses of lived experiences of students, teachers, and clinicians. *Advances in Nursing Science, 23*(3), 53–71.

Heinrich, K. (2001). Doctoral women as passionate scholars: An exploratory inquiry of passionate dissertation scholarship. *Advances in Nursing Science, 23*(3), 88–103.

Hudacek, S. (2000). *Making a difference: Stories from the point of care.* Indianapolis, IN: Sigma Theta Tau Press.

Lindholm, M., Uden, G., & Rastam, L. (1999). Management from four different perspectives. *Journal of Nursing Management, 7*, 101–111.

Little, C. V. (2000). Technological competence as a fundamental structure of learning in critical care nursing: a phenomenological study. *Journal of Clinical Nursing, 9*, 391–399.

Omery, A. (1987). Qualitative research designs in the critical care setting: Review and application. *Heart and Lung, 16*(4), 432–436.

Pallikkathayil, L., & Morgan, S. A. (1991). Phenomenology as a method for conducting clinical research. *Applied Nursing Research, 4*(4), 195–200.

Paterson, J. G. (1971). From a philosophy of clinical nursing to a method of nursology. *Nursing Research, 20*(2), 143–146.

Rasmussen, B. H., Jansson, L., Norberg, A. (2000). Striving for becoming at-home in the midst of dying. *American Journal of Hospice & Palliative Care, 17*(1), 31–43.

Roberts, D. C., & Cleveland, L. A. (2001). Surrounded by ocean, a world apart . . . The experience of elder women living alone. *Holistic Nursing Practice, 15*(3), 45–55.

Tarzian, A. J. (2000). Caring for dying patients who have air hunger. *Journal of Nursing Scholarship, 32*(2), 137–143.

Taylor, B. (1993). Phenomenology: One way to understand nursing practice. *International Journal of Nursing Studies, 30*(2), 171–179.

Todres, L., & Wheeler, S. (2001). The complexity of phenomenology, hermeneutics and existentialism as a philosophical perspective for nursing research. *International Journal of Nursing Studies, 38*, 1–8.

Tongprateep, T. (2000). The essential elements of spirituality among rural Thai elders. *Journal of Advanced Nursing, 31*(1), 197–203.

Van der Zalm, J. E., & Bergum, V. (2000). Hermeneutic phenomenology: Providing living knowledge for nursing practice. *Journal of Advanced Nursing, 31*(1), 211–218.

Vydelingum, V. (2000). South Asian patients' lived experience of acute care in an English hospital: A phenomenological study. *Journal of Advanced Nursing, 32*(1), 100–107.

Zerkwekh, J. V. (2000). Caring on the ragged edge: Nursing persons who are disenfranchised. *Advances in Nursing Science, 22*(4), 47–61.

RESEARCH ARTICLE

The Experience of Caring for a Family Member With Alzheimer's Disease

Howard Karl Butcher, Patricia A. Holkup, and Kathleen Coen Buckwalter

The purpose of this phenomenological study was to describe the experience of caring for a family member with Alzheimer's disease or related disorder (ADRD) living at home among a diverse sample of 103 family caregivers. The study involved secondary analysis of in-depth transcribed interview data using van Kaam's rigorous four-phase 12-step psychophenomenological method. A total of 2,115 descriptive expressions were categorized into 38 preliminary structural elements. Eight essential structural elements emerged from an analysis of the preliminary structural elements. The eight elements were then synthesized to form the following synthetic structural definition: Caring for a family member living at home with ADRD was experienced as "being immersed in caregiving; enduring stress and frustration; suffering through the losses; integrating ADRD into our lives and preserving integrity; gathering support, moving with continuous change; and finding meaning and joy."

Caring for a family member with Alzheimer's disease and related dementias (ADRD) is one of the most devastating and challenging experiences one can endure. ADRD are tragic, debilitating, chronic illnesses with unpredictable clinical courses that average nearly 10 years from diagnosis to death (Alzheimer's Association, 1996; National Advisory Council on Alzheimer's Disease, 1989). Approximately 70% of persons with ADRD, or more than 4 million persons, live at home and are cared for by a family member without pay (Alzheimer's Association, 1996; Taueber, 1992). The tragedy of ADRD is compounded by the toll it takes on their caregivers, who must cope with the long-term and disabling physical and behavioral problems associated with the care recipient's illness. Although caring for a family member with ADRD is often an anguishing experience, 80% of caregivers reported that they were willing to sacrifice "quite a bit" or "practically anything" to continue to care for the family member at home as long as possible (Archbold & Stewart, 1996). Because the incidence of Alzheimer's disease increases with age, the number of ADRD family caregivers is likely to increase dramatically due to increased life expectancy. The percentage of persons older than age 85 will nearly double from 1.2% in 1990 to 1.91% by 2010 (Malmgren, 1994). Although those persons 85 years or older are the fastest-growing segment of the U.S. population, it is estimated that 47% of the population older than 85 years of age may eventually become affected

Howard Karl Butcher, R.N., Ph.D., C.S., Assistant Professor, University of Iowa, College of Nursing; Patricia A. Holkup, R.N., M.A., Doctoral Student, University of Iowa, College of Nursing; Kathleen Coen Buckwalter, Ph.D., R.N., F.A.A.N., Associate Provost for Health Sciences, Office of the Provost, University of Iowa.

by ADRD (Hurley & Wells, 1999). Changing demographics combined with increasing concern over escalating health care cost are leading to growing social expectations that family should be responsible for providing care to their own family members (Estes, 1993; Kelley, Buckwalter, & Maas, 1999; Myers & Agree, 1994).

Much of the family ADRD caregiver research has focused on the caregiver burden experienced by family caregivers (Baumgarten et al., 1994; Browning & Schwirian, 1994; Chang, 1999; Farran, Keane-Hagerty, Tatarowicz, & Scorza, 1993; Kuhlman, Wilson, Hutchinson, & Wallhagen, 1991; Zarit, Todd, & Zarit, 1986). Researchers have focused on the negative consequences of caregiver burden (D. Cohen & Eisdorfer, 1988; Gallagher, Rose, Rivera, Lovett, & Thompson, 1989; Morrissey, Becker, & Rubert, 1990; Wright, 1991) including the demands and feelings of distress (Farran et al., 1993; Mastrian, Ritter, & Deimling, 1996; Phillips, et al., 1995; Seltzer, Vasterling, Yoder, & Thompson, 1997). Adverse feelings of sadness, anger, fatigue, guilt, grief, and depression have been found in ADRD caregivers (D. Cohen & Eisdorfer, 1988; Gallagher et al., 1989; Lindgren, Connelly, & Gaspar, 1999; Schultz, O'Brien, Bookwala, & Fleissner, 1995). Unresolved pressures and conflicts have been found to lead to decline in physical health in the caregiver (Davis, 1997; Kuhlman et al., 1991). There also is an emerging body of research on the impact of selected nursing interventions on caregiving (Buckwalter et al., 1992; Chang, 1999; Gerdner, Hall, & Buckwalter, 1996; Kuhlman et al., 1991).

The bulk of ADRD family caregiving research has been conducted by means of surveys, and closed-ended interview methods rely heavily on standardized psychometric instruments including various depression and anxiety scales, caregiver burden scales, symptom checklists, and structural diagnostic assessment tools. The quantitative emphasis in the body of family ADRD caregiving research has constrained the capacity of health care professionals to fully understand the caregiving experience and the shared meanings family members attribute to their experience as caregivers (Hasselkus, 1998; Kellet, 1997). Gubrium (1996) asserts that it is time "to hear from even more of the participating voices than we currently do" and "turn directly to lived experience and related and diverse situations and working with local discourses of caregiving" (p. 268).

Despite the considerable magnitude of caregiver research, there remains a lack of in-depth understanding of the nature and essence of the family ADRD caregiving experience grounded in the experiences and perceptions of caregivers themselves. A phenomenological approach to studying the caregiving experience provides a means to explicate the essence of the lived experience of providing care for a family member with ADRD.

PURPOSE OF THE STUDY

The aim of this phenomenological study was to describe the essential structure of the lived experience of caring for a family member with ADRD among a large and diverse sample of informal family Alzheimer's disease caregivers. The research question addressed in this study was, What is the lived experience of caring for a family member with Alzheimer's disease at home?

REVIEW OF THE LITERATURE

There are relatively few phenomenological studies or naturalistic studies of any type on family ADRD caregiving. In a classic qualitative study of ADRD family caregivers, Wilson (1989) used grounded theory to provide a "beginning knowledge basic to interpreting the meaning associated with their [caregivers] experience" (p. 44). Wilson's study of family caregivers ($N = 20$) uncovered three stages of the caregiving process: taking it on, going through it, and turning it over. Perry and Olshansky (1996) described a three-stage process in which family members come to terms caring for a family member with Alzheimer's disease. Family members ($N = 5$) first identified how the family member with Alzheimer's disease was different prior to disease onset, then redefined the identity of the family member with Alzheimer's disease, and last changed their relationship with the family member with Alzheimer's disease (Perry and Olshansky, 1996). Another grounded theory study of ADRD family caregivers ($N = 10$) yielded a five-stage model of gaining and relinquishing control of caregiving (Willoughby & Keating, 1991). The five stages described in the model were emerging recognition, taking control, losing control, adjusting to the psychiatric institution, and moving on. The interviews were conducted after the family member had been placed in a geriatric facility. In a grounded theory study of male ($N = 24$) ADRD perceptions of formal support, Coe and Neufeld (1999) identified four sequential stages: resisting, giving in, opening the door, and making the match. Male caregivers initially resisted formal help, preferring to manage the care themselves with some help from family and friends. Other grounded theory studies investigating aspects of ADRD family caregiving have focused on spousal decision making (Corcoran, 1994), the use of formal support community services (Winslow, 1998), and daughter caregiver stress (McCarty, 1996). Although grounded theory studies have served to uncover the social processes in the ADRD family caregiving experience, phenomenological studies are needed to describe the essence of the ADRD family caregiving experience.

In a phenomenological study analyzing books written by family caregivers, Lynch-Sauer (1990) identified two meta-themes (change and personal history) and eight core themes (putting patients in touch with their surroundings, predicting disconnection and attempting to prevent it, progressive asynchrony in sleeping and eating, loss of mutuality in the relationship, decline of a reciprocal relationship, progressive diminishment of diversity in relation to the patient, narrowing of horizons of the caregivers, and a search for personal connectedness). Pointing out that most of the research on family caregivers had focused on women as spouses or daughters, Parsons' (1997) phenomenological inquiry of ADRD family caregivers from a male perspective ($N = 8$) revealed eight themes describing the ADRD family caregiving process: enduring, vigilance, a sense of loss, aloneness and loneliness, taking away, searching to discover, the need for assistance, and reciprocity. Siriopoulos, Brown, and Wright (1999) used Giorgi's (1985) phenomenological method to discover the meaning of caregiving for eight husbands who were caring for wives diagnosed with ADRD. Five themes were identified: quality of previous relationship, loss, caregiver burden, coping and support methods, and effects of Alzheimer's disease.

Although these few phenomenological studies shed new understanding on the ADRD caregiving process, the goal of this study was to expand and deepen the understanding essence of caring for a family member with ADRD using van Kaam's (1966) revised and updated rigorous four-phase, 12-step psychophenomenological method (Anderson & Eppard, 1998) among a larger and more diverse sample of ADRD caregivers. Drebing (1999) recently pointed out that samples in caregiving research continue to be overrepresented by spousal caregivers. Typically, phenomenological studies focus on a homogenous sample such as either spousal, male, adult children caregivers, or caregivers of a particular ethnic group. Drebing asserted that there is an increasing need for qualitative research designs and larger sample sizes. This investigation responds to the need to include a larger and more diverse sample of caregivers.

The present investigation differs from other qualitative investigations because it uses secondary data from a multisite sample that is considerably larger than what is customary for phenomenological studies, thus allowing for greater diversity among the respondents. The 103 ADRD caregivers in this study lived in four states; 29 were male caregivers, and 37 caregivers were other than spouses.

METHOD

van Kaam's (1966) four-stage, 12-step phenomenological method is an appropriate scientific and rigorous method for analyzing phenomenological interviews from large data samples (Anderson & Eppard, 1998; Omery, 1993). Furthermore, it is one of the common descriptive phenomenological methods employed in nursing research (Beck, 1998; Omery, 1993; Parse, Coyne, & Smith, 1985). Mitchell (1992) used van Kaam's method to explore the meaning of being a senior for 600 participants. van Kaam's method has also been used to uncover the lived experience of health in 108 participants older than 80 years of age (Wondolowski & Davis, 1990) and in another study of 400 participants (Parse et al., 1985). One of the unique features of van Kaam's phenomenological method is the reporting of frequencies and percentages of participants for each of the preliminary structural elements and essential structural elements. The reporting of frequencies provides easier comparison and summary of the categorization of all data.

Overview of Study Design

The study involved a secondary phenomenological data analysis of 103 verbatim, transcribed, in-depth, open-ended, unstructured interviews describing the experience of caring for a family member with ADRD. Thorne (1994) contends that secondary phenomenological analysis "creates a powerful opportunity within the qualitative research tradition by those whose aptitudes are more remote from the data source" (p. 266). The secondary analysis of this data allowed for expansion of the original data through an in-depth and rigorous analysis of the baseline transcribed interviews. The baseline transcribed interviews came from a larger 4-year, longitudinal study designed to evaluate the efficacy of a 12-month, community-based psychoeducational nursing intervention. Based on the progressively lowered stress threshold (PLST) model (Hall & Buckwalter, 1987), the intervention aimed to lower stress through teaching home caregivers how to manage behavioral problems exhibited by their family members with ADRD (Buckwalter et al., 1992). Following Institutional Review Board approval at each institution, participants volunteered in response to radio and newspaper notices and word-of-mouth referrals in seven communities in Arizona, Iowa, Indiana, and Minnesota. All caregivers met the following criteria: (a) were nonpaid (informal) caregivers (either family or friends); (b) cared for an individual who has been diagnosed by a physician as having Alzheimer's disease, multiinfarct dementia, or mixed-type dementia, who is living in the community; (c) lived within 2 hours (one way) of the study sites; (d) provided 4 or more hours of supervision and/or care weekly; and (e) had not been exposed to any training based on the PLST model.

The baseline open-ended interviews were conducted before subjects responded to structured surveys and before the PLST intervention. The investigators at each study site trained the interviewers in the correct interview technique at the beginning of the study. Consistent with a phenomenological interviewing approach, the interviewer asked each caregiver to describe what caregiving was like for him or her in the context of caring for a family member with Alzheimer's disease living at home. The interviews were unstructured and open-ended, with the interviewer providing neutral probes when appropriate. The interviewer avoided introducing topics or discussion relating to the assessment of the care recipient or the intervention until after the interview was concluded. The in-depth interviews averaged 45 to 60 minutes in length. They were conducted and audiotaped in the caregivers' home setting and transcribed using a word-processing program.

Participants

Of the original 245 caregivers enrolled in the study, there were a total of 156 transcribed baseline interviews. Sixty-six of the original 245 participants did not have a baseline interview because baseline interviews were added after the study was piloted. The remaining missing interviews were either due to technical malfunction of the tape recorder or caregiver refusal to be recorded (Buckwalter, Hall, Kelly, Sime, & Richards, 1997). Each of the initial 156 transcribed baseline interviews was closely examined using Hinds, Vogel, and Clark-Steffen's (1997) criteria for evaluating the completeness and quality of qualitative data for secondary analysis. The criteria evaluated included the interview style and questions, the quality of interview with regard to eliciting the caregiver's experience, and the depth of caregiver's description. Of the initial 156 interviews, 103 were found to be of sufficient quality and depth appropriate for phenomenological data analysis. The vast majority (43) of the transcribed interviews eliminated from the analysis were two pages or less transcribed and not sufficient in depth of description of the ADRD caregiving experience. Two transcriptions were not verbatim transcriptions but rather the interviewer explaining what the participant stated, or the interviewer did not ask open-ended questions.

To assure that there was no selection bias between the original 245 participants and the 103 selected for inclusion in the phenomenological analysis, respondents selected for the phenomenological analysis were compared to those not selected on variables that might influence the discussion of caregiving. Variables were tested for both the caregiver and recipient where appropriate. Methods included ANOVA and nonparametric Wilcoxon methods for continuous variables and chi-square or Cochran-Mantel-Haenszel methods for categorical data. There were no statistical differences between the selected and unselected groups across all variables. Variables included proportion by gender; place of residence; education and income; mean age; mean hours for caregiving, respite, sleep, and other tasks; mean weight; number of prescriptions and medications; and mean scores for mood.

Of the 103 caregivers, there were 29 males and 74 females. Among the care receivers diagnosed with Alzheimer's disease living at home, 54 were males and 49 females. The family caregivers lived in four states: 44 from Minnesota, 5 from Arizona, 21 from Indiana, and 31 from Iowa. The care receivers had been living with the diagnosis of ADRD for an average of 4 years. Caregivers ranged in age from 36 to 86 years, with a mean of 66 years. Care receivers were between 46 and 94 years of age, with a mean of 76.5 years. Of the 103 caregivers, 93 were White, 4 were African American, 2 were Hispanic, 1 was Asian, and 3 identified themselves as "other." A total of 66 caregivers were spouses, 6 were sons, 21 were daughters, 2 were brothers, and 5 were sisters. Caregivers spent an average of 116.8 hours a week, or more than 16 hours a day, engaged in direct caregiving activities. Conversely, they experienced an average of only 3.3 respite hours or 4.9 hours of professional help a week.

Phenomenological Analysis

In recent writing, van Kaam provides specific directives for using what he now refers to as the "psychophenomenological method" (Anderson & Eppard, 1998). The phenomenological perspective, as explained by van Kaam (1966), views human experience as a dynamic, complex, continually moving entity. There are four stages in van Kaam's psychophenomenological research method: analysis, translation, transposition, and phenomenological reflection (Anderson & Eppard, 1998). In the first stage analysis the researcher carefully read each of the 103 descriptions in their entirety to obtain a general impression of the experiences structure. Each description was then reread with a focus on identifying descriptive expressions in the exact language of the informant using a selective highlighting approach described by van Manen (1990). Descriptive expressions are statements, phrases, or sentences that were particularly essential and revealing about the ADRD caregiving experience. Each descriptive expression was named and grouped together with other common compatible descriptive expressions, whereas text not descriptive of the caregiving experience was eliminated. This process was followed until all transcripts were analyzed.

Next, conforming elements were meaningfully related to one another across participants based on criteria of essentiality and compatibility. A total of 2,115 descriptive expressions were organized into 38 preliminary structural elements. The 38 preliminary structural elements were then synthesized into eight essential structural elements. van Kaam describes the synthesis of preliminary structural elements as a process of "conforming" or "coming together" of themes in common to form a sense of the whole (Anderson & Eppard, 1998, p. 401). Table 1 shows the final 38 preliminary structural elements organized by each of the eight essential structural elements. According to van Kaam, essential structural elements must be present implicitly or explicitly in a majority (50%) of the participants to be considered an "essential" element. All eight essential elements in this study were present in at least 65% of the participants (see Table 2). These techniques were facilitated through the use of the QSR NUD*IST Nvivo (1999) qualitative data analysis software, which manages narrative data by coding, indexing passages of text, labeling categories of text, and retrieving the labeled passages across all cases (Richards & Richards, 1994).

The 38 preliminary structural elements and eight essential elements were compared and reviewed for congruence by a judge experienced in phenomenological methods who also analyzed all 103 interviews using van Kaam's (1966) method. There was a high degree of congruence as to how researcher and judge grouped each of the preliminary structural elements together. Each of the 103 transcripts were read once again, this time in light of the structural elements to assure that the essential structural elements were forming the whole of the experience. Translation, the second stage, involved translating each essential element in the informant's words into the meaningful language of the discipline. The final wording of the 38 preliminary structural elements and essential structural elements were agreed on by the researcher and the judge. The third stage, transposition, involved submitting the translated essential elements to two independent expert judges for review to assure fidelity of the findings. Each judge reviewed how all 2,115 descriptive expressions were categorized in the 38 preliminary structural elements. The expert judges also reviewed the grouping of common preliminary structural elements into each of the eight essential structural elements. Although a preliminary structural element may have fit in more than one category, the final grouping of preliminary structural elements was based on the best fit on which there was a consensus among

TABLE 1 RESEARCH   FREQUENCIES AND PERCENTAGES OF PRELIMINARY STRUCTURAL ELEMENTS

Essential Structural Element	Preliminary Structural Element	Number of Passages	Percentage of Cases
Enduring stress and frustration	Caregiving is stressful	134	61.17
	Dealing with the memory loss	123	55.34
	Caregiving is frustrating	86	49.51
	Caregiving is never-ending	74	44.66
	Not having time for oneself	52	32.04
	Anger surfaces	38	23.30
	Dealing with family conflicts	28	16.50
	Everything takes longer	13	11.65
	Sometimes its embarrassing	14	10.68
	Feeling dismissed by health care professionals	12	6.80
Immersed in caregiving	Caring day to day	126	66.02
	Managing difficult symptoms	119	54.37
	Creating moments for activities	104	53.40
	Monitoring the stress of others	19	13.59
Finding meaning and joy	Finding positives in caring	99	55.34
	Fortifying commitment	86	48.54
	Creating joyful times	75	35.92
Integrating ADRD into our lives	Monitoring the degree of disability	61	42.72
	Seeking knowledge	53	33.01
	Realizing something is wrong	28	21.36
	Accepting the way things are	27	20.39
	Difficulty accepting the illness	17	13.59
Moving with continuous change	Taking on new responsibilities	80	48.54
	Anticipating and fearing the future	61	39.81
	Dealing with change	20	16.50
	Dealing with the unexpected	19	13.59
Preserving integrity	Caring for self	58	37.86
	Concerns about safety	66	35.92
	Recognizing one's limitations	22	17.48
	Having patience	18	15.53
Gathering support	Finding support from family	57	39.81
	Seeking support	69	34.95
	Finding support from friends	28	20.39
	Having faith in God	18	11.65
Suffering through the losses	The losses are painful	80	44.56
	Missing intimacy	58	30.10
	Losses bring grief and sadness	47	29.13
	It's like caring for a child	26	18.45
Total		2,115	

TABLE 2	PERCENTAGE OF PARTICIPANTS FOR EACH ESSENTIAL STRUCTURAL ELEMENT	
Essential Element	**Number of Passages**	**Percentage of Cases**
Enduring stress and frustration	574	93
Immersed in caregiving	368	93
Finding meaning and joy	260	78
Integrating ADRD into our lives	180	74
Moving with continuous change	186	71
Preserving integrity	164	69
Gathering support	172	67
Suffering through the losses	211	65

the researcher and all judges. The eight essential structural elements were then synthesized in the final synthetic description. In the last stage, phenomenological reflection, the judges' suggestions were integrated into the final synthetic description. The findings were then submitted to two advanced practice nurses who were experienced with working with Alzheimer's disease family caregivers and who had been involved as co-principal investigators in the original study for their review, comments, and confirmation. In addition, the final eight essential structural elements and the synthetic description were shared with a family caregiver participant in the study for comment.

FINDINGS

Eight essential structural elements emerged from the phenomenological analysis. Table 1 is a summary of the total number of descriptive expressions and total number of cases that have each preliminary essential element. Table 2 lists the total number of descriptive expressions and the percentage of participants having each of the eight essential structural elements. The final phase of presenting the findings in van Kaam's (1966) method is synthesizing the essential structural elements into one structural definition or "synthetic description" that captures the essence of the lived experience. In this study of 103 ADRD family caregivers, caring for a family member living at home with ADRD was experienced as being immersed in caregiving/enduring stress and frustration/suffering through the losses/integrating ADRD into our lives/preserving integrity/gathering support/moving with continuous change/and finding meaning and joy. Each of the eight essential structural elements are presented below with supporting verbatim descriptive expressions from participants.

Immersed in Caregiving

Immersed in caregiving describes the day-to-day activities caregivers engaged in to care for their loved one. Caregivers were engaged deeply in the day-to-day work of caregiving. In spite of the stress and frustration they described, they found ways to express a caring attitude toward their loved ones, respecting their dignity as well as keeping things as normal as possible. "I guess day by day does come to mind because it means I need to be aware of the fact that I'm the one who is here to take care of the meals." Caregivers also felt that it was important to keep their loved ones occupied with activities they were still capable of doing and enjoying. "Now if I have a little project going, I take her out and she will sit there." Another stated, "He will help me do a little cleaning or something." The caregivers were vigilant for the onset of difficult behaviors, searching for ways to manage those behaviors. "The minute I see that he might be getting a little frustrated, I fix it." Caregivers had to juggle the other roles and relationships they had in their lives. This involved monitoring how others were responding to the experience of living with or relating to the mental incapacity of their loved one. "She does not really bother him if she gets up in the night. As a matter of fact, if she gets up, he gets up with her sometimes."

Enduring Stress and Frustration

To endure is to carry on in the face of hardship. The caregivers in this investigation found their experiences to be both stressful and frustrating, yet they persevered in spite of the difficulties. Statements about stress and frustration were among the most frequent: "But there are days where I get really, almost hysterical; "I'm just kind of stressed out; I think I'm a little burned out;" "...is a very difficult thing to do. So I would say its tiring, its emotionally draining;" and another stated, "It has been nerve wracking, I have been exhausted at work for several days. I have to take several days off of work to sleep." Another stated, "In one sentence, it is hell. There are days when what I really want to do most is step in front of a truck."

Aspects of frustration and stress included the difficulties surrounding memory loss, in which a great deal of time and energy was spent looking for misplaced items and in repetitious reminding. "She forgets what she is doing while she is doing it." Caregivers reflected on how much time was spent caring for their loved one. "We get it done. It just takes us a long time," and "Everything takes much longer, not only for her to do it, but me to do it for her."

Caregiving was also seen as never-ending. One caregiver summed it up by stating, "Caregiving is all-consuming, it seems to me"; and another stated,

It is hard, working seven days a week, twenty-four hours around the clock for three or four months without time off. Just kind of stressed out. So it's the constant caregiving. You do not ever forget about it. You may be doing something else to try to enjoy yourself, but it is always in the back of your mind and you realize, as soon as I am done with this, I have to be concerned about my mother eating, is she locked out of the house...any number of things. So it is always there.

The most frequent expression of the ADRD caregiving experience was how frustrating it can be. "I think it is real frustrating and heartbreaking that she does not know I am her daughter. That is hard"; another said, "I get exasperated with her"; "It is a matter of a lot of time and frustration." Many of the participants identified feelings of anger that surfaced as a result of the stress and frustration. Worrying about how to handle the anger as well as the effect their anger might have on their loved one caused additional stress.

Sometimes I get angry. Then I have to blow my top and get rid of it that way. That is the part I hate. Sometimes I get so stressed, I get so angry. I get angry at myself for getting angry. It is hard to talk about.

Another source of frustration arose at the time when caregivers were first beginning to recognize something was wrong with their loved one. As they sought an answer to what was happening, several felt they had been dismissed by health care professionals.

I didn't get much from him. He was real busy he told me and I did not have an appointment that day. We had gone in for his MRI and the doctor had not even planned to see me that day. I said, "Well I am here, I want to see you," so he gave me five minutes, he told me very plainly.

Suffering Through the Losses

Caregivers spoke of their pain associated with the "heartbreaking" losses they had experienced as their loved ones became increasingly disabled with Alzheimer's disease. These losses included realizing that dreams for the golden years of retirement were no longer accessible to them. "It makes me sad a lot of the times. But I can remember all the good times. I guess it just makes you sad that is all I can say"; and another captured the essence of suffering when stating, "It makes you a prisoner. You know the slogan 'living death?' That's what it is for the caregiver."

The slow deterioration of their loved ones constituted a sad and extended leave-taking from the people they once were: "It is hard to watch her personality and the things that made her go away." They missed the intimacy of their former relationships with their family member. Seeing the person they had known for so long, who still was physically the same person but in many other ways so different, was an incongruity that at times seemed unreal. "Then all of a sudden I am there for him but he is not there for me. He had always been there for me." Another said, "It is almost like part of him has died." When speaking of the changed relationship they now had with their family member, several participants felt that although they still saw their loved ones as adults, they had to care for them like children.

I think the pain comes from watching someone who has been so healthy and so intelligent and witty and personable, turn into someone who is confused the majority of the time, whose judgment is gone and knowing that you have to care for that person as if they were a child yet you have to still treat them as an adult. That has been difficult.

Grief was apparent for many of the respondents, draining energy and causing feelings of depression. They described their grief as "heartbreaking" and "a sadness to see him losing some of those things that he was able to do before.... The loss is what makes me depressed."

Integrating ADRD Into Our Lives

The insidious entry of ADRD into these families' lives involved a gradual understanding of the meaning this devastating disease had for them and their loved ones. The first signs of something being wrong were subtle and difficult to identify when they were first noticed.

I was not sure when it really started but I know that we had a couple arguments and normally we did not argue and I got really upset and later on as time went on I realized there was something wrong.

Once they had become aware of the problem, some caregivers went through a period of shock and disbelief, finding it difficult to accept the disease. "That was the initial shock. Last year, I guess, was the worst here because I could not believe it was happening." In spite of the shock and grief, caregivers continued to monitor their loved ones' progressing disability. They wanted insight into the mental experience of their loved ones so they could meet their needs and know how to relate to them. "It is hard to gauge sometimes what she understands and what she does not understand." As caregivers came to terms with the reality and permanence of their loved ones' condition, many wanted to find out as much as they could about the disease. What they learned was helpful to them in their new roles. "The more I learned about the disease, the easier it became to be a caregiver. But I also realize that this is just the beginning." "We are learning a lot. It is all new to us and that series of Alzheimer's education; that really helped us."

Preserving Integrity

Integrity is being whole or complete. Many of the participants in this investigation exhibited ways of maintaining a sense of wholeness for their loved ones and for themselves in their roles as caregivers. Caregivers strove for a sense of integrity, being concerned about the safety, maintaining the dignity of their loved one, realizing their own limitation by caring for themselves. "She can be somewhat impulsive like I say, make bad choices for herself that could cause her harm." Another participant expressed concerns about safety, stating that "once in a while, when it has been an issue of safety, like the stove, I cannot back off." The caregivers recognized the importance of being patient in maintaining the integrity of their relationship with the care recipient. "You have to have a very gentle, very patient, subservient approach. Leave her in charge in the unreality situations," and "I am much more patient, much more giving. If I am not that rested, then I am impatient, and impatience gets impatience. I am very cognizant of the fact that it is not one person."

Recognizing their own limitations was a struggle for some caregivers. "But once I just decided OK I have to get other help, then that was really a big help." "I just cannot deal with it no more by myself." Similarly, they realized how necessary it was to take care of themselves. "I know I am going to have to take care of myself first of all if I am ever going to take care of him," and "So I take these mental health space days. I take the time, I think, to rejuvenate myself and say now I can start again."

Gathering Support

Gathering support describes the process by which family care sought information about ADRD, joined support groups, and/or sought physical and psychological support from friends and family members.

I belong to the Alzheimer's Association. I belong to the Wellness Foundation, the one that is out in New York, just to get the mailing, what they have progressed with. The Jewish Family Service. I got the magazine from them...I talk to a lot of people that have the same problems.

Many found support from their families and friends, for which they were grateful. "We have two kids. We are very fortunate; they have been very supportive and really a lot of help." Another respondent stated,

There are a lot of people here and they are all willing to help. They are all from different places so I have neighbors that are willing to help when he goes to day care. If I cannot be here when they bring him home...they have offered to be here for him.

Many relied on their faith for the strength to help them through the hardships of caring for a loved one with ADRD. "But I have a lot of faith and I guess that is what keeps me going and keeps me thankful he is not any worse." Another participant stated, "I just have to pray for help and strength to carry on every day."

Moving With Continuous Change

Although it was apparent that the caregivers' lives had changed drastically with the onset of ADRD, it was also obvious with the unpredictability of the disease their lives would continue to change toward a future that was unknown. The unpredictability was expressed in statements such as, "Well sometimes I get surprises when I least expect them" and "practically anything can set her off"; another stated, "I never really know what to expect." "It is pretty scattered. It just seems like you have to be with him every minute and to anticipate what is going to happen."

This ominous future was frightening to some caregivers as they anticipated the continued decline of their family member. "Well, I am anxious because I do not know what the future is going to bring. I just hope that we are all up to it, whatever it does bring"; "It is scary to think that...they tell me he is going to have to go to a nursing home, and I do not know when. I do not know how I will know when he has to." Another respondent stated, "I guess there is a fear of not knowing what the future holds and how much more time we have until things get to be really more of a problem than they are now." One of the caregivers summed up the moving with continuous change in this way:

I feel like we are kind of going down this path. It is not even a path; it is like a roller coaster ride. All of a sudden you take this huge drop. It evens out for a while and you think ok, we are doing all right. Then it takes another dip. You never know when it is going to happen, when you are going to take the next big slide.

Another change affecting caregivers came as each had to assume new responsibilities their loved ones could no longer meet. This involved learning new skills related to responsibilities such as financial management, power of attorney, homemaking and home repair, yard care, and automobile maintenance and purchasing. "All of a sudden I had the responsibility of everything: the car, the house, everything, even laying out his clothes." Respondents also revealed how difficult it was to deal with the changes. "Boy, that has changed fast so fast in the last three months that I am not sure of my description anymore...Right now with just getting staffing and getting stuff set up, everything has changed so fast"; and "It just changes your life completely"; whereas another said, "It effectively changes your life. Your priorities change. Your life style changes. Your attitude to the person you are giving care to changes. Your role changes."

Finding Meaning and Joy

To focus only on the hardships would provide an unbalanced and incomplete picture of the experience. Many caregivers identified positive aspects of caring. The experience provided an opportunity to cherish the relationship between caregiver and care recipient. "It gives us a bond that would not be there otherwise." With insight into their loved ones' certain decline, participants felt it was important to focus on and enjoy those aspects of their relationships that were still intact. "I know my Dad is not going to get better. So I am trying to enjoy whatever part I can were [sic] he is still himself." They created joyful times to share with their loved ones. "So we are down there practically every day and every day I try and sort of give her a treat"; and "We keep the baby five days a week four hours a day. Four hours a day and she plays with this baby and she loves it." Caregiving, although difficult, was met with a sense of commitment flowing from the quality of the relationship at earlier times. "I just feel that this is the least I can do for him, because we do care for each other." "It certainly is an added chore, but we love each other." Two of the participants captured the essence finding of meaning and joy amidst the burdens of caregiving in each of the following statements:

> Now we are in that stage between, where we are able to enjoy each other to a large extent. So we take advantage and make some good memories now. When you get past that, it is similar to somebody else having another disease who is dying except that it is a disease of the mind. But I would be very happy if he would progress with no pain and very little depression.
>
> Portions of your life are empty. I do not want to cry. I have done a lot of it...I think I feel blessed that I have him and he is still loving toward me...I try to save errands for when he is home because he likes to ride. He likes to eat, so we stop and have ice cream. He will go shopping with me. He will shop til I drop...He never wants anything, he never looks at anything, but he will stay with me. We use up days driving around...A trip without him would be meaningless.

DISCUSSION

The methodological innovativeness of this study expands and deepens understanding of the experience of caring for a family member with ADRD. Methodological innovativeness included the use of secondary qualitative data, phenomenological analysis of a large sample of family caregivers, and the use of a data grid to report the relative frequencies of all preliminary and essential elements. Hinds et al.'s (1997) assessment criteria for evaluating the quality and completeness of a secondary set of qualitative data served as a rigorous means to identify transcribed interviews for appropriate phenomenological data analysis, and van Kaam's (1966) method provides a means to uncover the essence of a human experience in a large data sample. In addition, the reporting of frequencies in van Kaam's method is useful in representing the data in a way that conveys an overall sense of the phenomenon without the loss of salient details. The listing of the preliminary essential elements and their frequencies adds another dimension to understanding the essence of the ADRD caregiving experience. The meaning of each essential element is illuminated by examining the common preliminary themes that were grouped together to form the essential structural element. The larger and more diverse sample of caregiver relationships in this study strengthens the transferability of the findings. The essential structural elements describe the essence of the experience of caring for a more diverse sample of family caregivers, which included spouses, sons, daughters, and sisters.

The synthetic description of the ADRD caregiving experience brought themes together in a way that is distinct from other descriptions of the ADRD caregiving experience in the research literature (C.A. Cohen et al., 1993; Farran, Keane-Hagerty, Salloway, Kupferer, & Wilkin, 1991; Loukissa, Farran, & Graham, 1999; Parson, 1997; Siriopoulos et al., 1999; Willoughby & Keating, 1991; Wilson, 1989). Consistent with the research findings in other qualitative studies of ADRD family caregivers, the most pervasive and difficult experiences in this sample of ADRD family caregivers involved dealing with stress, frustration, and the never-ending day-to-day care; managing difficult symptoms; protecting the care recipient from harm; and dealing with the repetition due to memory loss (Loukissa et al., 1999; Parsons, 1997; Siriopoulos et al., 1999). Respondents vividly described their pain and anguish over the loss of their loved one to the ravishes [sic] of Alzheimer's disease. Caregivers also detailed how much their lives had changed by having to take on all the new responsibilities in caring for their family member as well as taking over those responsibilities their loved one could not longer perform.

Yet, despite the suffering, loss, sadness, pain, stress, and frustration, most caregivers (78%) found positive aspects of and meaning in the caregiving process. Meaningful and joyous times were created through the recollection of earlier and happier memories, engaging in pleasant activities they could enjoy together, cherishing the preciousness of the immediate moment before Alzheimer's disease took even more of their loved ones away, and remaining loyal to their commitment to one another. Recently there has been an increasing focus on the positive aspects of caregiving (Farran, 1997; Kramer, 1997; Langner, 1995). Kramer (1997), in a critical review of 29 studies on "gains" among informal caregivers of older adults, noted that only two of the studies (C.A. Cohen et al., 1993; Farran et al., 1991) used qualitative methods to explore positive aspects of caregiving. She asserts, "given that this [positives aspects] is a relatively new area of inquiry, qualitative approaches...would offer a useful approach for development of comprehensive measures and exploring these issues" (p. 228). Farran et al. (1991) found that 90% of 94 caretakers reported positive aspects in caregiving. In a study of family caregivers of frail elders, Langner (1995) discovered that caregivers felt meaning and personal growth accompanied the pain and loss they experienced. Through the act of caregiving, they entered a process of rediscovering and redefining themselves.

The findings in this study support Farran and Keane-Hagerty's (1991) postulate that valuing positive aspects of relationships and caregiving, and the making of choices about their life and caregiving activities contributes to finding meaning. Meaning, for the participants in this phenomenological study, was found within the anguish of caregiving through their commitment to the care recipient, by identifying the positives in caring for another, and by creating moments of joyfulness together.

Note

1. This research was supported by funds from the NIH/NINR (R01-NR03434) and the Central Investment Fund for Research Enhancement at the University of Iowa. The authors acknowledge the assistance of Toni Tripp-Reimer, RN, PhD, FAAN for her methodological and editorial contributions and Linda Rubenstein, PhD for her statistical consultation.

Research article taken from: Butcher, H.K., Holkup, P.A., & Buckwalter, K.C. (2001). The Experience of Caring for a Family Member With Alzheimer's Disease. *Western Journal of Nursing Research, 23*(1), 33–55. (Reprinted with permission.)

References

Alzheimer's Association. (1996). *Facts about Alzheimer's disease.* Chicago: Author.

Anderson, J., & Eppard, J. (1998). van Kaam's method revisited. *Qualitative Health Research, 8,* 399–403.

Archbold, P.G., & Stewart, B.J. (1996). The nature of the family caregiving role and nursing interventions for caregiving families. In E.A. Swanson & T. Tripp-Reimer (Eds.), *Advances in gerontological nursing: Issues for the 21st century* (Vol. 1, pp. 133–156). New York: Springer.

Baumgarten, M., Hanley, J. A., Infante-Rivard, C., Battista, R. N., Becker, R., & Gauthier, S. (1994). Health of family members caring for elderly persons with dementia: A longitudinal study. *Annals of Internal Medicine, 120,* 126–132.

Beck, C. R. (1998). Phenomenology. In J. Fitzpatrick (Ed.), *Encyclopedia of nursing research* (pp. 431–433). New York: Springer.

Browning, J. S. & Schwirian, P. M. (1994). Spousal caregivers' burden: Impact of care recipient health problems and mental status. *Journal of Gerontological Nursing, 20*(3), 17–22.

Buckwalter, K. C., Hall, G. R., Kelly, A., Sime, A. M., & Richards, B. (1997). *PLST model: Effectiveness for rural ADRD caregivers* (Final Report No. R01-NR03434). Iowa City: University of Iowa.

Buckwalter, K. C., Hall, G. R., Kelly, A., Sime, A. M., Richards, B., & Gerdner, L.A. (1992). *PLST model effectiveness for rural ADRD caregivers* (Report No. R01NR03234). Bethesda, MD: National Institute of Health/National Institute of Nursing Research.

Chang, B. L. (1999). Cognitive-behavioral intervention for homebound caregivers of persons with dementia. *Nursing Research, 48,* 173–181.

Coe, M., & Neufeld, A. (1999). Male caregivers' use of formal support. *Western Journal of Nursing Research, 21,* 568–588.

Cohen, C. A., Gold, D. P., Shulman, K. I., Wortley, J. T., McDonald, G., & Wargon, M. (1993). Factors determining the decision to institutionalize dementing individuals: A prospective study. *The Gerontologist, 33*(6), 714–720.

Cohen, D., & Eisdorfer, C. (1988). Depression in family members caring for a relative with Alzheimer's disease. *Journal of the American Geriatrics Society, 36,* 885–998.

Corcoran, M. A. (1994). Management decisions made by caregiver spouses of persons with Alzheimer's disease. *American Journal of Occupational Therapy, 48,* 38–45.

Davis, L. L. (1997). Family conflicts around dementia home care. *Family Systems Medicine, 15*(1), 85–95.

Drebing, C. E. (1999). Trends in the content and methodology of Alzheimer caregiving research. *Alzheimer Disease and Associated Disorders, 13*(Suppl 1), S93–S100.

Estes, C. (1993). The aging enterprise revisited. *The Gerontologist, 33,* 292–298.

Farran, C. J. (1997). Theoretical perspectives concerning positive aspects of caring for elderly persons with dementia: stress/adaptation and existentialism. *The Gerontologist, 37*(2), 250–256.

Farran, C. J., & Keane-Hagerty, E. (1991). An interactive model of finding meaning through caregiving. In P.L. Chinn (Ed.), *An anthology on caring* (pp. 225–237). New York: National League for Nursing.

Farran, C. J., Keane-Hagerty, E., Salloway, S., Kupferer, S., & Wilken, C. S. (1991). Finding meaning: An alternative paradigm for Alzheimer's disease family caregivers. *The Gerontologist, 31*(4), 483–489.

Farran, C. J., Keane-Hagerty, E., Tatarowicz, L., & Scorza, E. (1993). Dementia care–receiver needs and their impact on caregivers. *Clinical Nursing Research, 2*(1), 86–97.

Gallagher, D., Rose, J., Rivera, P., Lovett, S., & Thompson, L. W. (1989). Prevalence of depression in family caregivers. *The Gerontologist, 29,* 449–456.

Gerdner, L. A., Hall, G. R., & Buckwalter, K. C. (1996). Caregiver training for people with Alzheimer's based on a stress threshold model. *Image: Journal of Nursing Scholarship, 28*(3), 241–246.

Giorgi, A. (1985). Introduction. In A. Giorgi (Ed.), *Phenomenology and psychological research* (pp. 1–7). Pittsburgh: Duquesne University Press.

Gubrium, J. F. (1996). Taking stock. *Qualitative Health Research, 5*(3), 267–269.

Hall, G. R., & Buckwalter, K. C. (1987). Progressively lowered stress threshold: A conceptual model for care of adults with Alzheimer's disease. *Archives of Psychiatric Nursing, 1*(6), 399–406.

Hasselkus, B.R. (1998). Meaning in family caregiving: Perspectives on caregiver/professional relationships. *The Gerontologist, 28,* 686–691.

Hinds, P. S., Vogel, R. J., & Clark-Steffen, L. (1997). The possibilities and pitfalls of doing a secondary analysis of a qualitative data set. *Qualitative Health Research, 7,* 408–423.

Hurley, A. C., & Wells, N. (1999). Past, present, and future directions for Alzheimer research. *Alzheimer Disease and Associated Disorders, 13*(Suppl 1), S6-S10.

Kellet, U.M. (1997). Heideggerian phenomenology: An approach to understanding family caring for an older relative. *Nursing Inquiry, 4,* 57–65.

Kelley, L. S., Buckwalter, K. C., & Maas, M. L. (1999). Access to health care resources for family caregivers of elderly persons with dementia. *Nursing Outlook, 47*(1), 8–14.

Kramer, G.J. (1997). Gain in the caregiving experience: Where are we? What next? *The Gerontologist, 37*(2), 218–232.

Kuhlman, G. J., Wilson, H. S., Hutchinson, S. A., & Wallhagen, M. (1991). Alzheimer's disease and family caregiving: Critical synthesis of the literature and research agenda. *Nursing Research, 40*(6), 331–337.

Langner, S. R. (1995). Finding meaning in caring for elderly relatives: Loss and personal growth. *Holistic Nursing Practice, 9*(3), 75–84.

Lindgren, C. L., Connelly, C. T., & Gaspar, H. L. (1999). Grief in spouse and children caregivers of dementia patients. *Western Journal of Nursing Research, 21*(4), 521–537.

Loukissa, D., Farran, C. J., & Graham, K. L. (1999). Caring for a relative with Alzheimer's disease: The experience of African-American and Caucasian caregivers. *American Journal of Alzheimer's Disease, 14*(4), 207–216.

Lynch-Sauer, J. (1990). When a family member has Alzheimer's disease: A phenomenological description of caregiving. *Journal of Gerontological Nursing, 16*(9), 8–11.

Malmgren, R. (1994). Epidemiology of aging. In C.E. Coffey & J.L. Cummings (Eds.), *The American Psychiatric Press textbook of geriatric neuropsychiatry* (pp. 17–33). Washington, DC: American Psychiatric Press.

Mastrian, K. G., Ritter, C., & Deimling, G. T. (1996). Predictors of caregiver health strain. *Home Healthcare Nurse, 4*(3), 209–217.

McCarty, E. F. (1996). Caring for a parent with Alzheimer's disease: Process of daughter caregiver stress. *Journal of Advanced Nursing, 23*(4), 792–803.

Mitchell, G.J. (1992). The meaning of being a senior: Phenomenological research and interpretation with Parse's theory of nursing. *Nursing Science Quarterly, 7,* 70–79. Morrissey, E., Becker, J., & Rubert, M. P. (1990). Coping resources and depression in the caregiving spouses of Alzheimer patients. *British Journal of Medical Psychology, 63*(Pt 2), 161–171.

Myers, G., & Agree, E. (1994, March). The world ages, the family changes: A demographic perspective. *Aging International,* 11–18.

National Advisory Council on Alzheimer's Disease. (1989). *First report of the advisory panel on Alzheimer's disease* (DHHS Pub. No. (ADM) 86–1664). Washington, DC: Superintendent of Documents, Government Printing Office.

Omery, A. (1993). Phenomenology: A method for nursing research. *Advances in Nursing Science, 5*(2), 49–63.

Parse, R. R., Coyne, A. B., & Smith, M. J. (1985). *Nursing research: Qualitative methods.* Bowie, MD: Brady.

Parsons, K. (1997). The male experience of caregiving for a family member with Alzheimer's disease. *Qualitative Health Research, 7*(3), 391–407.

Perry, J., & Olshansky, E. F. (1996). A family's coming to terms with Alzheimer's disease. *Western Journal of Nursing Research, 18*(1), 12–28.

Phillips, L.R., Morrison, E., Steffl, B., Chae, Y. M., Cromwell, S. L., & Russell, C. K. (1995). Effects of the situational context and interactional process on the quality of family caregiving. *Research in Nursing and Health, 18*(3), 205–216.

QSR NUD*IST Nvivo. (1999). [Computer software]. Victoria, Australia: Qualitative Solutions and Research Pty. Ltd.

Richards, T. J., & Richards, L. (1994). Using computers in qualitative research. In N.K. Denzin & Y.S. Lincold (Eds.), *Handbook of qualitative research* (pp. 445–462). Thousand Oaks, CA: Sage.

Schultz, R., O'Brien, A. T., Bookwala, J., & Fleissner, K. (1995). Psychiatric and physical morbidity effects of dementia caregiving: Prevalence, correlates, and causes. *The Gerontologist, 35*(6), 771–791.

Seltzer, B., Vasterling, J. J., Yoder, J. A., & Thompson, K. A. (1997). Awareness of deficit in Alzheimer's disease: Relation to caregiver burden. *The Gerontologist, 37*(1), 20–24.

Siriopoulos, G., Brown, Y., & Wright, K. (1999). Caregivers of wives diagnosed with Alzheimer's disease: Husbands' perspectives. *American Journal of Alzheimer's Disease, 14*(2), 79–87.

Taueber, C. (1992). *Sixty-five plus in America* (Series P23, C3, 186:P23/178). Washington, DC: U.S. Department of Commerce, Bureau of the Census.

Thorne, S. (1994). Secondary analysis in qualitative research: Issues and implications. In J. Morse (Ed.), *Critical issues in qualitative research methods* (pp. 263–279). Thousand Oaks, CA: Sage.

van Kaam, A. (1966). *Existential foundations of psychology.* New York: Image.

van Manen, M. (1990). *Researching the lived experience.* New York: State University of New York Press.

Willoughby, J., & Keating, N. (1991). Being in control: The process of caring for a relative with Alzheimer's disease. *Qualitative Health Research, 1*(1), 27–50.

Wilson, H. S. (1989). Family caregiving for a relative with Alzheimer's dementia: Coping with negative choices. *Nursing Research, 38,* 94–98.

Winslow, B. W. (1998). Family caregiving and the use of formal community support services: A qualitative case study. *Issues in Mental Health Nursing, 19*(1), 11–27.

Wondolowski, C., & Davis, D. K. (1990). The lived experience of health in the oldest old: A phenomenological study. *Nursing Science Quarterly, 4*(3), 113–118.

Wright, L. K. (1991). The impact of Alzheimer's disease on marital relationship. *The Gerontologist, 31*(2), 224–237.

Zarit, S. H., Todd, P. A., & Zarit, J. M. (1986). Subjective burden of husbands and wives as caregivers: A longitudinal study. *The Gerontologist, 26*(3), 260–266.

Grounded Theory as Method

Grounded theory is a qualitative research approach used to explore the social processes that present within human interactions. As a research approach, grounded theory differs from phenomenology in that the primary purpose is to develop a theory about the dominant social processes rather than to describe a particular phenomenon. The roots of grounded theory can be found in the interpretive tradition of symbolic interactionism, which speculates on issues related to human behavior. Through application of the approach, researchers develop explanations of key social processes or structures that are derived from or grounded in empirical data (Hutchinson, 2001). Grounded theorists assume that each group shares a specific social psychological problem that is not necessarily articulated (Hutchinson, 2001). Glaser and Strauss (1967) developed the method and published the first text addressing method issues: *The Discovery of Grounded Theory*.

Nursing has used the grounded theory to describe phenomena important to professional nursing (Beck, 1993; Benoliel, 1967; Hutchinson, 1992; Stern, 1981; Wilson 1977, 1986). Benoliel (1996) noted that grounded theory began to influence nursing knowledge development in the early 1960s. In her manuscript "Grounded Theory and Nursing Knowledge," she examined how the method has contributed to nursing's body of substantive knowledge from the 1960s through the 1990s. Benoliel (1967) suggested that the major focus of the contributions to nursing knowledge over these decades was on "adaptations to illness, infertility, nurse adaptation and interventions, and status passages of vulnerable persons and groups" (p. 406). Grounded theory is an extensively applied research approach and makes important contributions to nursing's development of a substantive body of knowledge, primarily due to its ability to develop middle-range theory, which can be tested empirically.

GROUNDED THEORY DEFINED

Grounded theory as a method of qualitative research is a form of field research. Field research refers to qualitative research approaches that explore and describe phenomena in naturalistic settings such as hospitals, outpatient clinics, or nursing homes. Unlike quantitative research, grounded theory does not begin with an existing theory but rather generates theory in a specific substantive area. The pri-

mary purpose of grounded theory research is the discovery of theory from method-
ical data generation. Precise procedural steps are applied to ultimately develop a
grounded theory, or theoretically complete explanation about a particular phenomenon (Benoliel, 1967; Stern, 1980; Strauss & Corbin, 1990). Strauss and
Corbin (1990) have explained grounded theory as follows:

> A grounded theory is one that is inductively derived from the study of the phe-
> nomenon it represents. That is, it is discovered, developed, and provisionally
> verified through systematic data collection and analysis of data pertaining to
> that phenomenon. Therefore, data collection, analysis, and theory stand in
> reciprocal relationship with each other. One does not begin with a theory, then
> prove it. Rather, one begins with an area of study and what is relevant to that
> area is allowed to emerge (p. 23).

The goal of grounded theory investigations is to discover theoretically complete explanations about particular phenomena. According to Strauss and Corbin
(1990), grounded theory involves "systematic techniques and procedures of analysis that enable the researcher to develop a substantive theory that meets the criteria for doing 'good' science: significance, theory-observation compatibility, generalizability, reproducibility, precision, rigor, and verification" (p. 31).

Through an inductive approach, researchers using the method generate theory
that can be either formal or substantive. *Substantive theory* is that developed for
a substantive, or empirical, area of inquiry (Glaser & Strauss, 1967). Examples
pertinent to nursing might include client care, hope describing a model of health
for homeless people (McCormack & Macintosh, 2001) or health warnings for
people with diabetes and hypertension (Weiss & Hutchinson, 2000). *Formal theory* is developed for a formal, or conceptual, area of inquiry (Glaser & Strauss,
1967). Examples might include socialization to professional nursing or authority
and power in nursing practice. Substantive and formal theories are considered to
be middle-range theories in that both types fall between the working hypotheses
and the all-inclusive grand theories (Glaser & Strauss, 1967).

Grand theories are complex, attempting to explain broad areas within a discipline as opposed to middle-range theory, which comprises primarily relational
concepts. "A grand theory consists of a global conceptual framework that defines
broad perspectives for practice and includes diverse ways of viewing nursing phenomena based on these perspectives" (Marriner-Tomey, 2002, p. 307). Grand theories are broadest in scope, frequently lack operationally defined concepts, and
are unsuitable to direct empirical testing (Fawcett, 1989). *Partial theories* are the
most limited in scope and utility, comprising summary statements of isolated
observation within a narrow range of phenomena. Some partial or micro theories
may be developed into middle-range theories with additional research (Fawcett,
1989).

Middle-range theories have a narrower scope than grand theories and encom-
pass limited concepts and aspects of the real world (Fawcett, 1989). Middle-range
theories have been purported to be most useful because researchers can empirically
test them in a direct manner (Merton, 1957).

An important concept for new grounded theorists to recognize is that researchers do not begin with theory. Instead, researchers identify essential constructs from generated data; from these data, theory emerges. Procedural steps in grounded theory are specific and occur simultaneously (Fig. 7.1). Because the information pertinent to the emerging theory comes directly from the data, the generated theory remains connected to or grounded in the data (Glaser & Strauss, 1967; Stern, 1980; Strauss & Corbin, 1990).

Stern (1980) differentiated grounded theory from other qualitative methodologies. There are five basic differences:

1. The conceptual framework of grounded theory is generated from the data rather than from previous studies.
2. The researcher attempts to discover dominant processes in the social scene rather than describe the unit under investigation.
3. The researcher compares all data with all other data.
4. The researcher may modify data collection according to the advancing theory; that is, the researcher drops false leads or asks more penetrating questions as needed.
5. The investigator examines data as they arrive, and begins to code, categorize, conceptualize, and write the first few thoughts concerning the research report almost from the beginning of the study.

Methodological issues raised by more recent attempts to refine the process of generating grounded theory continue to be addressed in the literature (Baker, Wuest, & Stern, 1992; Keddy, Sims, & Stern, 1996; Robrecht, 1995; Wuest, 1995). Baker et al. (1992) discussed method slurring between grounded theory and phenomenology, which mixed steps from both methods, and addressed the importance of being specific about method. Robrecht (1995) proposed "dimensional analysis, described by Schatzman in 1991 as a method for the generation of grounded theory" (p. 169). Within a feminist framework, the grounded theory method incorporates diversity and change (Wuest, 1995).

GROUNDED THEORY ROOTS

As a qualitative research method, grounded theory has been used extensively in the discipline of sociology. Based on the symbolic interactionist perspective of human behavior, the development of this qualitative research approach has been credited to Barney Glaser and Anselm Strauss, two sociologists at the University of California in San Francisco. Nurse–researchers have widely recognized the significance of grounded theory as a method to investigate phenomena important to nursing and have used this approach extensively.

Benoliel (1996) examined the roots of grounded theory in nursing and its development over the past several decades. She identified the knowledge generation that occurred during this period as the Decade of Discovery, 1960–1970;

Decade of Development, 1970–1980; Decade of Diffusion, 1980–1990; and Decade of Diversification, 1990 to present.

During the Decade of Discovery, 1960–1970, grounded theory emerged as a major research method within the field of sociology. As the method entered the Decade of Development (1970–1980), seminars for the continued development of grounded theorists emerged as well as funding for postdoctoral research training programs (Benoliel, 1996). The Decade of Diffusion (1980–1990) resulted in even further expansion of the research method, and nursing became visible as a group of researchers who could explain and implement grounded theory method. Nursing journals gave more attention to grounded theory and university centers evolved that focused on grounded theory research in nursing (Benoliel, 1996). The Decade of Diversification (1990 to present) has resulted in the dissemination of the knowledge gained through grounded theory research.

Grounded theory is an important research method for the study of nursing phenomena. The method explores the richness and diversity of the human experience and contributes to the development of middle-range theories in nursing. This chapter reviews fundamental themes of grounded theory and addresses methodological issues specific to engaging in this qualitative research approach. The chapter also reviews the systematic techniques and procedures of analysis essential to grounded theory investigations. Additional reading of primary sources is necessary to grasp the method in a comprehensive manner.

FUNDAMENTAL CHARACTERISTICS OF THE GROUNDED THEORY METHOD

Because Glaser and Strauss (1967) were the first to address grounded theory as a research method, they are consequently credited with the development and refinement of the method. Stern (1980) has written about the use of grounded theory in nursing and the importance of its use as a rigorous research method.

Grounded theory explores basic social processes. Symbolic interactionism theory, described by George Herbert Mead (1964) and Herbert Blumer (1969), provides theoretical underpinnings of grounded theory method. In symbolic interactionism theory, it is believed that people behave and interact based on how they interpret or give meaning to specific symbols in their lives, such as style of dress or verbal and nonverbal expressions. For example, the nurse's cap, which is seen less frequently, was a style of dress that gave meaning to some clients, which is apparent from statements such as, "How do I know you are my nurse if you do not wear your cap?" or "I liked it better when nurses wore caps—they looked more professional." Language can also have different meanings for different people. A common statement made by many nurses is, "I'm working on the floor today." Individuals familiar with the health care environment are likely to interpret that statement to mean that the nurse has been assigned to a specific unit in the hospital where he or she is providing nursing care to clients. Someone who is unfamiliar with the hospital setting or is from a different culture may interpret this statement differently. To them, "I'm working on the floor today" may mean cleaning or repairing the floor. Stern, Allen, and Moxley (1982) emphasized that

> it is also through the meaning and value of which these symbols have for us that we try to interpret our world and the actors who interact with us. In this way, we try to read minds, and to act accordingly. Learning the meaning and value of interactional symbols is everyone's lifetime study, and no easy task (p. 203).

The study and exploration of the social processes that present within human interactions in grounded theory are linked directly to symbolic interactionism.

Grounded theory methodology combines both inductive and deductive research methods (Glaser & Strauss, 1967; Stern, 1980; Strauss & Corbin, 1990). From an inductive perspective, theory emerges from specific observations and generated data. The theory then can be tested empirically to develop predictions from general principles such as a deductive research method. Hutchinson (2001) addressed an important difference between verificational research and grounded theory research. Her explanation is helpful in clarifying the inductive nature of grounded theory:

> In verificational research, the researcher chooses an existing theory or conceptual framework and formulates hypotheses, which are then tested in a specific population. Verificational research is linear; the researcher delineates a problem, selects a theoretical framework, develops hypotheses, collects data, tests the hypotheses, and interprets the results. On a continuum, verificational research is more deductive whereas grounded theory research is more inductive. Verificational research moves from a general theory to a specific situation, whereas grounded theorists aim for the development of a more inclusive, general theory through the analysis of specific social phenomena (p. 212).

Constant comparative analysis is another fundamental characteristic that guides data generation and treatment. *Constant comparative analysis* of qualitative data combines an analytic procedure of constant comparison with an explicit coding procedure for generated data. "The aim of this method is the generation of theoretical constructs that, along with substantive codes and categories and their properties, form a theory that encompasses and explains as much behavioral variation as possible" (Hutchinson, 2001, p. 228). *Core variables* that are broad in scope interrelate concepts and hypotheses that emerge during data analysis. *Basic social psychologic processes* (BSPs) illustrate the social processes that emerge from the data analysis. A later section on the application of the grounded theory method explains these fundamental characteristics in greater detail.

SELECTION OF GROUNDED THEORY AS A METHOD

The need for more middle-range theories in nursing that can be empirically tested is one reason for using grounded theory to conduct scientific investigations of phenomena important to nursing. Stern et al. (1982) further articulated the factors linking grounded theory to nursing: Nursing occurs in a natural rather than controlled setting, and the nursing process requires "constant comparison of collected and coded data, hypothesis generation, use of the literature as data, and collection of additional data to verify or reject hypotheses" (p. 201).

Grounded theorists embarking on a new investigation should ask themselves, Have I paid enough attention to this particular phenomenon in terms of the individual's viewpoint? Has empirical research and the published literature offered what seems to be an oversimplification of the concepts relevant to the phenomenon under investigation? Is there a need for a deeper understanding of specific characteristics related to a particular phenomenon? Has the phenomenon been previously investigated? Positive answers to these or similar questions can validate for grounded theorists that the method choice is appropriate. As in any type of research, grounded theorists must consider the issues of available resources, time frame, and personal commitment to the investigation.

ELEMENTS AND INTERPRETATION OF THE METHOD

Application of grounded theory research techniques to the investigation of phenomena important to nursing education, practice, and administration involves several processes. The following is a discussion on the development and refinement of the research question as well as on the sample, researcher's role, and ethical considerations in grounded theory investigations. Also described are the steps in the research process, including data generation, treatment, and analysis.

Research Question

The main purpose of using the grounded theory approach is to explore social processes with the goal of developing theory. The research question in a grounded theory investigation identifies the phenomenon to be studied. More specifically, the question lends focus and clarity about what the phenomenon of interest is (Strauss & Corbin, 1990). Furthermore, researchers need a research question or questions that will give us the flexibility and freedom to explore a phenomenon in depth. Also underlying this approach to qualitative research is the assumption that all of the concepts pertaining to a given phenomenon have not yet been identified, at least not in this population or place; or if so, then the relationships between the concepts are poorly understood or conceptually undeveloped (Strauss & Corbin, 1990).

The nature of grounded theory methodology requires that investigators refine the research question as they generate and analyze the study data. Because the study focus may change depending on the data generated, the original question merely lends focus to the study. A truly accurate research question is impossible to ask before beginning any grounded theory study (Hutchinson, 2001).

An example of a grounded theory question that begins an investigation and lends focus to the study is, How do nursing faculty address unsafe skill performance by nursing students? The question is broad but adds focus to the investigation by clarifying that the study will explore faculty evaluation and feedback techniques as they relate to unsafe student clinical performance. As data collection and analysis proceed, the focus of the study may change, given the emerging theory. Hypothetically, the focus of the study could change to, What is unsafe skill performance? Researchers must begin with a broad question that also provides focus. Researchers should expect that they will refine the question throughout the research process.

Sampling

Participants for a grounded theory investigation must be selected based on their experience with the social process under investigation. Just as it is impossible to finalize the research question before a grounded theory investigation, it is equally impossible to know how many participants will be involved. The sample size is determined by the data generated and their analysis. Grounded theorists continue to collect data until they achieve saturation of conceptual information and no new codes emerge. The researcher can gain closure by constant questioning and reexamination of the data (Hutchinson, 2001).

Researcher's Role

Stern (1980) emphasized that, in a naturalistic setting, it is impossible to control for the presence of the researcher. Investigators bring personal experience to a study to enhance understanding of the problem. According to Stern et al. (1982), in the conduct of naturalistic research, investigators do not attempt to remove themselves from the study. Rather, researchers openly recognize they have a role in the investigation. Stern et al. further delineated the grounded theorist's role as follows: "The grounded theory researcher works within a matrix where several processes go on at once rather than following a series of linear steps. The investigator examines data as they arrive, and begins to code, categorize, conceptualize, and to write the first few thoughts concerning the research report almost from the beginning of the study" (p. 205). The researcher is an integral part of the investigation and, consequently, must recognize the intimate role with the participants and include the implications of that role in the actual investigation and interpretation of the data.

Strauss and Corbin (1990) have identified skills needed for doing qualitative research: the ability "to step back and critically analyze situations, to recognize and avoid bias, to obtain valid and reliable data, and to think abstractly" (p. 18). Furthermore, "a qualitative researcher requires theoretical and social sensitivity, the ability to maintain analytical distance while at the same time drawing upon past experience and theoretical knowledge to interpret what is seen, astute powers of observation, and good interactional skills" (p. 18). To conduct a grounded theory investigation, researchers must possess excellent interpersonal and observational skills, compelling analytical abilities, and writing skills that facilitate communication in written word, with a high degree of accuracy, regarding what they have learned.

Ethical Considerations

Researchers must also consider the ethical implications of conducting a grounded theory investigation or, for that matter, any qualitative investigation. Obtaining informed consent, maintaining confidentiality, and handling sensitive information are a few examples of ethical considerations researchers must address. Because it is impossible to anticipate what sensitive issues might emerge during data collection in a grounded theory investigation, researchers must be prepared for unexpected concerns. Chapter 16 provides an extensive discussion of ethical considerations pertinent to qualitative investigations.

Steps in the Research Process

Stern (1980) described five steps in the process of grounded theory research that compose the fundamental components of the method. They are (1) the collection of empirical data, (2) concept formation, (3) concept development, (4) concept modification and integration, and (5) production of the research report.

Data Generation

Researchers may collect grounded theory data from interview, observation, or documents, or from a combination of these sources (Stern, 1980). Daily journals, participant observation, formal or semistructured interviews, and informal interviews are valid means of generating data. As concepts and categories emerge during data analysis, the required sampling of particular data sources continues until each category is saturated. No limits are set on the number of participants, interviewees, or data sources (Cutcliffe, 2000). Sampling in grounded theory research is consequently theoretical rather than purposeful (Glaser & Strauss, 1978). Participant selection and data generation sources are a function of the emerging hypothesis. Theoretical sampling is the process of data generation that requires the researcher to collect, code, and analyze data simultaneously. This process develops in response to the emerging theory and allows the research to develop richer data where needed.

Weiss and Hutchinson (2000) describe their data generation techniques in their study "Warnings About Vulnerability in Clients with Diabetes and Hypertension."

> Audio-recorded interviews, conducted and transcribed by the first author, lasted from 1 to 2 hours. Word Perfect computer software facilitated the analysis. Most interviews occurred in the client's home; interviews with providers occurred in their offices. Follow-up interviews to confirm and expand the initial interviews occurred with 2 participants and 2 health care providers (p. 524).

Hutchinson (1992) further explained that her data collection included participant observation at six Board of Nursing (BON) meetings and three administrative hearings as well as document analysis in which she read files on nurses who had appeared before the BON. This example should give readers a sense of the many methods researchers use to generate data in grounded theory investigations.

The researcher examines and analyzes the data gathered using field techniques, observational methods, documents, and publications through a system of constant comparison until the investigation generates a number of hypotheses. As investigators develop hypotheses, they consult the literature for previously developed theories that relate to the emerging hypotheses of the study in progress. The developed theory, consisting of related factors or variables, should be suitable for testing (Hutchinson, 2001; Stern, 1980; Strauss & Corbin, 1990).

Data Treatment

The choice of data treatment and collection methods is influenced primarily by researcher preference. Researchers generally tape-record interviews and transcribe them verbatim. Researchers should transcribe and type double-spaced field notes immediately. It is also helpful to leave at least a 2-inch margin on one side of the transcribed data sheets for coding purposes. The availability of computer programs for qualitative data analysis offers another option. Table 7.1 provides readers with an example of a field note and Level I coding.

Data Analysis: Generating Theory

The discovery of a core variable is the goal of grounded theory. "The researcher undertakes the quest for this essential element of the theory, which illuminates the main theme of the actors in the setting, and explicates what is going on in the data" (Glaser, 1978, p. 94). The core variable serves as the foundational concept for theory generation, and "the integration and density of the theory are dependent on the discovery of a significant core variable" (Hutchinson, 2001, p. 222). The core variable has six essential characteristics:

1. It recurs frequently in the data.
2. It links various data.
3. Because it is central, it explains much of the variation in all the data.
4. It has implications for a more general or formal theory.
5. As it becomes more detailed, the theory moves forward.
6. It permits maximum variation and analyses (Strauss, 1987, p. 36).

BSPs are core variables that illustrate social processes as they continue over time, regardless of varying conditions (Glaser, 1978). For example, in Weiss and Hutchinson's (2000) article "Warnings About Vulnerability in Clients with Diabetes and Hypertension," the basic social process consists of internal and external warnings related to adherence to health care directives. Emergence of the core variable is discussed later in the section Concept Development.

TABLE 7.1	SAMPLE FIELD NOTE	
Field Note	**Level I Coding**
2/18/98	
There are 7 students, 1 faculty member, and 3 staff members to care for 35 orthopedic clients. Each student has been assigned 1 client. The students are juniors in a baccalaureate nursing program. This is their <u>1st clinical experience</u> and their 4th week on the unit. The instructor is working with a student as she prepares an intramuscular injection. <u>The student's hands are trembling.</u> The student drops the uncapped syringe on the floor, bends down, picks up the syringe to prepare to use the contaminated syringe to prepare the injection. <u>The instructor asks her what is wrong with the way she is proceeding.</u> <u>The student does not know. Tears are welling up in</u> <u>the student's eyes. The instructor's face is flushed and</u> <u>she seems frustrated.</u> The instructor <u>explains</u> what is wrong, <u>tells</u> the student she is unprepared for the experience, and <u>asks</u> a staff member to give the injection. The staff member comments she doesn't have time. <u>The student leaves the medication room crying. The instructor takes her to a conference room to discuss the incident.</u>	Fear Questioning Overwhelming Frustration Telling Asking Privacy

Concept Formation

Grounded theory requires that researchers collect, code, and analyze data from the beginning of the study. "The method is circular, allowing the researchers to change focus and pursue leads revealed by the ongoing data analysis" (Hutchinson, 2001, p. 223). Figure 7–1 illustrates the ongoing nature of data analysis in grounded theory.

Coding

During the conduct of a grounded theory investigation, the processes of data collection, coding, and analysis occur simultaneously. As they collect data through interviews, participant observation, field notes, and so forth, researchers begin to code data. They then examine data line by line, identify processes, and conceptualize underlying patterns. Coding occurs at three levels.

Level I Coding *Level I coding* requires that grounded theorists look for process. As they receive data, investigators apply a system of open coding; that is, they examine the data line by line and identify the processes in the data. It is critical to code each sentence and incident using as many codes as possible to ensure

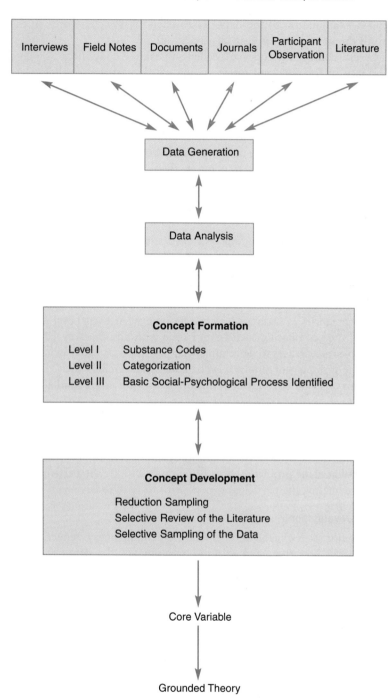

FIGURE 7-1. Grounded theory and connections among data generation, treatment, and analysis.

a thorough examination of the data. Researchers write code words in the wide margins of the field notes for easy identification.

In Level I coding, the codes are called substantive codes because they codify the substance of the data and often use the words participants themselves have used (Stern, 1980, p. 21). The two types of substantive codes are (1) those from the language of the people who were observed or interviewed and (2) implicit codes constructed by researchers based on concepts obtained from the data (Mullen & Reynolds, 1978).

From the beginning of the study, grounded theorists attempt to discover as many categories as possible and to compare them with new indicators to uncover characteristics and relationships. They discard early codes if those codes lack foundation in the data and may add more codes as data gathering progresses (Mullen & Reynolds, 1978).

Level II Coding   *Level II coding* or *categorizing* requires use of the constant comparative method in the treatment of data. Researchers code the data, compare them with other data, and assign the data to clusters or categories according to obvious fit. Categories are simply coded data that seem to cluster and may result from the condensing of Level I codes (Hutchinson, 2001; Stern, 1980). Deciding on specific categories is facilitated by questioning what each Level I code might indicate and then comparing each Level I code with all other Level I codes. This process enables researchers to determine what particular category would be appropriate for the grouping of similar Level I codes. Researchers then compare each category with every other category to ensure the categories are mutually exclusive.

Level III Coding   *Level III coding* describes BSPs, which essentially compose the title given to the central themes that emerge from the data. Questions suggested by Glaser and Strauss (1967) to describe BSPs include the following: What is going on in the data? What is the focus of the study and the relationship of the data to the study? What is the problem that is being dealt with by the participants? What processes are helping the participants cope with the problem?

Concept Development

Three major steps expand and define the emerging theory: reduction, selective sampling of the literature, and selective sampling of the data. Through these processes, the core variable emerges (Stern et al., 1982).

Reduction   During data analysis, an overwhelming number of categories emerge that researchers need to reduce in number. Comparing categories allows researchers to see how they cluster or connect and can be fit under another broader category (Stern et al., 1982). Category reduction is an essential component determining the primary social processes or core variables that trace the action in the social scene being investigated. The result of this reduction is a clustering of categories that, when combined, form a category of broader scope.

Selective Sampling of the Literature   Stern (1980) has suggested that attempting a literature search before the study begins is unnecessary and perhaps may even be detrimental to the study. Reviewing the literature may lead to prejudgments and affect premature closure of ideas, the direction may be wrong, and available data or materials may be inaccurate (Stern, 1980).

Selective sampling of the literature is suggested and generally follows or occurs simultaneously with data analysis. The literature review helps researchers become familiar with works published on the concepts under study and fills in the missing pieces in the emerging theory. Referring to the example—How do nursing faculty address unsafe skill performance by nursing students?—that illustrated the development of the research question, investigators may review the published literature on the teaching of clinical skills, evaluation of those skills, or perhaps literature on what constitutes unsafe performance. Depending on what additional data emerge, researchers will also need to review literature pertinent to those new concepts.

As theory begins to develop, researchers conduct a literature review to learn what has been published about the emerging concepts. They use the existing literature as data and weave the literature into a matrix consisting of data, category, and conceptualization. Literature, carefully scrutinized, helps expand the theory and relate it to other theories (Stern et al., 1982). The literature can fill in gaps in the emerging theory and add completeness to the theoretical description.

Selective Sampling of the Data   As the main concepts or variables become apparent, comparison with the data determines under which conditions they occur and if the concepts or variables seem central to the emerging theory. Researchers may collect additional data in a selective manner to develop the hypotheses and identify the properties of the main categories. Through selective sampling, saturation of the categories occurs (Stern et al., 1982).

Emergence of the Core Variable   Through the process of reduction and comparison, the core variable for the investigation emerges. "The concept of core variable refers to a category which accounts for most of the variation in a pattern of behavior and which helps to integrate other categories that have been discovered in the data" (Mullen & Reynolds, 1978, p. 282). Draucker and Stern (2001) studied "Women's Responses to Sexual Violence by Male Intimates." The core variable of their grounded theory investigation was described as "forging ahead in a dangerous world," which "reflects the women's descriptions of life after violence as a struggle to get on with their lives in a social world they know through first hand experience to be unsafe" (p. 385).

Following the emergence of the core variable, researchers begin the steps of concept modification and integration. Through the use of theoretical codes, the conceptual framework moves from a descriptive to a theoretical level.

Concept Modification and Integration

Concept modification and integration are accomplished as researchers continue to analyze data. Theoretical coding provides direction, and memoing preserves the researcher's thoughts and abstractions related to the emerging theory.

Theoretical Coding   *Theoretical coding* gives direction to the process of examining data in theoretical rather than descriptive terms (Stern, 1980). According to

Stern (1980), this means applying a variety of analytical schemes to data to enhance their abstraction. Moving from descriptive to theoretical explanations, researchers examine all the variables that may affect data analysis and findings (Stern, 1980). During concept modification and integration, researchers use memoing to maintain their ideas pertinent to the emerging theory.

Memoing   Memoing preserves emerging hypotheses, analytical schemes, hunches, and abstractions. Researchers must sort memos into cluster concepts to tie up or remove loose ends. They write memos on file cards or paper or store them in computer files. During the process, it becomes clear how concepts fully integrate with one another and which analytical journey extends beyond the focus of the research report. Investigators set aside memos that do not fit until they write another focus of the study. Sorted memos become the basis for the research report (Stern, 1980).

Production of the Research Report

The research report for a grounded theory investigation presents the theory, which is substantiated by supporting data from field notes. The report should give readers an idea of the sources of the data, how the data were rendered, and how the concepts were integrated. A good report reflects the theory in ways that allow an outsider to grasp its meaning and apply its concepts.

EVALUATION OF GROUNDED THEORIES

Strauss and Corbin (1990) identified four criteria for judging the applicability of theory to a phenomenon: (1) fit, (2) understanding, (3) generality, and (4) control. If theory is faithful to the everyday reality of the substantive area and is carefully induced from diverse data, then it should fit that substantive area. If a researcher collected insufficient data and attempted closure too soon, then it is impossible to meet this criterion. Because it represents a reality, the grounded theory derived should be comprehensible to both the study participants and to practitioners with experience in the specific area studied. If the data on which the theory is based are comprehensive and the interpretations conceptual and broad, then that theory should be abstract enough and include sufficient variation so that it may apply to a variety of contexts related to the phenomenon under study, thus meeting the criterion of generality. The theory also should provide control with regard to action toward the phenomenon (Strauss & Corbin, 1990).

SUMMARY

Grounded theory plays a significant role in the conduct of qualitative research. The fundamental characteristics and application of the approach include issues related to refinement of the research question; determination of the sample; and data generation, treatment, and analysis. Applied to the profession of nursing, grounded theory can increase middle-range substantive theories and help explain theoretical gaps among theory, research, and practice. Chapter 8 continues with the grounded theory method as it has been applied in nursing education, practice, and administration.

REFERENCES

Baker, C., Wuest, J., & Stern, P. N. (1992). Method slurring: The grounded theory/phenomenology example. *Journal of Advanced Nursing, 17,* 1255–1360.

Beck, C. T. (1993). Teetering on the edge: A substantive theory of postpartum depression. *Nursing Research, 42*(1), 42–48.

Benoliel, J. Q. (1967). *The nurse and the dying patient.* New York: Macmillan.

Benoliel, J. Q. (1996). Grounded theory and nursing knowledge. *Qualitative Health Research, 6*(3), 406–428.

Blumer, H. (1969). *Symbolic intervention, perspective and method.* Englewood Cliffs, NJ: Prentice Hall.

Cutliffe, J. R. (2000). Methodological issues in grounded theory. *Journal of Advanced Nursing, 31*(6), 1476–1484.

Draucker, C. B., & Stern, P. N. (2001). Women's responses to sexual violence by male intimates. *Western Journal of Nursing Research, 22*(4), 385–406.

Fawcett, J. (1989). *Analysis and evaluation of conceptual models of nursing* (2nd ed.). Philadelphia: F. A. Davis.

Glaser, B. (1978). *Theoretical sensitivity.* Mill Valley, CA: Sociology Press.

Glaser, B. G., & Strauss, A. (1967). *The discovery of grounded theory: Strategies for qualitative research.* New York: Aldine.

Hutchinson, S. A. (1992). Nurses who violate the Nurse Practice Act: Transformation of professional identity. *Image, 24*(2), 133–139.

Hutchinson, S. (2001). Grounded theory: The method. In P. L. Munhall (Ed.), *Nursing research: A qualitative perspective* (pp. 209–243). Sudbury, MA: Jones and Bartlett.

Keddy, B., Sims, S. L., & Stern, P. N. (1996). Grounded theory as feminist methodology. *Journal of Advanced Nursing, 23,* 448–453.

Marriner-Tomey, A., & Alligood, M. R. (2002). *Nursing theorists and their work* (5th ed). St. Louis: C. V. Mosby.

McCormack, D., & MacIntosh, J. (2001). Research with homeless people uncovers a model of health. *Western Journal of Nursing Research, 23*(7), 679–697.

Mead, G. H. (1964). *George Herbert Mead on social psychology.* Chicago: University of Chicago Press.

Merton, R. K. (1957). *Sociological theory: Uses and unities.* New York: Free Press.

Mullen, P. D., & Reynolds, R. (1978). The potential of grounded theory for health education research: Linking theory and practice. *Health Education Monographs, 6*(3), 280–294.

Robrecht, L. C. (1995). Grounded theory: Evolving methods. *Qualitative Health Research, 5*(2), 169–177.

Schatzman, L. (1991). Dimensional analysis: Notes on an alternative approach to the rounding of theory in qualitative research. In D. R. Maines (Ed.), *Social organization and social process: Essays in honor of Anselm Strauss* (pp. 303–314). New York: Aldine.

Stern, P. N. (1980). Grounded theory methodology: Its uses and processes. *Image, 12*(7), 20–23.

Stern, P. N. (1981). Solving problems of cross-cultural health teaching: The Filipino childbearing family. *Image, 13*(2), 47–50.

Stern, P. N., Allen, L. M., & Moxley, P. A. (1982). The nurse as grounded theorist: History, processes, and uses. *Review Journal of Philosophy and Social Science, 7,* 142, 200–215.

Strauss, A. (1987). *Qualitative analysis for social scientists.* New York: Cambridge University Press.

Strauss, A., & Corbin, J. (1990). *Basics of qualitative research: Grounded theory procedures and techniques.* Newbury Park, CA: Sage.

Weiss, J., & Hutchinson, S. A. (2000). Warning about vulnerability in clients with diabetes and hypertension. *Qualitative Health Research, 10*(4), 521–537.

Wilson, H. S. (1977). Limiting intrusion-Social control of outsiders in a healing community. *Nursing Research, 26*(2), 103–111.

Wilson, H. S. (1986). Presencing-Social control of schizophrenics in an antipsychiatric community: Doing grounded theory. In P. L. Munhall & C. J. Oiler (Eds.), *Nursing research: A qualitative perspective* (pp. 111–114). Norwalk, CT: Appleton-Century-Crofts.

Wuest, J. (1995). Feminist grounded theory: An exploration of the congruency and tensions between two traditions in knowledge discovery. *Qualitative Health Research, 5*(1), 125–137.

Grounded Theory in Practice, Education, and Administration

Chapter 8 examines method issues pertaining to grounded theory investigations as described in Chapter 7 in relationship to studies published in the areas of nursing practice, education, and administration. Two important questions guided the direction of this chapter: When should grounded theory be used? and How has the method been used to study issues in nursing education, administration, and practice? The chapter reviews three published studies using the guidelines for evaluating completed grounded theory research presented in Box 8.1. The chapter also provides readers with an overview of selected studies that highlight how nurse–researchers have used grounded theory in nursing practice, education, and administration (Table 8.1).

CRITIQUE GUIDELINES

Strauss and Corbin (1990) indicated that "a qualitative study can be evaluated accurately only if its procedures are sufficiently explicit so that readers of the resulting publication can assess their appropriateness" (p. 249).

> If a grounded theory researcher provides this information, readers can use these criteria to assess the adequacy of the researcher's complex coding procedure. Detail given in this way would be supplemented with cues that could, in longer publications, at least be read as pointing to extremely careful and thorough tracking of findings of conscientious and imaginative theoretical sampling (Strauss & Corbin, 1990, pp. 253–254).

Furthermore, they suggested that, in reality, "there may be no way that readers can accurately judge how the researcher carried out the analysis" (Strauss & Corbin, 1990, p. 253). Therefore, guiding criteria for evaluating grounded theory investigations are provided. Criteria can assist reviewers of grounded theory studies to search out the critical elements of the method (see Box 8.1). When reviewers are critiquing any published investigation, it is important to recognize that journal restrictions, page limitations, or other external forces beyond the author's control may have necessitated deletion of certain material, resulting in a limited

Box 8.1

GUIDELINES FOR CRITIQUING RESEARCH USING GROUNDED THEORY METHOD

Focus/Topic

1. What is the focus or the topic of the study? What is it that the researcher is studying? Is the topic researchable? Is it focused enough to be meaningful but not too limited so as to be trivial?

2. Has the researcher identified why the phenomenon requires a qualitative format? What is the rationale for selecting the grounded theory approach as the qualitative approach for the investigation?

Purpose

1. Has the researcher made explicit the purpose for conducting the research?

Significance

1. Does the researcher describe the projected significance of the work to nursing?

2. What is the relevance of the study to what is already known about the topic?

Method

1. Given the topic of the study and the researcher's stated purpose, how does grounded theory methodology help to achieve the stated purpose?

2. Is the method adequate to address the research topic?

3. What approach is used to guide the inquiry? Does the researcher complete the study according to the processes described?

Sampling

1. Does the researcher describe the selection of participants and protection of human subjects?

2. What major categories emerged?

3. What were some of the events, incidents, or actions that pointed to some of these major categories?

4. What were the categories that led to theoretical sampling?

5. After the theoretical sampling was done, how representative did the categories prove to be?

Data Generation

1. Does the researcher describe data collection strategies?

2. How did theoretical formulations guide data collection?

(continues)

Box 8.1

Data Analysis

1. Does the researcher describe the strategies used to analyze the data?
2. Does the researcher address the credibility, auditability, and fittingness of the data?
3. Does the researcher clearly describe how and why the core category was selected?

Empirical Grounding of the Study: Findings

1. Are concepts grounded in the data?
2. Are the concepts systematically related?
3. Are conceptual linkages described and are the categories well developed? Do they have conceptual density?
4. Are the theoretical findings significant? If yes, to what extent?
5. Were data collection strategies comprehensive and analytical interpretations conceptual and broad?
6. Is there sufficient variation to allow for applicability in a variety of contexts related to the phenomenon investigated?

Conclusions, Implications, and Recommendations

1. How does the researcher provide a context for use of the findings?
2. Are the conclusions drawn from the study appropriate? Explain.
3. What are the recommendations for future research?
4. Are the recommendations, conclusions, and implications clearly related to the findings?

From Strauss, A., & Corbin, J. (1990). *Basics of qualitative research: Grounded theory procedures and techniques.* Newbury Park, CA: Sage. Adapted with permission.

critique of the research. Readers interested in more detailed discussion of method in a published study should contact the author.

APPLICATION TO PRACTICE

An excellent example of grounded theory research related to the practice arena is the study "A Metaphor for HIV-Positive Mexican and Puerto Rican Women" by Valdez (2001). This research study provides an example of the use of grounded theory in the investigation of phenomena important to nursing practice. Valdez's (2001) article conveys the intensity and rigor of grounded theory method while sharing detailed findings from her research.

Text continues on page 130

TABLE 8.1   SELECTIVE SAMPLING OF GROUNDED THEORY RESEARCH STUDIES

Author	Date	Domain	Phenomenon of Interest	Method
McCormack & MacIntosh	2001	Practice	To understand how homeless persons in three New Brunswick cities describe their health experiences and the strategies they use to attain, maintain, or regain health	Grounded Theory
Skillen, Olson, & Gilbert	2001	Practice	To conduct thematic analysis of unanalyzed semistructured interview segments from data that emerged during an earlier exploratory descriptive study on organizational factors and work hazards	Grounded Theory

Sample	Data Generation	Findings
11 homeless persons in shelters	Private tape-recorded interviews with a common interview guide that included questions related to participants' understanding of health, health status, behaviors and activities related to health maintenance, and participants' perceptions of their success in maintaining their health.	A model of health emerged that included two central components, person and health. Person is influenced directly by family values and beliefs and indirectly by societal values and beliefs. Health is the outcome and is reached through two mediating factors of lifestyle behaviors and sector services. The first pathway to health contains the mediating factor of lifestyle behaviors, the second contains the mediating factor of sector services, and the third contains both mediating factors. Pathway strategies of choosing, accessing, and appraising appropriateness of methods influence the active participation of the person that directs the action with the model. Implication of the study include that a fragmented system of help hinders access to services intended to promote health in this population.
56 staff and managerial public health nurses	Tape-recorded interviews, transcribed verbatim	The framework that resulted from this secondary analysis describes the ideologies of female public health nurses (PHNs) related to their workplace environmental risks. Four categories of the overarching theme, framing personal risk in work environments, emerged: becoming aware, recognizing influences, comparing with others, and knowing rights and freedoms. Two subthemes also emerged: framing for no action and framing for action. When framing for no action, PHNs were either unconcerned or wanted to avoid trouble. When framing for action, PHNs found humor, took responsibility, used voice, collected support, and struggled for action.

(continues)

Author	Date	Domain	Phenomenon of Interest	Method
Williamson & Folaron	2001	Practice	To explore the risks and responses of street prostitutes to customer-related violence	Grounded Theory
Draucker & Stern	2000	Practice	To devise a theoretical framework that describes the problem of sexual violence by male intimates.	Grounded Theory
Hallberg & Carlsson	2000	Practice	To describe, from the perspective of patients with fibromyalgia themselves, their experiences of having to live with chronic pain and how they manage their situation	Grounded Theory
Hallberg, Passe, & Ringdahl	2000	Practice	To describe the experience of coping with demanding auditory situations in everyday life from the perspective of individuals with severe-profound hearing impairment	Grounded Theory
Higgins, Dunn, & Theobald	2000	Practice	To describe participants' perceptions of recovery after angioplasty.	Grounded Theory

Sample	Data Generation	Findings
13 female street prostitutes, aged 18 to 40	Tape-recorded interviews, transcribed verbatim	Various bodily traumas were described, severe drug addictions along with anticipatory survival strategies.
23 women who have experienced such violence at some time in their adult lives	Open-ended interviews, audiotaped and transcribed verbatim	The core variable, forging ahead in a dangerous world, reflects the women's descriptions of life after violence as a struggle to get on with their lives in a social world they know through firsthand experience to be unsafe. The theoretical framework includes three variations of forging ahead (getting back on track, starting over again, and surviving the long, hard road). The framework also outlines three common processes used to forge ahead: telling others, making sense of the violence, and creating a safer life.
22 female patients	Open-ended in-depth interviews, transcribed verbatim	Three descriptive categories were grounded in the data, labeled subjective pain language, diversified pain coping, and pain communication. These descriptive categories were from the higher-order or core concept preoccupied with pain.
11 women and 6 men with post-lingual severe-profound hearing impairment	Audiotaped interviews, transcribed verbatim	Six theoretical constructs labeled coaching, belonging to two worlds, self-efficacy, hardiness, and directing coping strategies were grounded in the data. The core category was identified as "finding flow and entering a positive circle."
8 men and 3 women	Audiotaped interviews, transcribed verbatim	Three major categories were identified: awareness of the problem, coping response, and appraisal of the situation. Participants also noted whether they had a "good" or "bad" recovery.

(continues)

TABLE 8.1	SELECTIVE SAMPLING OF GROUNDED THEORY RESEARCH STUDIES (CONTINUED)			
Author	**Date**	**Domain**	**Phenomenon of Interest**	**Method**
Instone	2000	Practice	To describe how school-aged children with HIV infection adjusted to their illness and information from parents or guardians	Grounded Theory
Miller	2000	Practice	To discover factors that influenced the healthcare-seeking behavior of women cardiac patients	Grounded Theory
Paterson & Thorne	2000	Practice	To describe how people with long-standing type 1 diabetes make everyday self-care decisions with emphasis on decision making related to unanticipated blood glucose levels	Grounded Theory

The title and introduction clearly identify the focus of this qualitative investigation by Valdez. The statement of purpose further emphasizes the rationale for a qualitative design and the focus of the study. Valdez's (2001) intent is to describe culture-guided health practices, health-seeking behaviors, and folk care activities used by HIV-positive Hispanic women. Valdez (2001) intended to discover the relationship between the customs of Hispanic women and HIV/AIDS among this population. She justifies the need for the study, noting that Hispanic women are believed to have the highest risk of contracting HIV. By studying the habits of these women, the researcher hopes to raise awareness about the incidence of HIV/AIDS and how it relates to a specific aggregate of society. Knowing what influences women to make certain health care choices will allow professionals to focus their interventions appropriately. The data gathered from this research will benefit health care professionals and emphasizes the need to be culturally sensitive and understand the practices of diverse customs.

Sample	Data Generation	Findings
12 children and 13 parents	Audiotaped interviews, transcribed verbatim	A specific process of interaction between the parents and the children emerged and was described as "When not told for so long." Disclosure regarding illness was reflected in children's drawings and suggested emotional distress, disturbed self-image, and social isolation.
10 women with cardiac disease, 2 women at risk for cardiac disease, 3 nurse practitioners, and 1 cardiologist	Audiotaped interviews, transcribed verbatim	A core process of cardiac cue sensitivity was identified. The stages included cue apprehension, cue assimilation, and medical consultation. Cues included signs, symptoms, or self-risk appraisal.
22 individuals with diabetes	Data triangulation was used and included a "think-aloud" technique, formal interviews, and a final focus group interview.	Decision making was differentiated by familiar and unfamiliar situations. The primary focus in familiar situations was related to course of action. In unfamiliar situations, identifying cause was important.

A qualitative format is important for this study, allowing participants to describe their customs and beliefs in full detail. The philosophical underpinnings of grounded theory methodology are addressed. Valdez (2001) relates the work of Glaser and Strauss and states that symbolic interactionism "provided the philosophical foundations for GT and guided the research question, interview questions, data collection, and method of data analysis" (p. 520). Further, Valdez (2001) emphasized the fact that behavioral, cultural, and environmental factors place Hispanic women at greater risk for heterosexual transmission of HIV/AIDS. Investigations related to health beliefs, customs, and traditions were lacking, adding further support for this study and its qualitative format. "Knowledge of these beliefs, customs, and tradition as they affect Hispanic women's lifestyles and health-seeking behaviors may bring forth information to provide better health care to this group and information to cure" (Valdez, 2001, p. 519).

Grounded theory methodology was used "to discover underlying social forces that shaped behaviors of HIV Hispanic women" (Valdez, 2001, p. 520). Valdez (2001) used a semistructured interview technique to generate data for her study. According to Valdez (2001):

> The semistructured interview consisted of a series of open-ended questions designed to elicit measures used by HIV Hispanic women to stay healthy. The women were told that the purpose of the interview was to get a sense of what they did to stay healthy and what health practices they used to live with this disease. Issues of emotional/psychological response, diagnosis, disclosure, and future plans were addressed. The interest was in gathering data about what persons do or do not do to identify, develop, and relate concepts that proved theoretical relevance. (p. 520)

The data collection techniques applied in this study are consistent with a grounded theory investigation. Valdez (2001) also included relevant demographic information in her investigation. Theoretical sampling along with the fulfillment of specific background criteria was used to access participants for this investigation. HIV-positive Mexican and Puerto Rican women were chosen from a community-based organization in the state of Texas. Out of 22 people invited to participate in the study, nine ultimately agreed to be interviewed. The participants represented a segment of the Hispanic population appropriate to inform the research. The selection process for sampling supported a qualitative paradigm. Issues of confidentiality and disclosure were discussed when the women arranged their interviews. Participants were informed regarding the purpose of the study. "Issues of emotional/psychological response, diagnosis, disclosure, and future plans were addressed" (Valdez, 2001, p. 520).

Since Valdez (2001) was proficient in both English and Spanish, interviews were conducted based on the participant's language preference. To ensure confidentiality, the interviews were conducted in the home setting or in a private room in a community-based organization. Semistructured interviews that were audiotaped and transcribed verbatim were utilized. Transcriptions and translation of the audiotapes were completed. Demographic information was accounted for using basic statistical measures. The researcher before, during, and after the hour-long interviews took notes. "Interviewing continued until all categories were saturated and no new data emerged" (Valdez, 2001, p. 522).

Data analysis was consistent with grounded theory methodology. Valdez (2001) used the constant comparative technique to simultaneously collect, code, and analyze her data. Valdez describes her techniques in detail. This is extremely helpful to the reader, making clear how grounded theory methodology was applied in this investigation and allowing the reader to understand how issues of reliability and validity were addressed. According to Valdez (2001):

> ...Before subsequent interviews, the transcripts were coded and analyzed as they were completed. Transcripts were read and recoded several days later and the results were compared with the first coding. Repeated coding, yield-

ing the same results, established consistency of the data. Coded data were checked by a second coder for agreement and added reliability (Miles & Huberman, 1994). Common themes were identified and recorded in the respondents' own words in theoretical memos. Emerging themes and categories were clarified with each participant and an expert researcher in grounded theory and the area of study. Using the constant comparative technique (Glaser & Strauss, 1967), codes were clustered into themes, and themes were clustered into categories. Participants in subsequent interviews further validated the emerging categories and provided additional data (Valdez, 2001, p. 522).

Valdez (2001) discusses her findings in full detail. She found that many factors are involved in the health practices of Hispanic women. "The theoretical framework *La Protectora* (The Protectress), emerged as the researcher linked the categories" (Valdez, 2001, p. 522).

Trustworthiness was demonstrated when the participants agreed with the interpretation made by Valdez (2001). Member checks and persistent observation were among the tools used to maintain credibility of the findings.

Consistent with the purposes of grounded theory, a model emerged from the data to describe the health-seeking behaviors of HIV-positive Mexican and Puerto Rican women. The framework *La Protectora* (The Protectress) was described by five main categories: "The Revelation of Death, *Ofrecer*, Living, Revealing, and Duality. Subcategories, Dealing and Surviving, emerged from Living; Protecting and Advocating emerged from Revealing; Intensifying and Actualizing emerged from Duality" (p. 523).

In an effort to explain health-seeking practice, *La Protectora* emerged as the framework to illustrate the sociological process of HIV-positive Hispanic women. The findings of this study describe important cultural values that impact on the care and treatment of Hispanic women with HIV/AIDS. Valdez (2001) concludes by noting that her research explains the psychological response of women coping with HIV. She discusses her findings within the context of the literature and relates implications for future nursing research. The findings indicated that women delayed medical care. The chief motivator for maintaining health in the woman's life was raising her children. "A strong belief in a higher power, the use of prayer, reading the Bible, and going to church was expressed by all of the women, despite differences in religion. Investigation into how religion and spirituality affect decision making and living with HIV is necessary" (Valdez, 2001, p. 533).

Valdez (2001) suggests that the nursing implications of the study are to increase awareness of health beliefs among all HIV-positive women. The findings noted by Valdez (2001) are limited to her study but reflect the need to repeat the investigation with different groups of women. Overall, Valdez (2001) has contributed significantly to the body of nursing research in general but specifically to research related to women and HIV/AIDS. Her use of grounded theory methodology makes an important contribution to nursing theory development.

APPLICATION TO EDUCATION

Nursing education continues to be an important area for the conduct of research. An example of the contribution grounded theory can make to nursing education is a study by Scholes, Endacott, and Chellel (2000) entitled "A Formula for Diversity: A Review of Critical Care Curricula." This study illustrates a good presentation of findings from a grounded theory investigation.

The purpose of Scholes et al.'s (2000) study was to "explore the way critical care programmes were configured and how different levels of performance were articulated, the impact this had on the stated learning outcomes and the implication of these findings for practitioners and educationalists" (p. 383). Since the article focuses on core competencies for critical care practice in the UK, the authors provide an overview of how critical care courses have been developed in the UK and the policy changes that have had an impact on these programs. This is important introductory material, allowing the reader to understand the focus of the study and its importance to nursing education.

Scholes et al. (2000) report using an adapted grounded theory approach as the methodology for their research. They further explain that the research was divided into four key phases, which included:

Phase 1: a telephone survey with critical care lecturers ($N = 84$). This served three purposes: to request the course documents, to ensure that the correct procedures for the release of the curricula were followed, and to give lecturers the opportunity to set their curriculum in context.

Phase 2: an overview of all the curriculum documents returned to the research team ($N = 105$) from 30 different institutions.

Phase 3: detailed analysis of 44 programmes from 15 different institutions.

Phase 4: a survey of critical care managers ($N = 81$) to illuminate their issues and concerns about the courses.

In addition, "A comprehensive literature review ran through the project and was driven by the findings from the four phases of the study" (Scholes et al., 2001, p. 383).

The data collection techniques reflect the process of theoretical sampling that is consistent with grounded theory methodology. Although the researchers have detailed for the reader their data collection and analysis techniques, they do not connect them to grounded theory methodology. The authors have described their data analysis strategies in detail. They do not address issues of credibility, auditability, or fittingness of the data. It seems that the authors were attempting to find conceptual linkages between critical care programs. Their data collection was comprehensive and systematic. The study does not propose a theory or identify a core variable. The reader assumes that the adapted grounded theory is applied to data collection and analysis. The study would be strengthened if the authors had made a clearer connection between grounded theory methodology and their study.

The authors conclude that although critical care courses should have something in common, there was little consistency in the "learning outcomes (academic and practice competencies), theoretical and practice assessments, course configuration and academic credits across the sample" (Scholes et al., 2001, p. 388). The study has implications for nursing education in the UK, and the basic principles of the investigation could be applied to other academic issues.

APPLICATION TO ADMINISTRATION

Severinsson and Borgenhammar's (1997) study "Expert Views on Clinical Supervision: A Study Based on Interviews" provides an example of grounded theory applied to nursing administration. They described the study purpose early in the article: "The aim of this study is to analyze views on clinical supervision held by a number of experts, and to reflect on the effects and value of clinical supervision in relation to public health" (p. 177). Severinsson and Borgenhammar have grounded the importance of the work in a comprehensive literature review and a sound rationale.

The sample for the investigation included seven well-known researchers from four Nordic countries: Norway, Denmark, Finland, and Sweden. They are experts on "working conditions" and hold positions as associate professors and professors. Their fields are psychiatry, psychotherapy, psychosocial medicine, social medicine, social work, education, theology, and nursing. Three are women and four are men. The sampling procedure appeared to be purposeful, although the authors did not specify this in the article. Given the description provided, however, readers may assume that Severinsson and Borgenhammar selected participants specifically for their experience and ability to discuss the research topic.

The researchers conducted data analysis using the methodology of grounded theory construction. They followed three procedures to inductively generate categories grounded on data: (1) open coding (labeling phenomena for the discovery of structure), (2) axial coding (identification of patterns), and (3) selective coding (identification of core category).

A table in the article illustrated the authors' interpretations of the experts' views on how clinical supervision affects clients and professionals, thus giving readers a sense of how data analysis proceeded. The authors did not address credibility, auditability, and fittingness in the article; such discussion would have added to the presentation of the study and enhanced the meaning of the data.

Severinsson and Borgenhammar discussed the conclusions, implications, and recommendations in relationship to the data and literature presented. The results showed that clinical supervision is an integration process guiding a person from novice to expert by establishing a relationship of trust between supervisor and the individual being supervised. The study indicated that implementation of systematic clinical supervision may positively affect quality of care and client recovery, may create improved feelings of confidence in one's work, and may prevent burnout among staff. The reported negative aspect was the possibility of high "opportunity costs; that is, the time loss for client care by nurses participating in organized systematic supervision" (Severinsson & Borgenhammar, 1997, p. 175).

SUMMARY

Grounded theory as a qualitative research approach provides an excellent method of investigation for phenomena important to nursing. This chapter reviewed application of the method to areas important to nursing practice, education, and administration and offered new grounded theorists examples of research that apply the method described in Chapter 7. Recognizing the need for middle-range theory development in nursing, investigators should continue to apply this rigorous qualitative method to the investigation of phenomena important to nursing practice, education, and administration.

REFERENCES

Draucker, C. B., & Stern, P. N. (2000). Women's responses to sexual violence by male intimates. *Western Journal of Nursing Research, 22*(4), 385–406.

Glaser, B. G., & Strauss, A. (1967). *The discovery of grounded theory: Strategies for qualitative research.* New York: Aldine.

Hallberg, L. R.-M. & Carlsson, A. G. (2000). Coping with fibromyalgia: A qualitative study. *Scandinavian Journal of Caring Science, 14,* 29–36.

Hallberg, L. R.-M., Passe, U., & Ringdahl, A. (2000). Coping with post-lingual severe-profound hearing impairment: A grounded theory study. *British Journal of Audiology, 34,* 1–9.

Higgins, M., Dunn, S., & Theobald, K. (2000). The patients' perception of recovery after coronary angioplasty. *Australian Critical Care, 13*(3), 83–88.

Instone, S. L. (2000). Perception of children with HIV infection when not told for so long: Implications for diagnosis disclosure. *Journal of Pediatric Health Care, 14,* 235–243.

McCormack, D., & MacIntosh, J. (2001). Research with homeless people uncovers a model of health. *Western Journal of Nursing Research, 23*(7), 679–697.

Miles, M., & Huberman, A. (1994) *Qualitative data analysis.* Thousand Oaks, CA: Sage.

Miller, C. L. (2000). Cue sensitivity in women with cardiac disease. *Progress in Cardiovascular Nursing, 15,* 82–89.

Paterson, B., & Thorne, S. (2000). Expert decision making in relation to unanticipated blood glucose levels. *Research in Nursing & Health, 23,* 147–157.

Severinsson, E. I., & Borgenhammar, E. V. (1997). Expert views on clinical supervision: A study based on interviews. *Journal of Nursing Management, 5,* 175–183.

Scholes, J., Endacott, R., & Chellel, A. (2000). A formula for diversity: A review of critical care curricula. *Journal of Clinical Nursing, 9,* 382–390.

Skillen, L. D., Olson, J. K., & Gilbert, J. A. (2001). Framing personal risk in public health nursing. *Western Journal of Nursing Research, 23*(7), 664–678.

Strauss, A., & Corbin, J. (1990). *Basics of qualitative research: Grounded theory procedures and techniques.* Newbury Park, CA: Sage.

Valdez, M. R. (2001). A metaphor for HIV-positive Mexican and Puerto Rican women. *Western Journal of Nursing Research 23*(5), 517–535.

Williamson, C., & Folaron, G. (2001). Violence, risk, and survival strategies of street prostitution. *Western Journal of Nursing Research, 23*(5), 463–475.

RESEARCH ARTICLE

A Metaphor for HIV-Positive Mexican and Puerto Rican Women

Maria del Rosario Valdez

Human Immunodeficiency Virus (HIV) represents an overwhelming disruption for His-panic women. This Grounded Theory (GT) (Glaser & Strauss, 1967) study sought to explore how culture guided health practices and to identify health and folkcare activities used by HIV+ Hispanic women. La Protectora (The Protectress), a theoretical framework, emerged to describe the process by which cultural beliefs guided Hispanic women's health practices and how they dealt with life after their affirmation of HIV status. Five main categories emerged to describe the process. Knowledge about how culture influ-ences HIV+ Hispanic women obtain and/or make decisions about health care will con-tribute to a foundation for theory development and subsequent theory testing.

The face of Acquired Immunodeficiency Syndrome (AIDS) in the United States is chang-ing, with the problem of Human Immunodeficiency Virus (HIV) in women of growing magnitude and concern. As a result of the 1993 expanded AIDS case definition and improved survival from new combination-drug therapies, the number of people living with AIDS increased in all groups (Centers for Disease Control and Prevention [CDC], 2001a). Through 1999, the proportion of reported U.S. AIDS cases occurring among women increased from 7% to 23%. Most women (40%) were infected through het-erosexual exposure to HIV (CDC, 2001b). The growing proportion of women living with AIDS reflected the shift in populations affected by the epidemic. Women of color have dramatically been affected. African American and Hispanic women together represent less than one fourth of all women in the United States, yet they account for more than three fourths (77%) of AIDS cases reported among women in the U.S. (CDC, 2000, 200b). Hispanic women are believed to be at greatest risk for HIV infection due to behavioral, cultural, and environmental factors (Barken et al., 1998; Chu, Peterman, Doll, Buehler, & Curran, 1992; Diaz, Buehler, Castro, & Ward, 1993).

CULTURALLY AT RISK

A change in the trend of new HIV infections and AIDS diagnoses exists in the United States. The incidence of HIV/AIDS in homosexual and bisexual men is leveling off (CDC, 1999). Women of color are most dramatically affected in this trend change as heterosexual transmission escalates globally and accounts for 80% of HIV infection (CDC, 2000, 2001b; World Health Organization [WHO], 2000). The large and growing Hispanic population is heavily affected by the HIV/AIDS epidemic. In 1998 and 1999, Hispanics represented 13% of the U.S. population (including residents of Puerto Rico), but accounted for 20% and 19%, respectively, of the total number of new U.S. AIDS

Maria del Rosario "Rosie" Valdez, Ph.D, RNC, Assistant Professor, Intercollegiate College of Nurs-ing/Washington State University College of Nursing.

cases reported for those years. The AIDS incidence rate per 100,000 population (the number of new cases of a disease that occur during a specific time period) among Hispanics in 1999 was 25.6, almost three times the rate for Whites (7.6), but lower than the rate for African Americans (66.0). Fifty-seven percent of Hispanics reported with AIDS in 1999 were born in the United States, of which 43% were born in Puerto Rico. Men continue to account for the largest proportion (79%) of AIDS cases reported among Hispanics in the United States, with women representing 21% of the cases. Heterosexual contact accounts for the highest proportion (47%) (CDC, 2001a; National Institutes of Health [NIH], 2000).

Behavioral, cultural, and environmental factors have been suggested as sources for the higher risk of heterosexual transmission among Hispanic women. Higher risk for heterosexual transmission has been suggested because Hispanic women have lower condom use (Marin, Tschann, Gomez, & Kegeles, 1993); greater reluctance to suggest condom use to male partners (Marin & Marin, 1992), and less confidence about avoiding HIV than non-Hispanic White women (Marin et al., 1993). A high level of bisexuality among Hispanic men (CDC, 1993) and the decreased concern about becoming infected among bisexual men further increases risk (CDC, 1999).

In a cross-sectional survey of African American and Hispanic men at a New York-based sexually transmitted disease (STD) clinic, Lehner and Chiasson (1998) found that of the 3,069 male subjects, 415 reported having sex with men. Of those 415 men, 13% (n = 55) were classified as homosexual, 35% (n = 145) were classified as bisexual, and 52% (n = 215) were classified as heterosexual. They concluded that HIV transmission from bisexual men in African American and Hispanic communities played a larger role in heterosexual transmission than was previously thought.

Salgado de Snyder, Diaz-Perez, and Maldonado (1996) found that Hispanic men who have sex with men (MSM) do not regard themselves as homosexual or even bisexual. As long as they assume the dominant role (insertive as opposed to receptive), continue to engage in heterosexual sex, and fulfill their masculine roles, there is no stigma attached to this behavior. They also found that extramarital sexual activity among males in Hispanic society is culturally sanctioned. These findings emphasized the increased risk of heterosexual transmission to Hispanic women and the need to take into account the cultural, ethnic, and behavioral diversity of these men and their sexual partners.

A complex system of beliefs, customs, and traditions based on cultural values and attitudes exists among Hispanics (Clark, 1970; Gonzalez-Swafford & Gutierrez, 1983). Health is viewed as the result of good luck and a reward for good behavior, a gift from God, and not to be taken for granted. Health is maintained by acting properly, eating the proper foods, and working a proper amount of time. Wearing religious medals and amulets, praying, and keeping relics in the home help prevent illness, whereas exemplary behavior, herbs, and spices, can enhance prevention (Kay, 1981; Spector, 2000). Illness is caused by an imbalance in a person's body or as punishment for wrongdoing. Five categories describe the imbalances that can cause illness: body imbalance (diseases of hot and cold), dislocation of body parts or organs, diseases of magic or supernatural causes, diseases of emotional origin, and *envidia* (envy) (Spector, 2000). *Curanderismo*, a medical system of healers, is used exclusively or in combination with institutionalized care throughout the Hispanic population. Healers (*curanderos*) are sought out for social, physical, and psychological purposes (Spector, 2000).

Few researchers have studied the health needs, health status, health beliefs, health-seeking behaviors, and/or family roles of Hispanics (Giachello, 1985; Zambrana, 1987). The majority of the HIV/AIDS research has focused on women's attitudes toward health, sexual practices, knowledge, and perceived risks of HIV for the prevention of AIDS (Nyamathi, Bennett, Leake, Lewis, & Flaskerud, 1993; Nyamathi, Leake, Flaskerud, Lewis, & Bennett, 1993). Most of the research has also been conducted with populations at greater risk for HIV transmission (Kline, Kline, & Oken, 1992), and very little has been devoted to the lifestyles, health-seeking behaviors, and concerns of those affected (Nyamathi & Flaskerud, 1992). No studies explain the health-seeking behaviors of HIV+ women or how cultural beliefs guide health practices of HIV+ Hispanic women. Knowledge of these beliefs, customs, and traditions as they affect Hispanic women's lifestyles and health-seeking behaviors may bring forth information to provide better health care to this group and information to cure.

PURPOSE

The purpose of the study was to explore how culture guided health practices and to identify health-seeking behaviors and folk care activities of HIV+ Hispanic women. The questions that guided this study were as follows: (a) What health-seeking practices do HIV+ Hispanic women incorporate into their everyday lives? And (b) How do HIV+ Hispanic women incorporate traditional Western medical practices with their folk care activities?

DESIGN

Grounded theory (GT) methodology as described by Glaser & Strauss (1967) was used to discover underlying social forces that shaped behaviors of HIV+ Hispanic women and the meanings of these situations for the purpose of generating theory. Symbolic interactionism (SI), described by sociologists Mead (1934) and Blumer (1969), provided the philosophical foundations for GT and guided the research question, interview questions, data collection, and method of data analysis (Stern, 1985; Stern, Allen, & Moxley, 1982; Hutchinson, 1993). Instruments included the researcher, a semistructured interview guide, and a demographic data form.

The semistructured interview consisted of a series of open-ended questions designed to elicit measures used by HIV+ Hispanic women to stay healthy. The women were told that the purpose of the interview was to get a sense of what they did to stay healthy and what health practices they used to live with this disease. Issues of emotional/psychological response, diagnosis, disclosure, and future plans were addressed. The interest was in gathering data about what persons do or do not do to identify, develop, and relate concepts that proved theoretical relevance.

Participants

Participants were recruited from HIV+ Hispanic women attending a community-based organization (CBO) in Texas. The CBO was a prevention and education organization focusing on HIV/AIDS outreach. Their major focus was to provide assistance with utilities, rent, food, and clothing to HIV/AIDS-affected women. They also provided counseling and support groups. Their services were also extended to men affected by HIV. For the purpose of this study, *Hispanic* was defined as Mexican American, Mexican National, Columbian, Honduran, Salvadoran, Cuban, and/or Puerto Rican, which were the city's dominant Hispanic groups. The final sample consisted of Mexican American, Mexican National, and Puerto Rican women.

Theoretical sampling (Glaser & Strauss, 1967) was used to identify participants present at the CBO's group meetings and from attendance rosters. The women, once identified and asked by the CBO case managers of their willingness to participate, were approached by the researcher and asked to participate in the study. Appointments were made to interview at a later date. Twenty-two women had been approached by the time data collection ceased. Thirteen of these women refused to participate for fear of loss of confidentiality and/or were not interested. The nine women who agreed to participate comprised the final sample.

The initial interview lasted approximately 1 hour. Two of the Puerto Rican participants were interviewed a second time for approximately 30 minutes for data clarification due to unfamiliarity with some of the terminology used. All of the participants were approached to clarify emergent themes and categories. The women were interviewed individually in either English or Spanish. Five women (56%) were interviewed in Spanish, and four (44%) were interviewed in English. Of those interviewed in Spanish, two were monolingual. Interviews were conducted at the participants' homes or in a private room at the CBO. All of the interviews were audiotaped.

The participants ranged in ages from 19 to 41 years, with a mean age of 31 years. Educational level ranged from 6 to 16 years, with a mean of 11 years. Of the sample, three were married, two were single, two were divorced, and two were widowed. Of the two that were widowed, both had lost their husbands to AIDS and one woman had lost both her husband and a child to AIDS. Time of HIV diagnosis ranged from 2 weeks to 6 years, with a mean of 2 years 10 months. One woman had an AIDS diagnosis; the other women were in the earlier stages of the disease. All of the women were in heterosexual relationships at the time of diagnosis, and eight (89%) related HIV transmission from husband or long-term partner. One was the victim of date rape. Eight (89%) had their HIV status revealed to them during pregnancy; one was diagnosed during treatment for a long-term gynecological problem. All of the participants had children. The mean number of children living with the participants was three, with ages ranging from 2.5 months to 18 years. Four of these children (ages 4, 9, 14, and 18 years) knew of their mother's diagnosis. One participant also had three children, ages 17, 20, and 22 years, who were not living at home. One participant's (victim of date rape) pregnancy ended in a miscarriage. She and her husband later chose to get pregnant, although they also had custody of his two children from a previous marriage. Their mother had died of AIDS. Six women (67%) were of Mexican origin and three (33%) were identified as Puerto Rican. Of the Mexican origin women, four were Mexican American (MA) and highly acculturated. Two of these women's parents were born in Mexico and the grandparents of the other two women were born in Mexico. The other two were Mexican nationals and less acculturated. The three Puerto Rican women had been in the United States less than 5 years and were less acculturated. Five of the women were Catholic, two identified as Christians, and two were Jehovah's Witnesses. Seven participants identified Supplemental Security Income (SSI) as their means of support and two were waiting for approval of benefits. One woman worked part-time. All of the participants had access to health care.

Data Analysis

The researcher, who was MA and fluent in English and Spanish (written and verbal), interviewed all of the participants and performed the verbatim transcriptions and translations as part of her dissertation. Translations were back translated by a doctoral-prepared MA, who was a nurse researcher and expert in Hispanic culture. Notes were made before, during, and after each interview to record observations and impressions of the social context and were added to the interview after transcription. Sociodemographics were descriptive and reported by mean and range. Using the logic of GT (Glaser & Strauss, 1967), before subsequent interviews, the transcripts were coded and analyzed as they were completed. Transcripts were read and recoded several days later and the results were compared with the first coding. Repeated coding, yielding the same results, established consistency of the data. Coded data were checked by a second coder for agreement and added reliability (Miles & Huberman, 1994). Common themes were identified and recorded in the respondent's own words in theoretical memos. Emerging themes and categories were clarified with each participant and an expert researcher in grounded theory and the area of study. Using the constant comparative technique (Glaser & Strauss, 1967), codes were clustered into themes, and themes were clustered into categories. Participants in subsequent interviews further validated the emerging categories and provided additional data. The theoretical framework, *La Protectora* (The Protectress), emerged as the researcher linked the categories. Interviewing continued until all categories were saturated and no new data emerged. To validate that the emergent theory of La Protectora was a correct interpretation of the findings, a final member check was done with seven (78%) of the participants. Two participants refused to take part in the final member check. Trustworthiness was demonstrated when the members agreed with the interpretation of the findings. Convinced that the theory was a reasonably accurate statement of the matters studied and the data were believable as validated by the participants, the research ended.

FINDINGS

The purpose of this study was to explore health-seeking behaviors of HIV+ Hispanic women. La Protectora, a theoretical framework and model (Figure 1), emerged to describe the health-seeking behaviors of HIV+ Mexican and Puerto Rican women, how they respond to their affirmation of HIV status, and how they become empowered women wanting to live with HIV. Five main categories emerged that describe the process: The Revelation of Death, *Ofrecer* (which means "to offer" according to the *Larousse Diccionario Moderno* [1983]), Living, Revealing, and Duality. Subcategories, Dealing and Surviving, emerged from Living; Protecting and Advocating emerged from Revealing; and Intensifying and Actualizing emerged from Duality.

Revelation of Death

The first category, Revelation of Death, the catalyst of the theoretical framework (the first block), represents the women's initial responses to their affirmation of HIV status. Response to the revelation of status is similar to Kubler-Ross' (1973) stages of dying. Janie, a 36-year-old mother of four, living with HIV for approximately 3 years, described her reaction, "I wanted to go into a little closet and hide in there and cry all day. The first thing I did was to call my sister and tell her I wanted to die. I kept saying, 'maybe it's not true.'" Judy, a 36-year-old mother of three, living with her disease for only 8 months, summed up her reaction, "I feel like a prisoner given a life sentence waiting to die. But he knows why he's going to die. He knows he did a crime. But, I didn't...yet, I was given the same sentence." Olivia, a 30-year-old mother of three, living with the disease for 5 years, described her reaction, "I became very depressed. My

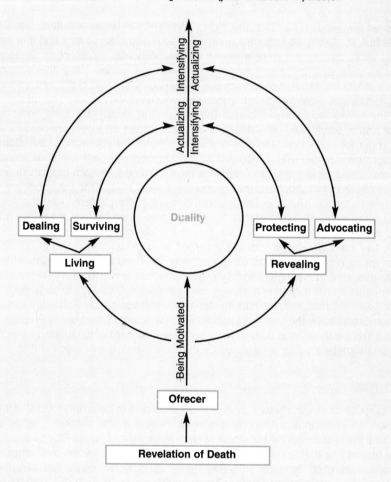

mother came and took care of me and my children. I couldn't even wash my face. I didn't get out of bed." All of the women experienced some or all of the stages of dying at their own pace and in their own sequence. Because eight of the women were pregnant and one had small children at diagnosis, the child or children became the motivation that took the women to the next step of the framework, Ofrecer.

Ofrecer

Ofrecer (second block) represents the negotiating and an offer to change between the women and their God as they struggle with their mortality and the possibility of their children's positive status. The women promise to do good, live for their child, and reveal their status to benefit others. The woman's exchange is not for more time for herself but for the life of her child. She prays and implores her God to spare her child of a positive status and, ultimately, the same death sentence. Yolanda, a 19-year-old mother of a 2 1/2-month-old infant, described her experience, "The results came back and he was negative. I told God that I would tell others of my status if He let my son be OK. God has blessed me and answered my prayers." Maria, a 40-year-old mother of five, living with the disease for 6 years, summed up her negotiation with God since diagnosis, "I have lived 6 years since my baby was born and this makes me happy but, I want to live more. I want to live as long as I can for my children. Without Him, nothing would be possible." Janie, not pregnant at diagnosis, summed up her negotiation, "I prayed to keep going and to be there for my children." Ana, who had lost her husband and first child to AIDS, summed up her negotiation, "I lost my child and then my husband to this disease, and then I asked God to protect me and my other baby. She is negative."

Being Motivated

Being motivated is a triggering to the next level of the framework and model. It is the outcome of Ofrecer and triggers the next three categories, Living, Revealing, and Duality. Some life event occurred during Ofrecer that motivated the Hispanic woman to see her life with HIV differently. Having a family and needing to live for them, her child's negative status, and/or having lived longer than presumed are examples of some of the life events. The woman feels that God has listened, accepted, and granted her offer to change. She moves into the next level meeting challenges and wanting to live with this disease. Meeting the stressors of HIV, she draws from her maternal strength as she progresses through the categories of Living and Revealing.

Living

Living depicts the woman's decision to live her life with HIV. Her life was challenged before diagnosis by concerns for food, clothing, and shelter for her family. Now, her life is further taxed by the demands, effects, and treatments of the disease, She must learn to juggle and keep strict medication schedules, doctor's appointments, and group meetings in her already stressed life. Olga, a 27-year-old mother of three, living with this disease for 2 years, expressed it as such,

> More of the stress is put on women because we're left to raise the children. Even if he was here, I would still raise them. You know, it's all put on the woman, whether you have HIV or not. But having HIV, that's just more stress. Stress is what takes you with HIV.

As the HIV+ woman makes decisions about her life, she proceeds through the subcategories Dealing and Surviving.

Dealing

Dealing describes how the Hispanic woman struggles to access and use traditional health care. The Hispanic women who sought health care were faced doubly with prejudice for being women of lower socioeconomic status (SES), and now HIV+. Prejudice was demonstrated to the women by their health care providers' language, demeanor, and the services or lack of services provided. Some women chose to forgo health care, others gained strength in acquiring health care, and others sought comfort in traditional folkways because of this prejudice. Judy, in need of dental care, chose to forgo seeing the dentist rather than deal with the lack of professionalism,

He's some dentist at the Ryan White clinic...I've seen gay guys go in there with the ugliest teeth and he treats them with the utmost respect. When I go he's always rude, he goes...you're never gonna take care of your teeth, we're not gonna fix them. But yet, he'll fix those guys teeth...no questions asked. I told him, I came into this world toothless and I'll leave this world toothless.

Yolanda (victim of date rape) and her new husband—both HIV+—chose to get pregnant and have a child despite their diagnosis. Yolanda and her husband read about the latest interventions and treatments during pregnancy and made an informed decision to get pregnant. They sought early treatment at a local obstetrical (OB) clinic. Yolanda's experience was one of total disappointment,

Even doctors turn their backs on us. They're educated and even though like that they're afraid of the HIV. Because I know when I was pregnant, they changed my doctor like nine times. Because they just came in and when they read the chart and they read the HIV positive, they just turned and got out of the room. Later the nurse came to release me...she didn't even check my belly or nothing. Another doctor just came in with gown, gloves, mask. I just told him, don't touch me, you're dumb, you're stupid. They just kicked me out of the clinic. Yes, I had to go back for my baby. Most of the time after that, I took care of my pregnancy in the emergency room. That doctor didn't want to see me around. If doctors are not educated, it would be hard to educate all the people too.

Despite her disappointment and disgust with the health care providers at this particular clinic, she continued her prenatal care for the safety of her pregnancy and ultimately her child.

Despite the inadequacies of services, all of the women took responsibility for their health care, and they all followed their medical regimens. In response to the question, "What did you do to stay healthy today?", all of the participants responded, "take my medicine." The women were well versed on types, dosages, and effects of their medications. They could give rationale for taking various medications based on their particular laboratory values, T-cell counts, and viral loads. Maria expressed the importance of taking the medications, "The medicines sometimes make me feel worse but I know that they will help me live longer."

Some of the women combined traditional folk ways with Western medicine to ease the problems of living and dealing with this disease. Alternative modalities of care were used for alleviating symptoms brought on by the disease. Herbs helped manage some of the side effects of medications and symptoms of the disease; herbs were used in teas, therapeutic baths, their hair, and for massages. Specific herbs and teas were chosen for their calming and soothing effects. Selection and use was based on past experience; encouragement or recommendation of family, friends, and the curandero/a; and/or through personal research.

Diagnosis and affirmation of status were such a devastation and burden that the women sought comfort in a higher source. Some turned to prayer, others to the Bible, and yet others to the Church. A curandero/curandera was sought to heal them physically and spiritually. Maria incorporated prayer, church, and spiritual healing with her medical regimen,

Since I have this "virus," I go see Don Jesus at least once a week. He is a viejito *[an old one], a* curandero. *I can't always get to the clinic so I go to him to help me pray. He gives me strength. I get so tired waiting at the clinic, that I just hate to go, but I go because Don Jesus says, "God will help us if we help ourselves." So, I feel that I must try to keep my visits at the clinic and take the medicine. Sometimes, I think that medicines just makes me feel worse. But I take it and go see Don Jesus a little more.*

Living in an already complicated world compounded by the devastation of this disease, these women found order in their lives by making the most of each day and by making the best of their available resources. They dealt with their lives as best they could by meeting each day face on and drawing from their inner strengths, their faith, and their families.

Surviving

Surviving describes the woman's day-to-day survival and her look to the future. Day to day she provides and cares for her family while struggling with her own physical and emotional well-being. For every one of the participants, getting up was the biggest daily struggle they faced. Each woman's day was dependent on how she managed to get up, which was an effort both physically and emotionally. One could almost feel Yolanda's exhaustion as she described her effort in getting up in the morning, "I'm just...so tired that I can't get up in the day and I just don't seem to wake up. And, sometimes even carrying my baby is hard for me. He's too heavy. It makes me tired." Judy, diagnosed at 6 months pregnant, summarized how she met each morning, "I just grin and bear it. It's mind over matter. I just get up."

Despite the woman's constant hardship and periodic inability to get out of bed, most of them had a very good outlook of the future. Judy attributed her future to her baby girl,

She's the girl I always wanted. I feel that if I had had a boy, I wouldn't have to live as long because I've already seen two of my sons grow up and I know those sons would take care of my little boy. But she's a little girl.

Revealing

Revealing depicts the struggles and fears these HIV+ women face with disclosure. The women had faced the initial revelation with devastation and disbelief. They even dealt with the revelation to their husbands or partners. Disclosure to their mothers was a little more difficult, however, they sought to disclose to their mothers first and then to a sister. Disclosure to other family members was left to this person. Most expressed strong support from their families. Some expressed denial and distancing on the part of some family members.

Disclosure did not extend to most of the children. A few of the women told their children that they "were sick and should be careful if mother hurt herself and bled." They could not tell their children, however, that they had HIV. Despite lack of disclosure to their children, most had made arrangements for them upon their death including leaving significant family members with detailed instructions on the children's care and leaving lengthy letters to each one to be given to them upon their death. Some hoped that they would live long enough to let their children grow to an age more able to tolerate the news. These HIV+ women experience Protecting and Advocating as they decide to reveal their status.

Protecting

Protecting depicts these women's struggles to protect their families from the ramifications of disclosure. Judy, who discussed exposure from her boyfriend and father of her child, described her struggle,

> *You gotta keep it to yourself. They think only women who do drugs or who are prostitutes have HIV, not a normal, ordinary citizen like me has HIV. She's dirty, she did drugs, she's a whore.*

Despite personal fear, some of the women expressed more fear for their children and families. Olga's fear to disclose was based on its effect on her 9-year-old son, "I'm afraid for my son. A lot of kids go to school with my son. How would that make my son feel? What would they do to him?"

Some of the women found it necessary to change their lives to make family and friends more comfortable. Changes were as drastic as not playing, touching, or being alone with nieces and nephews. Judy described her brother's reaction, "He doesn't leave the children over anymore. He won't leave them alone in the room with me." Food preparation for gathered family and friends was a concern for Olivia as she expressed her desire to be compassionate of other's feelings,

> *The congregation knows and they don't turn me away. When they come for dinner, I am considerate of their feelings. I know that you don't get it that way, but to ease their minds, my mother cooks everything.*

Advocating

Advocating depicts the empowerment these women demonstrate as they reveal their status for the purpose of reaching, teaching, and empowering other women with this disease. Judy describes her commitment to reach other women, "I speak when they ask me to speak." Some of the women expressed surprise that they did not know the extent to which HIV affected families. Yolanda expressed, "We go to retreats and talk to families about how to get help. We never knew there were so may families that had the HIV." This motivated them to speak out publicly about the disparate services available for women and their families, "My husband and I went on TV to talk about how we live with HIV. We told them that this is no longer a 'gay' disease but, a disease of families...an every-person disease."

Duality

Duality, the core of the model, represents the empowerment that develops as these women make choices as they live with HIV. The circle was chosen to depict the women's center—their wombs—whereas a single-ended arrow climbs out and gives birth to the two subcategories Intensifying and Actualizing. The subcategories sit on either side of the arrow to depict the unified strength and empowerment that develops as these women made positive choices to live for and protect their children and families. The woman's empowerment began as she changed by her willingness to live with HIV and the exchanges that she negotiated with God. Meeting basic needs was necessary at first for personal and family survival. She met higher level needs as she helped other women. Intensification of her mother role and actualization as a woman with HIV are the woman's dual empowerment. This dual empowerment moves her toward the final attainment of La Protectora.

Intensifying

Intensifying depicts the intensification of the mother role. As these women struggled in their decision to live for their child and/or children and to survive with this disease, they drew from their maternal strength. They drew from this same maternal strength as they protected and provided for their families. They replenished that strength as they made positive decisions. This same maternal strength moved them toward wanting to help and empower other women to live with this disease for the sake of their children. Positive in their convictions, they found ways to reach out to other women. Olga's maternal strength was demonstrated as she expressed her view, "We're fighting for our children. We need the focus put on us now." Yolanda also demonstrated her maternal strength as she expressed, "This disease is not just of gay men, it is of families and we must get help for all these families."

Actualizing

Maslow (1970) redefined self-actualizing as a person's need to be and do that which the person was born to do, his or her calling. Actualizing is characterized by those behaviors that call the HIV+ woman to be more than the subservient woman she has a history of being. For example, she was called to reveal her status, to educate, and encourage other women to seek early treatment. She told her story to groups in the hope of bringing about change. The HIV+ woman may not achieve all higher level needs and reach self-actualization as originally professed by Maslow, but in her quest to live with this disease, she self-actualizes as a woman with HIV. She struggles to learn more about her disease to make informed decisions about her own care. She finds the inner strength to reach out, educate, and empower other women. Olga's sense of self-actualization was evident by her comment, "This is how it's done. This is how it begins. We've got to network to everyone." Judy's actualization was evident as she described her experience at a local jail. "When we come and tell about being HIV positive, the women stay and listen. They walk out when the professionals talk about HIV."

Double-ended arrows between Intensifying and Actualizing and the subcategories of Dealing, Surviving, Protecting, and Advocating demonstrate a strengthening that occurs within the Mexican/Puerto Rican woman and the categories as she makes positive choices. The inner circling around Duality demonstrates closure in the Mexican/Puerto Rican woman's decision to live for herself and her family. The outer circling around Duality signifies the Mexican or Puerto Rican woman's move from a focus on herself to a focus on others and participation in activities that promote and aid other women. She moves from a subservient role to an emancipated role for the benefit of herself, her family, and other affected women and their families.

DISCUSSION

The findings of this study enrich the understanding of HIV as a life-altering chronic disease and demonstrate the complexity of the process as HIV+ Mexican and Puerto Rican women make decisions in response to their affirmation of HIV status. The primary focus of this study was to explore how culture guided HIV+ Hispanic women's health-seeking practices to uncover specific health and folk care activities. La Protectora emerged as the theoretical framework to explain the basic sociological process as HIV+ Mexican and Puerto Rican women response to their affirmation of status. The metaphor was chosen to describe women strong in their convictions, taking control of their lives, and willing to live with HIV. Descriptions of their experiences and beliefs as they struggle to live with HIV/AIDS richly contribute to the research.

Previous research (Chu, Hanson, & Jones, 1996; Raveis, Siegel, & Gorey, 1998) noted that high rates of pregnancy were found at diagnosis of women infected with HIV and that women exhibited significant delay in seeking care after testing positive. Psychological responses to learning their serostatus were the most pervasive factors associated with delaying care. This study provides some insight into how Mexican and Puerto Rican women respond to their affirmation of HIV status, their mortality, and the birth of a child. Because most of the women were pregnant at diagnosis, the pregnancy became the motivator for the women to live and seek care. For the woman who was not pregnant, her children and family became her motivators. The women did not delay care but rather overcame any and all obstacles to obtain health care to live for their children and families. Although one woman lost her first child and her husband to AIDS, her other child became her motivator to live.

These Mexican and Puerto Rican HIV+ women saw themselves as women first. When asked, "What is it like being a Hispanic women with HIV?'" all of them said the question should be, "What is it like being a woman with HIV?" The inequalities they faced were recognized as women's issues rather than cultural issues. How they lived their lives, cared for their families, and faced the prejudice of being HIV+ were based on being women. They assumed a proactive role as they lived with and took responsibility for their disease. The woman's focus on herself and participation in activities to promote her personal well-being were different from findings in previous research (Amaro, 1995; Anastasio, McMahan, Daniels, Nicholas, & Paul-Simon, 1995). In this study, the women were motivated to change their self-sacrificing orientation by overcoming obstacles and taking ownership of their disease. They became interested in their own health care and struggled to learn more about this disease to make informed decisions about care. They networked with other women and health care providers to share ideas and for personal growth. Once they felt that they were strong, they found the inner strength to reach out, educate, and empower other women. They continued to get stronger in their role as women with HIV. Their story is one of power and strength.

The metaphor, La Protectora, emerged to describe these HIV+ Mexican and Puerto Rican women as they faced their mortality and the psychological responses to their affirmation of HIV status. La Protectora emerged as the women faced everyday stressors and gained strength by their decisions. The process was fluid, not static. The women shifted through the categories at various times as they faced the stressors of living with HIV.

The metaphor was chosen to describe the embodiment of the Protectress that the HIV+ women took on when they chose to live with HIV, similar to Our Lady of Guadalupe, a protective religious figure esteemed in the Hispanic culture. The Virgin, a figure of hope, is believed to protect person and home from evil and harm (Spector,

2000). She is often called upon to intercede in time of need. These findings suggest that because of their motivation to live for their child, HIV+ Mexican and Puerto Rican women will assume the role of a Protectress to assure survival of herself and her child. These findings are limited to the Mexican and Puerto Rican women in this study and provide insight into a woman's reaction to her affirmation of status.

During Ofrecer, the Mexican and Puerto Rican women negotiated with their God to spare their children of a positive HIV status. This was similar to Kubler-Ross' (1973) [sic] "Bargaining" is similar to the Hispanic cultural practice of making a *promesa*, or promise, to overcome a punishment for wrongdoing (Spector, 2000). Their offer to change was made directly with their God. All of the children born to the women during diagnosis and who implored their God were negative. The one woman who had lost her first child to AIDS admitted to a spiritual change in her life after the loss of her first child and husband. She did not want the same outcome for her second child, so she too offered to change for the benefit of her second child.

These women did not follow the traditional cultural beliefs of making promises, visiting shrines, and offering candles to saints. They also did not implore the aid of the Virgin, Our Lady of Guadalupe, first. This moving away from the traditional shows a woman not willing to leave her life either to chance or in the hands of another. She is only willing to negotiate with the One she thinks can make a difference, namely her God. The recognition that she has to help herself to survive moves her closer to the role of the Protectress. A strong belief in a higher power, the use of prayer, reading the Bible, and going to church was expressed by all of the women, despite differences in religion. Investigation into how religion and spirituality affect decision making and living with HIV is necessary.

Traditional folk health care practices were followed to some extent by all of the women. The practices most commonly used (teas and herbs) were more palliative than curative. Teas and herbs were used primarily for experienced symptomology and side effects not necessarily specific to HIV. The women's ages, acculturation, length of time in the United States, language, and education all seemed to affect the extent to which they used traditional folk ways with their health care regimens. All of the women expressed comfort in meeting with the curandera (folk healer) at the CBO. One woman even sought the care of a neighborhood curandero for added comfort. Seeking the aid of a healer is not congruent with the beliefs of Jehovah, yet both women who identified themselves as Jehovah's Witnesses found comfort in attending the curandera's sessions.

Interviews were done in English and Spanish. Concern for the emergent theses in translations is necessary. The emergent themes and categories were not affected by the translations because they were validated with each participant and in subsequent interviews. The emergent themes were also not affected by the unfamiliarity of terms used by the two Puerto Rican women. The final member check validated the interpretation of the findings. The facts that the researcher was MA, with a mastery with [sic] the Spanish language and familiarity with the social context of the culture, facilitated the interviews of a very sensitive topic. This also added to the researcher's ability to understand the context of terms and themes as they emerged during the interviews and to elicit more rich data.

The women in this study were all economically disadvantaged, had children, and were only representative of the Mexican and Puerto Rican ethnic groups. They all expressed transmission from their husbands and/or partners in an apparent monogamous relationship. Some life event after diagnosis with HIV motivated them to live and care for themselves with this disease, which proves different from previous research. These characteristics and the small sample size ($n = 9$) limit the findings to this group. Further testing is needed with larger and more diverse groups.

Research article taken from: Valdez, M. R. (2001). A metaphor for HIV-positive Mexican and Puerto Rican women. *Western Journal of Nursing Research, 23*(5), 517–535. (Reprinted with permission.)

References

Amaro, H. (1995). Love, sex, and power. Considering women's realities in HIV prevention. *American Psychology, 50*(6), 437–447.

Anastasio, C., McMahan, T., Daniels, A., Nicholas, P. K., & Paul-Simon, A. (1995). Self-care burden in women with human immunodeficiency virus. *Journal of Association of Nurses in AIDS Care, 6*(3), 31–42.

Barkan, S. E., Melnick, S. L., Preston-Martin, S., Weber, K., Kalish, L. A., Miotti, P., et al. (1998). The Women's Interagency HIV Study. WIHS Collaborative Study Group. *Epidemiology, 9*(2), 117–125.

Blumer, H. (1969). *Symbolic interaction.* Englewood Cliffs, NJ: Prentice Hall.

Centers for Disease Control and Prevention (1993). *HIV/AIDS surveillance report: U.S. AIDS cases reported through September 1993.* Atlanta, GA: Center for Infectious Diseases, Division of HIV/AIDS.

Centers for Disease Control and Prevention (1999). *Need for sustained HIV prevention among men who have sex with men (August, 1999).* Atlanta, GA: Center for Infectious Diseases, Division of HIV/AIDS.

Centers for Disease Control and Prevention (2000). *HIV/AIDS surveillance report: U.S. AIDS cases reported through December 1999, Vol. 11, No. 2.* Atlanta, GA: Center for Infectious Diseases, Division of HIV/AIDS.

Centers for Disease Control and Prevention (2001a). *HIV/AIDS among Hispanics in the United States (January 2001).* Atlanta, GA: Center for Infectious Diseases, Division of HIV/AIDS.

Centers for Disease Control and Prevention (2001b). *HIV/AIDS among U.S. women: Minority and young women at continuing risk (January, 2001).* Atlanta, GA: Center for Infectious Diseases, Division of HIV/AIDS.

Chu, S. Y., Hanson, D. L., & Jones, J. L. (1996). Pregnancy rates among women infected with human immunodeficiency virus. Adult/Adolescent HIV Spectrum of Disease Project Group. *Obstetrics and Gynecology, 87*(2), 195–198.

Chu, S. Y., Peterman, T. A., Doll, L. S., Buehler, J. W., & Curran, J. W. (1992). AIDS in bisexual men in the United States: Epidemiology and transmission to women. *American Journal of Public Health, 82*(2), 220–224.

Clark, M. (1970). *Health in the Mexican-American culture: A community study* (2nd ed.). Los Angeles: University of California Press.

Diaz, T., Buehler, J. W., Castro, K. G., & Ward, J. W. (1993). AIDS trends among Hispanics in the United States. *American Journal of Public Health, 83*(4), 504–509.

Garcia-Pelayo, R. (Ed.). (1983). *Larousse Diccionario Moderno.* Mexico: Ediciones Larousse. Larousse Modern Dictionary, Larousse Edition, Mexico City: Mexico.

Giachello, A. L. (1985). Hispanics and healthcare. In P. Cafferty & W. McCready (Eds.), *Hispanics in the United States: A social agenda.* New Brunswick, NJ: Transaction Books.

Glaser, B. G., & Strauss, A. K. (1967). The discovery of grounded theory: Strategy for qualitative research. Hawthorne, NY: Aldine.

Gonzalez-Swafford, M. J., & Gutierrez, M. G. (1983). Ethno-medical beliefs and practices of Mexican-Americans. *Nurse Practitioner, 8*(10), 29–30, 32, 34.

Hutchinson, S. (1993). Grounded theory: The method. In P. L. Munhall & C. J. Oiler (Eds.), *Nursing research: A qualitative perspective* (pp. 180–212). Norwalk, CT: Appleton-Century-Crofts.

Kay, M. A. (1981). Health and illness in a Mexican-American barrio. In E. H. Spicer (Ed.), *Ethnic medicine in the southwest* (pp. 99–166). Tucson, AZ: University of Arizona Press.

Kline, A., Kline, E., & Oken, E. (1992). Minority women and sexual choice in the age of AIDS. *Social Science & Medicine, 34*(4), 447–457.

Kubler-Ross, E. (1973). On death and dying. In E. Wyschogrod (Ed.), *The phenomenon of death* (pp. 14–40). New York: Harper & Row.

Lehner, T., & Chiasson, M. A. (1998). Seroprevalence of human immunodeficiency virus type 1 and sexual behaviors in bisexual African-American and Hispanic men visiting a sexually transmitted disease clinic in New York City. *American Journal of Epidemiology, 147*(3), 269–272.

Marin, B. V., & Marin, G. (1992). Predictors of condom accessibility among Hispanics in San Francisco. *American Journal of Public Health, 82*(4), 592–595.

Marin, B. V., Tschann, J. M., Gomez, C., & Kegeles, S. (1993). Acculturation and gender differences in sexual attitudes and behaviors: Hispanic vs. non-Hispanic White unmarried adults. *American Journal of Public Health, 83*(12), 1759–1761.

Maslow, A. (1970). *Motivation and personality*. New York: Harper & Row.

Mead, G. (1934). *Mind, self, and society*. Chicago: University of Chicago Press.

Miles, M., & Huberman, A. (1994) *Qualitative data analysis*. Thousand Oaks, CA: Sage.

National Institutes of Health [NIH] (2000). *Fact sheet: HIV infection in minority populations (May, 2000)*. Bethesda, MD: U.S. Department of Health and Human Services, National Institute of Allergy and Infectious Diseases.

Nyamathi, A., Bennett, C., Leake, B., Lewis, C., & Flaskerud, J. (1993). AIDS-related knowledge, perceptions, and behaviors among impoverished minority women. *American Journal of Public Health, 83*(1), 65–71.

Nyamathi, A., & Flaskerud, J. (1992). A community-based inventory of current concerns of impoverished homeless and drug-addicted minority women. *Research in Nursing & Health, 15*(2), 121–129.

Nyamathi, A., Leake, B., Flaskerud, J., Lewis, C., & Bennett, C. (1993). Outcomes of specialized and traditional AIDS counseling programs for impoverished women of color. *Research in Nursing & Health, 16*(1), 11–21.

Raveis, V. H., Siegel, K., & Gorey, E. (1998). Factors associated with HIV-infected women's delay in seeking medical care. *AIDS Care, 10*(5), 549–562.

Salgado de Snyder, V. N., Diaz-Perez, M. J., & Maldonado, M. (1996). AIDS: Risk behaviors among rural Mexican women married to migrant workers in the United States. *AIDS Education Preview, 8*(2), 134–142.

Spector, R. E. (2000). *Cultural diversity in health and illness* (5th ed.). Englewood Cliffs, NJ: Prentice Hall.

Stern, P. N. (1985). Using grounded theory method in nursing research. In M. M. Leininger (Ed.), *Qualitative research methods in nursing* (pp. 149–160). Philadelphia: W.B. Saunders.

Stern, P. N., Allen, L., & Moxley, P. (1982). The nurse as grounded theorist: History, process and uses. *Review Journal of Philosophy and Social Science, 7*(1–2), 200–215.

World Health Organization (2000). *AIDS epidemic update: December, 1999* [Online]. Retrieved from the World Wide Web: http://www.UNAIDS.org.

Zambrana, R. (1987). A research agenda on issues affecting poor and minority women: A model for understanding their health needs. *Women and Health, 12*(3–4), 137–160.

Ethnography as Method

If publication of manuscripts in nursing journals can be viewed as the measure of interest in and commitment to ethnographic ways of knowing, then it is clear that ethnography has gained a stable place in the development of nursing knowledge. Nurse–researchers use ethnography to study the culture of parish nursing (Chase-Ziolek, 1999); operating room practice (Graff, Roberts, & Thornton, 1999); parenting of grandchildren (Haglund, 2000); and self-care practices of individuals with multiple chemical sensitivities (Lipson, 2001). These are just a few examples of areas of study published recently. To gain a clear understanding of why there is a demonstrated commitment to ethnographic research, it is important to look at the foundations of ethnography as a method.

Social scientists share an interest in and a commitment to discovery. Anthropologists, as a particular group of social scientists, are committed to the discovery of cultural knowledge. Early in the history of the social sciences, individuals interested in culture found that the ways of traditional science were inadequate to discover the nuances of people who live together and share similar experiences. This inadequacy led to the beginnings of *ethnography*, a means of studying groups of individuals' lifeways or patterns. Sanday (1983) has reported that ethnographic methods are not new. The ancient Greek Herodotus was an ethnographer who recorded variations in the cultures to which he was exposed. According to Sanday, Franz Boas's (1948) ethnographic examination of the Eskimo culture signaled the contemporary beginning of ethnographic study.

Anthropology is synonymous with the term *ethnography*. The product of anthropologists' work is ethnography (Muecke, 1994). As early as the 1960s, references can be found regarding the value of an ethnographic approach as a means to study nursing culture (Boyle, 1994; Leininger, 1970; Ragucci, 1972). Early nurse–ethnographers embraced the methods of anthropology to study phenomena they perceived were irreducible, unquantifiable, or unable to be made objective. Leininger (1985) went beyond the borrowing of ethnographic methods to develop what she called "ethnonursing research." This chapter explores the research method called ethnography and discusses common elements of ethnographic methodology, its uses, interpretations, and applications.

ETHNOGRAPHY DEFINED

According to Spradley (1980), "Ethnography is the work of describing culture" (p. 3). The description of culture or the cultural scene must be guided by an intense desire to understand other individuals' lives so much that the researcher becomes part of a specific cultural scene. To do this, Malinowski (1961) believed that researchers must learn the "native's point of view" (p. 25). Spradley, however, warned that ethnography is more than the study of the people; rather, "ethnography means learning from people" (p. 3). Spradley also pointed out that "the essential core of ethnography is this concern with the meanings of actions and events to the people [ethnographers] seek to understand" (p. 5).

Beyond Spradley's (1980) discussion of ethnography lies a long-standing debate about what constitutes ethnography. Muecke (1994) suggested "there is not a single standard form of ethnography" (p. 188). Boyle (1994) proposed that "the style and method of ethnography are a function of the ethnographer, who brings her or his own scientific traditions, training, and socialization to the research project" (p. 182). This debate has led to a certain amount of confusion about ethnography as a method and further fueled arguments around the relative value of ethnography as rigorous science (Savage, 2000). Despite the disagreements around the method, ethnographic methods have and will continue to provide important information about the meanings, organization, and interpretations of culture.

According to Muecke (1994), the four major ethnographic schools of thought are (1) classical, (2) systematic, (3) interpretive or hermeneutic, and (4) critical. Classical ethnography requires that the study "include both a description of behavior and demonstrate why and under what circumstances the behavior took place" (Morse & Field, 1995, p. 154). This type of work requires considerable time in the field, constantly observing and making sense of behaviors.

The objective of *systematic ethnography* is "to define the structure of culture, rather than to describe a people and their social interaction, emotions, and materials" (Muecke, 1994, p. 192). The difference between classical and systematic ethnography lies in scope. Classical ethnography aims to describe everything about the culture. Systematic ethnography takes a focused look at the structure of the culture-what organizes the study group's lifeways. Systematic ethnography is the framework used by Spradley, whose method of ethnographic inquiry is explored fully in this chapter.

The aim of *interpretive* or *hermeneutic ethnography* is to "discover the meanings of observed social interactions" (Muecke, 1994, p. 193). According to Wolcott (cited in Muecke, 1994), "Ethnography is quintessentially analytic and interpretive, rather than methodological" (p. 193). Interpretive ethnographers are interested in studying the culture through analysis of inferences and implications found in behavior (Muecke, 1994).

Critical ethnography is another type of ethnography Muecke (1994) described. It relies on critical theory (Fontana & Frey, 1994). Critical ethnographers do not believe there is a culture out there to be known but, rather, that researchers and members of a culture together create a cultural schema. Ethnographers subscribing to this tradition account for "historical, social and economic situations" (Fontana & Frey, 1994, p. 369) when reporting. Germain (2001) adds that "critical ethnography...is distinguished from conventional approaches by its focus on issues of injustice and social oppression" (p. 279). "Inherent in a critical approach is the understanding that through communicative practices and reflection, researchers and participants discern an absolute truth of the culture" (Manias & Street, 2001, p. 235).

These four types of ethnographies represent a philosophic position. "All research proceeds from philosophy, articulated or not" (Germain, 2001, p. 279). Therefore, it is essential that researchers define their position before embarking on an ethnographic study. A researcher's philosophic stance determines what he or she will study as well as the framework for data collection and analysis.

In addition to the four types of ethnographies described, it is important to add the work of Leininger (1985). Leininger identifies a specific approach to ethnography she calls ethnonursing that allows nurses to "study explicit nursing phenomena from a cross-cultural perspective" (p. 38). The goal is "to discover nursing knowledge as known, perceived and experienced by nurses and consumers of nursing and health services" (p. 38). The most significant contribution of Leininger's work is its complete focus on nursing as the phenomenon of interest.

ETHNOGRAPHY ROOTS

There is much debate about the historical beginnings of ethnography. Sanday (1983) proposed that ethnography began with Herodotus. Rowe (1965) has suggested that the Renaissance marked the initiation of ethnography as a research method. Still others have indicated that Malinowski's (1922) study of the Trobriand Islanders marked the beginning of ethnography. Atkinson and Hammersley (1994) offered that the contemporary beginning of ethnography occurred late in the nineteenth century as individuals began to acknowledge cultural differences or "deviations from norms" (p. 249) and became interested in studying these deviations. "The application of ethnographic method by Western anthropologists and sociologists to the investigation of their own societies has been a central feature of twentieth-century social science" (Cole, cited in Atkinson & Hammersley, 1994, p. 250). Atkinson and Hammersley (1994) identified two key phases in the development of ethnography in the twentieth century: "the work of the founders of modern anthropology and that of the Chicago school of sociology" (p. 250).

Boas, Malinowski, and Radcliffe-Brown, the founders of modern anthropology (Atkinson & Hammersley, 1994), were committed to anthropology as a science. These ethnographers had the idea to chronicle their descriptions of primitive cultures. "The prime motivation on the part of all three founders was the rejection of speculation in favor of empirical investigation, a theme that has always been a central characteristic of empiricism, but not exclusive to it" (Atkinson & Hammersley, 1994, p. 250).

The Chicago school's most striking feature was its limited "questioning of the relevance of natural science as a methodological model for social research" (Atkinson & Hammersley, 1994, p. 250). One of the most important influences of the Chicago school was the attempt by many scientists in the school to connect scientific and hermeneutic philosophies with pragmatic philosophies such as the one espoused by Dewey (Atkinson & Hammersley, 1994). According to Woods (1992), these University of Chicago scientists laid the foundation for field research. They saw the city as a "social laboratory" (Woods, 1992, p. 338) that exemplified all forms of human behavior and activity. It was here that the idea of "native" was expanded to include social groups of local importance.

Beyond these early developments, ethnography has expanded and developed to meet the needs of scientists using its varied forms. As Atkinson (1999) points out,

> ...ethnography has always contained within it a variety of perspectives. As a whole, it has never been totally subsumed within a framework of orthodoxy and objectivism. There have been varieties of aesthetic and interpretive standpoints throughout nearly a century of development and change (p. 465).

Today, it is the quest to discover cultures and behaviors different from the researcher's that drives the use of this method. It is an exciting, interactive, decidedly qualitative approach that appeals to its followers. As Hughes (1992) pointed out, "What is quintessentially distinctive about anthropology [and thus ethnography] is just [its] *species-centeredness* and holistic character" (p. 442).

FUNDAMENTAL CHARACTERISTICS OF ETHNOGRAPHY

Six characteristics are central to ethnographic research. Three could be claimed by other qualitative methods: (1) researcher as instrument, (2) fieldwork, and (3) the cyclic nature of data collection and analysis. The other three arguably could be said to be exclusive to ethnography: (4) the focus on culture, (5) cultural immersion, and (6) the tension between researcher as researcher and researcher as cultural member, also called reflexivity. These characteristics should be considered foundational to ethnographic research.

Researcher as Instrument

The study of culture requires an intimacy with the participants who are part of a culture. Ethnography as a method of inquiry provides the opportunity for researchers to conduct studies that attend to the need for intimacy with members of the culture, which is precisely why the ethnographer becomes the conduit for information shared by the group. When anthropologists speak of researcher as instrument, they are indicating the significant role ethnographers play in identifying, interpreting, and analyzing the culture under study. The primary way that researchers become the instrument is through observation and the recording of cultural data.

More than just observing, researchers often become participants in the cultural scene. Atkinson and Hammersley (1994) suggested that "participant observation is not a particular research technique but a mode of being-in-the-world characteristic of researchers" (p. 249). Participant observation demands complete commitment to the task of understanding. The ethnographer becomes part of the culture being studied to feel what it is like for the people in the situation (Atkinson & Hammersley, 1994; Boyle, 1994; Sanday, 1983).

Ethnographic researchers, despite becoming part of the cultural scene, will never fully have the insider's (emic) view. The emic view is the native's view, which reflects the cultural group's language, beliefs, and experiences. The only way ethnographers can begin to access the emic view is by collecting cultural group members' journals, records, or other cultural artifacts.

The strength of participant observation is the opportunity to access information from the outsider's (etic) view. The etic view is the view of the outsider with interpretation. The essence of ethnography is determining what an observed behavior is or what a ritual means in the context of the group studied. Ethnography is the description and interpretation of cultural patterns.

Fieldwork

All ethnographic research occurs in the field. Researchers go to the location of the culture of interest. For example, Lundberg (1999) was interested in studying the culture of immigrant Thai women married to Swedish husbands. Specifically, the researcher was interested in the meanings and practices of health held by these individuals. The author perceived this topic to be important for nursing. Lundberg participated in the informants' lives by going to their homes, attending social activities, and assisting in general daily life activities, including interacting with their families. Physically situating oneself in the environs of the study culture is a fundamental characteristic in all ethnographic work.

Cyclic Nature of Data Collection and Analysis

In ethnographic research, a question about the differences in human experience found in a culture usually different from one's own leads researchers to investigate those differences. As Agar (1982, 1986) has pointed out, one of the problems for ethnographers is that no clear boundaries exist between the similarities and differences in human experience. Therefore, data collected by ethnographers in the field to describe the differences and similarities lead to still other questions about the culture. Answering those questions leads to more questions. As Spradley (1980) and Spradley and McCurdy (1972) have indicated, the study ends not because a researcher has answered all of the questions or completely described the culture, but because time and resources do not allow continuation.

Focus on the Culture

Unique to ethnography is the focus on the culture. Ethnography is the only research method whose sole purpose is to understand the lifeways of individuals connected through group membership. As Boyle (1994) stated, "Ethnography focuses on a group of people who have something in common" (p. 161). It is essential that ethnographic researchers strive to discover and interpret the cultural meanings found within a connected group. Unfortunately, culture is hard to define (Roper & Shapira, 2000). From a behavioral/materialistic perspective, culture is the way a group behaves, what it produces, or the way it functions (Roper & Shapira, 2000). From a cognitive perspective, "it is the ideas, beliefs and knowledge that are used by a group of people as they live their lives" (p. 3). According to Roper and Shapira, the application of the two perspectives will help to demonstrate "what people know and believe and what they do" (p. 3).

Cultural Immersion

Another characteristic of ethnography is the depth and length of participation ethnographers must have with the culture under study. The researcher's participation has been called *cultural immersion*, which requires that researchers live among the people being studied. For example, if a nurse–researcher is interested in studying the culture of families coping with human immunodeficiency virus in a family member, the researcher would need to immerse himself or herself in the lives of the families studied. The researcher would observe how each family functions inside and outside of the home, studying as many facets of their lives as the participants will allow. Participant observation would take months, if not 1 year or more, to complete. Based on observation and most likely participation, the nurse–researcher would draw conclusions about the culture based on his or her discoveries while collecting data.

Reflexivity

Reflexivity describes the struggle between being the researcher and becoming a member of the culture. Although it is important for the researcher to remain objective and stay focused on the research, on some level the researcher becomes a member of the culture. Through this type of participation, researchers must realize that they alter the culture and have the potential to be less objective than is typical in the conduct of research. Because of the prolonged involvement as a researcher and participant in the group, it is extremely difficult to maintain a *completely* detached view.

This tension between researcher as pure researcher and researcher as participant has been discussed in many forums. How does one discover the emic—the insider's view—without becoming a part of the culture? The struggle for objectivity in collecting and analyzing data while being so intimately involved with the group is a characteristic unique to ethnography. More than just objectivity is of concern, however. Also of concern is the researcher's knowledge that just being present in the culture on some level affects its character.

SELECTION OF ETHNOGRAPHY AS METHOD

One of the goals of ethnography is to make explicit what is implicit within a culture (Germain, 1986). "Ethnography aims to get at the implicit or latent (backstage) culture in addition to the explicit, public, or manifested (front-stage) aspects of culture" (Germain, 2001, p. 284). Cultural knowledge requires an understanding of the people, what they do, what they say, how they relate to one another, what their customs and beliefs are, and how they derive meaning from their experiences (Goetz & LeCompte, 1984; Spradley, 1980; Spradley & McCurdy, 1972; van Maanen, 1983). With these goals in mind, nurses interested in exploring cultures or subcultures in nursing or nurse-related cultures have the world available to them for study. Within the profession of nursing, there are many undiscovered cultures. An example of cultural practices within nursing that is implicit and has been made explicit through research (Wolf, 1988) is nursing rituals. Wolf discovered the rituals that nurses use to enable and protect them in their work with clients. Similarly, in Wanta's (1998) study of "behavioral, cognitive and affective responses of a group of people asked to prepare for the possibility of their own sudden illness, injury, or death while in the prime of their life and apparently healthy" (p. 23) provides a look of how what is implicit is made explicit within a culture. The use of the ethnographic approach provides nurses with the opportunity to explore the holistic nature of society and to ask questions relevant to nursing practice. The naturalistic setting in which ethnographic research is carried out supplies nurses with the view of the world as it is, not as they wish it to be. Fundamentally, entrance into the naturalistic setting in which the research participants live without interference from outside sources is a rich data source for exploring many nursing practice issues.

Nurses conducting ethnographic research must accept reflexivity as part of the research design. Reflexivity allows nurses to explore cultures within the paradigm of nursing, which values the affective and subjective nature of humans. The duality of being both researcher and participant provides opportunities to capitalize on insights derived from datum sources. "'Meaning' is not merely investigated, but is constructed by [the researcher] and informant through active and reciprocal relationships and the dialectical processes of interaction" (Anderson, 1991, p. 116). Anderson (1991) added that "field work is inherently dialectical; the researcher affects and is affected by the phenomena (s)he seeks to understand" (p. 117). Reflexivity therefore leads to a greater understanding of the dynamics of particular phenomena and relationships found within cultures.

When choosing ethnography as the approach to study a particular culture or subculture, the nurse should ask several important questions. Do I have the time to conduct this study? Do I have the resources to carry it out? Will the data collected have the potential to bring new insights to the profession? If the nurse–researcher answers *yes* to these questions, then his or her study has the potential to contribute significantly to the nursing profession.

In addition to answering the preceding questions, nurses interested in ethnography should know why the approach may be useful. Spradley (1980) identified four primary reasons for using ethnography to study a particular culture. The first is to document "the existence of alternative realities and to describe these realities in [the terms of the people studied]" (p. 14). Much of what individuals know about other cultures they interpret based on their own culture. This way of thinking is limiting in that it promotes the idea that one truth—and thus, one reality—exists. For ethnographers, a description of alternative realities provides a rich and varied landscape of human life. Coming "to understand personality, society, individuals, and environments from the perspective of other than professional scientific cultures...will lead to a sense of epistemological humility" (Spradley, 1980, p. 15).

A second reason, according to Spradley (1980), for using the ethnographic approach is to discover grounded theories. Through a description of the culture, researchers are able to discover theories that are indigenous to the culture (Grant & Fine, 1992). Foundational to grounded theorists' research is a belief that the only useful theory is one that is grounded in the beliefs and practices of individuals studied. The principle that research should be based on the beliefs and practices of individuals (cultural groups) studied is also foundational to the work of ethnographers. The major difference between the conduct of ethnographic and grounded theory research is that ethnographers wishing to develop grounded theory will advance the description and interpretation of cultural observations to a level that yields a description of basic social-psychological process. For a full discussion of grounded theory, see Chapter 7.

Germain (2001) supports the development of theory as a natural outcome of ethnographic study. She offers that "ethnography contributes descriptive and explanatory theories of culture and cultural behaviors and meaning. Within the ethnography may be identified other middle-range theories such as typologies and hypotheses for further study" (p. 281).

A third reason for choosing ethnography is to better understand complex societies. Early anthropologists believed that the ethnographic method was ideally suited to the study of non-Western cultures. Today, anthropologists see the value of using ethnography to study subgroups of larger cultures—both Western and non-Western. Examples can be found in nursing in the works of Haglund (2000) and Wanta (1998).

The fourth reason Spradley (1980) offered for using the ethnographic approach is to understand human behavior. Human behavior has meaning, and ethnography is one way to discover that meaning. Such discovery becomes particularly important when nurses look at the clients' health and illness behaviors. Understanding why cultural groups such as Hispanics, elderly people, abused women, or the Amish behave in health and illness situations can assist nurses who care for these groups to better provide interventions so they may enhance the strategies already in use by the groups.

When nurses decide they will use ethnography to study a culture of interest, a parallel consideration will be whether they will conduct a micro- or macro-ethnographic study. Leininger (1985) called these study types "mini" or "maxi," respectively. Regardless of the terminology, the intent has to do with the scale of the study. A *micro-* or *mini-ethnography* is generally of a smaller scale and is narrow or specific in its focus. Schulte's (2000) ethnographic study of the culture of public health nurses in a large, Midwestern, urban health department is an example of a micro-ethnography. The study focused on one organization, a particular group of employees, and occurred during a 6-month period. Therefore, the study was considered a micro-ethnography because of its description of only one group, public health nurses, within one health department, and with a limited time in the setting.

Increasingly, nurse researchers are using the term *focused ethnography* to identify their small-scale ethnographies. Focused ethnographies have as their focal point a distinct problem that is studied within a single context with a limited number of individuals.

> Focused ethnographies share with classical ethnographies a commitment to conducting intensive participant observation activities within a naturalistic setting, asking questions to learn what is happening, and using other available sources of information to gain as complete an understanding as possible of people, places and events of interest (Roper & Shapira, 2000, p. 7).

Morin, Patterson, Kurtz, & Brzowski's (1999) study of "mothers' responses to care given by male nursing students before and after birth" (p. 83) is an example of a focused ethnographic study. The researchers interviewed women who had given birth in "one small community hospital located in the mid-Atlantic region of the United States" (p. 84). The number of participants in the study was small and was limited to one 14-bed maternal child unit, so the research focused on one small faction of a specific social group receiving care from male nursing students.

A *macro-* or *maxi-ethnography* is a study that examines the culture in a broader context, extends over a longer period, and is most often reported in book form. Magilvy and Congdon's (2000) and Lipson's (2001) ethnographies are examples of this type of study. These researchers observed a significant number of individuals over a period of several years with a larger scope.

Spradley (1980) further delineated the scope of ethnographic studies by placing them on a continuum. On one end are micro-ethnographic studies that examine a single social situation (nurses receiving report on one unit); multiple social situations (critical care nurses participating in a report on three intensive care units); or a single social institution (the American Cancer Society of Philadelphia). Moving on the continuum closer to macro-ethnographic studies, Spradley included multiple social institutions (American Cancer Societies of Northeastern Pennsylvania); a single community study (Chinatown in San Francisco); multiple communities (Hispanic communities in East Los Angeles); and a complex society (tribal life in Africa).

ELEMENTS AND INTERPRETATIONS OF THE METHOD

A number of individuals have described ethnographic research methods. Early ethnographic reports were written by individuals who documented their observations of the cultures they encountered. Although many of these individuals were not trained anthropologists, they gave rich and vivid accounts of the lives of the people they met. Sanday (1983) pointed out that these recorders were not participants in paradigmatic ethnography. *Paradigmatic ethnography* consists of the range of activities completed by a trained ethnographer, including observing, recording, participating, analyzing, reporting, and publishing experiences with a particular cultural group. Sanday offered three traditions within paradigmatic ethnography: (1) holistic, (2) semiotic, and (3) behavioristic.

The *holistic ethnographic interpretation* is the oldest tradition. The commitment of researchers in this tradition is to "the study of culture as an integrated whole" (Sanday, 1983, p. 23). According to Sanday, the ethnographers who ascribed to this approach included Benedict (1934), Mead (1949), Malinowski (1922), and Radcliffe-Brown (1952). Although all four ethnographers varied in their focus, their underlying commitment was to describe as fully as possible the particular culture of interest within the context of the whole. For instance, "Mead and Benedict were interested in describing and interpreting the whole, not in explaining its origin beyond the effect of the individual on it" (Sanday, 1983, p. 25). Radcliffe-Brown and Malinowski were not committed to the "characterization of the cultural whole but to how each trait functions in the total cultural complex of which it is part" (Sanday, 1983, p. 25). Although the focus of both sets of ethnographers was different, the underlying commitment to viewing the culture as a whole was preserved.

The *semiotic interpretation* focuses on gaining access to the native's viewpoint. Like the researchers committed to holistic interpretation, the major anthropologists in this tradition did not share epistemologies. The two major followers of this tradition are Geertz (1973) and Goodenough (1970, 1971). According to Sanday (1983), Geertz views the study of culture not as a means to defining laws but as an interpretative enterprise focused on searching for meaning. Furthermore, Geertz believes that the only way to achieve cultural understanding is through *thick descriptions*, large amounts of data (descriptions of the culture) collected over extended periods. According to Geertz, the analysis and conclusions offered by ethnographers represent fictions developed to explain rather than to understand a culture.

Goodenough (1970, 1971) is an ethnographer who embraces the semiotic tradition. He does so through what has been described as *ethnoscience*, "a rigorous and systematic way of studying and classify emic (local or inside) data of a cultural group's own perceptions, knowledge, and language in terms of how people perceive and interpret their universe" (Leininger, 1970, pp. 168–169). "Ethnoscience [is] viewed as a method of developing precise and operationalized descriptions of cultural concept" (Morse & Field, 1995, p. 29). Ethnoscience also is called ethnosemantics or ethnolinguistics to emphasize the focus on language.

According to Sanday (1983), Geertz's commitment is to the "notion that culture is located in the minds and hearts of men" (p. 30). Culture is described by writing out systematic rules and formulating ethnographic algorithms, which make it possible to produce acceptable actions such as the "writing out of linguistic rules that makes it possible to produce acceptable utterances" (Sanday, 1983, p. 30).

"The differences between Geertz and Goodenough are not in aim but in the method, focus, and mode of reporting" (Sanday, 1983, p. 30). Both ethnographers are committed to the careful description of culture. Geertz's method and reporting are viewed as more of an art form compared with Goodenough's method in which the focus is on rigorous, systematic methods of collecting data and reporting findings.

The third interpretation is the *behaviorist approach*. Ethnographers using this approach are most interested in the behavior of members of a culture. The main goal "is to uncover covarying patterns in observed behavior" (Sanday, 1983, pp. 33–34). This approach is deductive. Ethnographers subscribing to this interpretation look specifically for cultural situations that substantiate preselected categories of data. Use of this interpretation deviates radically from the intent of the other two interpretations, which rely solely on induction.

Leininger (1978, 1985), a nurse–anthropologist, developed her own interpretation of ethnography: ethnonursing. *Ethnonursing*, according to Leininger, is "the study and analysis of the local or indigenous people's viewpoints, beliefs, and practices about nursing care behavior and processes of designated cultures" (Leininger, 1978, p. 15). The goal of ethnonursing is to "discover nursing knowledge as known, perceived and experienced by nurses and consumers of nursing and health services" (Leininger, 1985, p. 38). The primary function of Leininger's approach to ethnography is to focus on nursing and related health phenomena. This approach has been an important contribution to the nursing field. Many nurse-ethnographers subscribe to Leininger's philosophy and apply her suggested method of inquiry.

SELECTING ETHNOGRAPHY

When individuals choose to conduct an ethnographic research study, usually they have decided there is some shared cultural knowledge to which they would like access. The way individuals access cultural knowledge is by making *cultural inferences*, which are the observer's (researcher's) conclusions based on what the researcher has seen or heard while studying another culture. Making inferences is the way individuals learn many of their own group's cultural norms or values. For instance, if a child observes another child being scolded for talking in class, the observer—without being told—concludes that talking in class can lead to an unpleasant outcome. Therefore, the child learns through cultural inference that talking in class is unacceptable. Ethnographers follow this same process in their observations of cultural groups. According to Spradley (1980), ethnographers use generally three types of information to generate cultural inferences: cultural behavior (what people do); cultural artifacts (the things people make and use); and speech messages (what people say).

A significant part of culture is not readily available. This information, called *tacit knowledge*, consists of the information members of a culture know but do not talk about or express directly (Hammersley & Atkinson, 1983; Spradley, 1980). In addition to accessing explicit or easily observed cultural knowledge, ethnographers have the responsibility of describing tacit knowledge.

Understanding the Researcher's Role

To access explicit and tacit knowledge, researchers must understand the role they will play in the discovery of cultural knowledge. Because the researcher becomes the instrument, he or she must be cognizant of what the role of instrument entails. The role requires ethnographers to participate in the culture, observe the participants, document observations, collect artifacts, interview members of the cultural group, analyze, and report the findings. This role requires a significant commitment to the research that should not be taken lightly.

The step-by-step method of collecting, analyzing, and presenting ethnographic research, according to Spradley (1980), is presented to educate readers. Although Spradley is not the only ethnographic approach available, it is presented because of its explicitness, clarity, and utility for inexperienced ethnographic researchers.

Spradley (1980) has identified eleven steps in the conduct of ethnographic research. Box 9.1 summarizes these steps. The processes for data generation, treatment, analysis, and interpretation are discussed within the framework of the steps identified.

Box 9.1

STEPS FOR CONDUCTING ETHNOGRAPHIC RESEARCH

1. Do participant observation.
2. Make an ethnographic record.
3. Make descriptive observations.
4. Make a domain analysis.
5. Make a focused observation.
6. Make a taxonomic analysis.
7. Make selected observations.
8. Make a componential analysis.
9. Discover cultural themes.
10. Take a cultural inventory.
11. Write an ethnography.

Gaining Access

One of the first considerations when initiating an ethnographic study is to decide on the *aim*. Based on the *aim* of the inquiry, researchers can decide the scope of the project. Will the aim be to focus on a particular group or a particular problem of a group? Will you use a focused, micro- or mini-ethnography approach? Will you examine a single social situation? Multiple social situations? A single social institution? Multiple social institutions? A single community study? Multiple communities? Complex societies?

Once researchers have decided on the scope of the project, their next step is to gain access to the culture. Because ethnography requires the study of people, the activities in which they are involved, and the places in which they live, to conduct the study, researchers will need to gain access to the culture. This may be the most difficult part of the study. Because researchers are not usually members of the group studied, individuals in the culture of interest may be unwilling or unable to provide the access required. In other instances, researchers may be studying social situations that do not require a group's permission. For instance, if researchers are interested in the culture of individuals who come to the local pharmacy to obtain their medications, permission may not be required. However, if they are interested in studying the culture of health professionals in an outpatient clinic, permission is necessary.

Access is easiest when researchers have clearly stated the study purpose and have shared how they will protect the participants' confidentiality. In addition, offering to participate in the setting may enhance researchers' ability to gain entry to the social situation. If, for example, a researcher wishes to study the culture of health professionals working in an outpatient clinic, his or her willingness to participate by offering "volunteer" services while in the setting may improve the chances of obtaining admission. As a "volunteer," the researcher not only has the opportunity to make observations but will become part of the culture after remaining on the scene for an extended period. Each organization or institution will have its policies and procedures, some more clearly delineated than others. It is strategically important that you ascertain early what those involved require both formally and informally to gain access. Gaining access using the appropriate procedures will begin to build the trust needed to be successful in the field.

Making Participant Observations

Actual fieldwork begins when researchers start asking questions about the culture chosen. Initially, the ethnographer will ask broad questions. Using the outpatient clinic as an example, the researcher might ask: Who works in the clinic? Who comes to the clinic for care? What is the physical set-up of the clinic? Who provides the care to clients who come to the clinic?

In addition to asking questions, the researcher will begin to make observations. Three types of observations are descriptive, focused, and selective (Spradley, 1980).

Descriptive observations start when the researcher enters the social situation. The ethnographer is trying to begin to describe the social situation, get an overview of the situation, and determine what is going on. After completing this type of observation, the researcher will conduct more focused descriptive observations. These observations are generated from questions the researcher asked during the initial descriptive phase. For example, while in the clinic the researcher discovers that nurses are responsible for health teaching. A *focused observation* is required to look specifically at the types of health teaching done by the nurses in the setting. Based on this focused observation, the researcher conducts a more *selective observation*. For example, the researcher observes that only two out of the seven nurses in the clinic conduct any health teaching with clients with acquired immunodeficiency syndrome (AIDS). A selective interview or observation involving the two nurses will address additional questions about why clinic staff members behave as they do.

Neophyte ethnographers should not be led to believe that they conduct observations and interviews in the linear manner just described. Rather, broad, focused, or selective questions may arise out of any observation. Furthermore, the intent of an observation is not to merely "look at" something. Rather, through observation, researchers look, listen, ask questions, and collect artifacts.

At any given time, ethnographers may be more or less involved in the social situation. For example, when the outpatient clinic is busy, the researcher as volunteer may be quite involved as a participant in the culture. At times of lesser traffic, the researcher may spend more time observing. Explicit rules for when to participate and when to observe are unavailable. Researchers, the *actors* (members of the culture studied), and the activity determine the degree of participation in the social situation.

Roper and Shapira (2000) offer that "relying on personal observations alone can be misleading" (p. 70). It will be essential that all interpretations of observations be validated through other collected information. The researcher must be always aware of the fact that all individuals view social situations through their own cultural lenses. Therefore, cross comparison of data is fundamental.

Making the Ethnographic Record

On completion of each observation, ethnographers are responsible for documenting the experience. Documents generated from the observations are called *field notes*. Researchers may manage field notes by handwriting and storing them manually or by using computer programs to store and categorize data. A number of data storage, retrieval, and analysis software programs are available (see Chapter 3). Researchers who do not have a computer or are more comfortable documenting their observations in writing may use handwritten notes they organize in file boxes. These notes will chronicle what the researchers have seen and heard, answers to questions they asked, and created or collected artifacts.

In the clinic, for example, the researcher may observe the physical layout. Based on the observation, the researcher may ask questions related to what happens in each room. A floor plan (artifact) may become part of the record. The researcher may also take photographs to document the colors of the clinic or the decorations used. These artifacts may offer important insights as the study continues.

It is important throughout the study—but especially in the beginning—not to focus too soon and also not to assume that any comment, artifact, or interaction is incidental. Researchers should document experiences to create a thick or rich description of the culture. In the outpatient example, the researcher should document the colors of the clinic. This observation may seem incidental; however, if a staff member later reports that it is important to maintain a calm atmosphere in the clinic because of the types of clients seen, then the choice of the color blue for the walls may be an artifact that supports this belief system.

In addition to recording explicit details of a situation, ethnographers also will record personal insights. A wide-angle view of the situation will provide the opportunity to detail what participants have said and to share what may be implicit in the situation. Using a wide-angle lens to view a situation provides ethnographers with a larger view of what is actually occurring in a social situation. For example, if an ethnographer is interested in observing a change-of-shift report and attends the report with the purpose of investigating the nurses' interactions, the researcher may miss valuable information regarding the report. With a wide-angle approach, the ethnographer would observe all individuals, activities, and artifacts that are part of the social situation, rather than merely focus on the interactions between the nurses in the report. Attention to all parts of the social situation will contribute to a richer description of the cultural scene. Once the researcher has a good grasp of the *wide-angle view*, then more focused and selective observations can take place.

Spradley (1980) has offered three principles researchers must consider as they document their observations: "the language identification principle, the verbatim principle, and the concrete principle" (p. 65). The *language identification principle* requires that ethnographers identify in whose language the text is written. Spradley (1980) has pointed out that the most frequently recorded language is the *amalgamated language* (see Example 9–2), that is, the use of the ethnographer's language as well as the informants' language. For example, a nurse–ethnographer recording his or her observations of a clinic day might choose to mix the answers to questions with personal observations. Such mixing may create problems when data analysis begins because the researcher can lose sight of the cultural meaning of the observation. To minimize the potential of this happening, entries should identify the person making the remarks. Example 9–1 illustrates the correct way

---

Example 9–1

Field Note Entry No. 1   *January 2, 2002*

Ethnographer: Today when I visited the clinic, I noticed that the walls were painted blue. I asked the receptionist who had done the decorating.

Receptionist: "We had several meetings with the decorator."

---

to record field notes. In Example 9–2, the record does not describe how the researcher obtained specific information. It is difficult to decipher whether the notes are the researcher's interpretations or whether the researcher obtained the information directly from the informants.

Although Example 9–1 is a limited notation, readers can get a sense of how researchers should report field notes to facilitate analysis. In this example, the receptionist's response gives the ethnographer clear information about the decorating. That the receptionist used the word *we* in Example 9–1 gives the researcher insight into the interactions occurring among staff members. Although Example 9–2 offers significant information, the researcher will find it difficult, after long months of data collection, to return to this note and distinguish his or her insights from factual information obtained from the informants.

The reporting of the receptionist's comments in Example 9–1 reflects the *verbatim principle*, which requires ethnographers to use the speaker's exact words. To adhere to this principle, researchers may use audiotaping, which not only offers ethnographers verbatim accounts of conversation but also affords them an extensive accounting of an interaction that will provide the material for intensive analysis. Documenting verbatim statements also provides researchers with a view of native expressions. In Example 9–1, the use of verbatim documentation allows the researcher to gain insight into the language. The receptionist's use of the word *we* to describe the activities with the decorator may provide valuable insights into the culture of the clinic. The *concrete principle* requires that ethnographers document without interpretation what they have seen and heard. Generalizations and interpretations may limit access to valuable cultural insights. To reduce interpretation, researchers should document observations with as much detail as possible. Example 9–3 offers an example of concrete documentation without interpretation or generalization. In this example, documentation is clear. The researcher has recorded facts and conversation verbatim.

Making Descriptive Observations

Every time ethnographers are in a social situation, they generally will make descriptive observations without having specific questions in mind. General questions, which guide this type of observation, are *grand tour questions*. For exam-

---

Example 9–2

Field Note Entry No. 1   *January 2, 2002*

Today I observed the clinic waiting area. The area is painted in a pale blue. The chairs are wood and fabric. The fabric is a white-and-blue print, which contrasts with the wallpaper. The waiting area is very busy. The colors have an effect on the clients. They come in looking very harassed, then they fall asleep. A decorator helped with the colors.

Example 9–3

Field Note Entry No. 1   *January 2, 2002*

The clinic waiting area is painted ocean blue. The ladder-back chairs are light brown wood with upholstered seats. The fabric on the seats is an ocean blue-and-white checkered pattern. There are two small 2 ft by 3 ft by 2½ ft brown wooden tables between the six chairs in the waiting room. There are two chairs along one wall with a table in the corner. Then, two chairs along the second wall with another table in the corner. The third wall has the two remaining chairs. The room is an 8 ft by 9 ft rectangle. Each table has a ginger jar lamp. The lamp base and shade are white. The fourth wall has a door and window in it. The draperies on the window are floor length and match the pattern on the chairs.

Individuals enter the clinic, state their names to the receptionist, sit in the chairs, and close their eyes. Some patients snore.

Ethnographer: "The colors in this room are great. Everything seems to go together so well. Who did the decorating?"

Receptionist: "We had several meetings with the decorator."

---

ple, a grand tour question that might initiate a study of a particular clinic is, How do people who live in this neighborhood receive health care? Remembering that the primary foci of all observations include the actors, activities, and artifacts will assist in the development of grand tour questions.

Spradley (1980) has identified nine major dimensions to any social situation:

1. *Space* refers to the physical place or places where the culture of interest carries out social interactions. In the outpatient clinic example, space would include the physical layout of the care delivery site.
2. *Actors* are people who are part of the culture under investigation. In the clinic example, the nurses, physicians, maintenance workers, secretarial/receptionist staff, and family members of clients in the clinic would be the actors.
3. The *activities* are the actions by members of the culture. In the clinic example, activities would include the treatments provided to clients and conversations between cultural group members.
4. *Objects* in the clinic example would include artifacts such as implements used for care, pamphlets read by clients, staff records, and meeting minutes. Any inanimate object included in the space under study may give insight into the culture.
5. Any single action carried out by group members is an *act*. An example of an act observed in the clinic would be the locking of the medicine cabinet.
6. An *event* is a set of related activities carried out by members of the culture. In the clinic example, the ethnographer one day may observe the staff giving a birthday party for a long-time client.

7. It is important that the researcher document the *time* he or she made observations and when activities occurred during those times. In addition to recording time, the researcher must relate the effect time has on all nine dimensions of social situations.

8. *Goal* relates specifically to what group members hope to achieve. In the clinic example, in painting the clinic blue, the staff may relate that their intention was to have a calming effect on clients, who often must wait long periods.

9. The researcher should also record *feelings* for each social situation, including the emotions expressed or observed. For example, during the staff-given birthday party for a long-time client, the ethnographer might observe tears from the client, cheers by the staff, and anger by a family member. Recording feelings provides a rich framework from which to make cultural inferences.

The nine dimensions can be useful in guiding observations and questions related to social situations. It is beneficial to plot the nine dimensions in a matrix (Spradley, 1980) to contrast each dimension. For example, in addition to describing the space where the culture carries out its interactions, researchers should relate space to object, act, activity, event, time, actor, goal, and feelings. What does the space look like?

> What are all the ways space is organized by objects? What are all the ways space is organized by acts? What are all the ways space is organized by activities? What are all the ways space is organized by events? What spatial changes occur over time? What are all the ways space is used by actors? What are all the ways space is related to goals? What places are associated with feelings? (Spradley, 1980, pp. 82–83).

Critical ethnographers would add the dimensions of social and political climate to Spradley's (1980) list. It is extremely important that researchers consider issues of power, social class, and politics to get a full view of the culture. In the clinic example, the researcher might ask the following questions: Why are women the primary care providers? Does the male doctor ultimately make all the decisions? If so, why? Once researchers have collected data on all dimensions and have related each piece of data to other information, they can begin to focus further observations.

Making a Domain Analysis

Throughout data collection, ethnographers are required to analyze data. Analyzing data while in the field helps to structure later encounters with the social group of interest. Ethnographic data "analysis is a search for patterns" (Spradley, 1980, p. 85). These patterns make up the culture.

To begin to understand cultural meaning, ethnographers must analyze social situations they observe. A social situation is not the same as the concept of culture but, rather, "refers to the stream of behavior (activities) carried out by people (actors) in a particular location (place)" (Spradley, 1980, p. 86). Analysis of the social situation will lead to discovery of the cultural scene. *Cultural scene*, an ethnographic term, refers to the culture under study (Spradley, 1980). The first step in analysis is to do a domain analysis. Ethnographers doing a domain analysis focus on a particular situation.

In the outpatient clinic example, the category—people in the clinic—is the first domain the researcher must analyze. The researcher should ask, Who are the people in the clinic? Reviewing the field notes, the people in the clinic should be easy to identify (Fig. 9–1). Spradley (1980) has suggested it is important to identify the semantic relationships in the observations made. For example, *x* is a kind of *y*: Nurses are kinds of people in the clinic. Furthermore, the researcher can do another analysis to explore the types of nurses who work in the clinic. Hammersley and Atkinson (1983) have approached analysis somewhat differently. They have recommended researchers generate concept categories, refining them further into subcategories. Regardless of the method used, it is essential that researchers work to discover the cultural meaning for people, places, artifacts, and activities. Creating as extensive a list as possible of categories will assist in discovery. To maintain inclusiveness, return to the dimensions described earlier in this chapter. Generating domain analyses leads ethnographers to ask additional questions and make further observations to explore the roles and relationships of the cultural group members.

Making Focused Observations

Based on the completed domain analysis, ethnographers will need to make new observations and collect additional material. The domain analysis should be the trigger for the next round of observations. Researchers identify the domain cate-

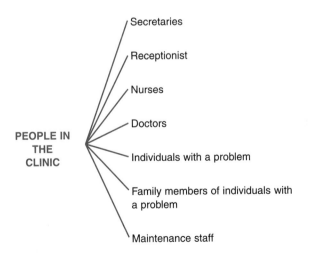

FIGURE 9–1

gories that need development and then return to the research site. In the clinic example, based on the identification of different types of nurses in the clinic, the ethnographer would want to focus on the different types of nurses and discover their specific roles and activities. This information could provide important insight into the culture of the situation.

Making a Taxonomic Analysis

The taxonomic analysis is a more in-depth analysis of the domains researchers have previously selected. Researchers are searching for larger categories to which the domain may belong. In the clinic example, nurses in the clinic is a category identified in the domain analysis. Nurses are a type of people in the clinic. In addition, there are types of nurses. Nurses can be categorized based on their educational backgrounds: licensed practical nurses (LPNs), registered nurses (RNs), nurse practitioners (NPs), and clinical nurse specialists (CNSs). These categories may be broken down further based on the focus of clients for whom the nurses care in the particular culture under study (Fig. 9–2).

On completion of this analysis, ethnographers will look for relationships among the parts or relationships to the whole. Based on these new categories, researchers will make additional observations and ask more questions. In the clinic example, the researcher might ask, Why do the RNs have the primary responsibility for care of the clients with AIDS and sexually transmitted diseases (STDs)? Are there different types of AIDS clients and are they cared for by specific RNs? Are AIDS clients treated differently from the clients with STDs? Are other nurses

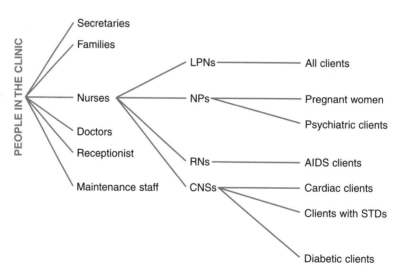

FIGURE 9–2

consulted regarding the care of these two groups of clients? Are the nurses able to select the types of clients for whom they care?

Clearly, the researcher has generated a number of questions from this taxonomic analysis of the concept *nurse*. In addition to using a reductive exercise, ethnographers should try to discover whether there are larger categories for which they have not accounted. In the clinic example, are the people in the clinic part of a larger system? If the clinic is affiliated with a hospital or a community based organization, then the answer is *yes*. The nurse–ethnographer will then need to ask further questions based on this association and conduct focused interviews to validate whether the previously derived larger or smaller categorizations are accurate.

Making Selected Observations

Through selective observations, researchers need to further refine the data they have collected. Selective observations will help to identify the "dimensions of contrast" (Spradley, 1980, p. 128). Spradley has offered several types of questions that will help researchers discern the differences in the dimensions of contrast. The *dyadic question* seeks to identify the differences between two domains. The question is, In what way are these two things different? In the clinic example, one of the questions the researcher should ask is, In what ways are NPs and CNSs different? *Triadic contrast questions* seek to identify how three categories are related. The researcher in the clinic example might ask, Of the three—NPs, CNSs, and RNs—which two are more alike than the third? *Card sorting contrast questions* allow ethnographers to place the domains on cards and sort them into piles based on their similarities. By identifying the similarities, the contrasts become easily recognizable. Asking these questions of the available data will lead ethnographers to the setting to ask still other questions.

Making a Componential Analysis

"Componential analysis is the systematic search for attributes associated with cultural categories" (Spradley, 1980, p. 131). Boyle (1994) has indicated that componential analysis has two objectives: to specify the conditions under which participants name something and to understand under what conditions the participants give something a specific name. Componential analysis is language driven.

During this stage of analysis, researchers are looking for units of meaning. Each unit of meaning is considered an attribute of the culture. Again, researchers are searching for missing data. During componential analysis, they examine each domain for its component parts and ask questions to identify the dimensions of contrast. Based on the identification of missing data, the researchers will make selected observations. Table 9.1 is an example of simple componential analysis that illustrates dimensions of contrast based on the sorting of people who work in

TABLE 9.1	DIMENSIONS OF CONTRAST		
		Dimensions of Contrast	
Domain	Licensed	Supervised Personnel	Health Care Provider
Doctors	Yes	No	Yes
Nurses	Yes	Yes	Yes
Receptionist	No	Yes	No
Maintenance staff	No	Yes	No
Secretaries	No	Yes	No

the outpatient clinic. In the clinic example, the ethnographer is able to determine that unlicensed personnel do not provide health care. This analysis helps the researcher to begin to identify a hierarchical structure. He or she must validate hypotheses through selective interviews and observations. The purpose of using this process is to search for contrasts, sort them out, and then group them based on similarities and differences. This activity provides ethnographers with important information regarding the culture under study.

To fully carry out a componential analysis, ethnographers should move through the process in a sequential manner. The eight steps of the procedure are (1) select a domain for analysis (people who work in the clinic); (2) inventory previously discovered contrasts (some members are licensed, have supervisors to whom they report, and provide health care); (3) prepare the worksheet (this is called a *paradigm*); (4) classify dimensions of contrast that have binary values (licensed, yes or no); (5) combine related dimensions of contrast into ones that have multiple values (doctors and nurses are licensed personnel who provide health care); (6) prepare contrast questions for missing attributes (Are doctors the owners of the clinic because they appear not to have a reporting relationship?); (7) conduct selective observations and interviews to discover missing data and confirm or discard hypotheses; (8) prepare a complete paradigm (Spradley, 1980). "The final paradigm can be used as a chart in [the] ethnography" (p. 139). Although every attribute will not be discussed on the chart, important ones can be, allowing ethnographers to present a large amount of information in a concise and clear manner (Spradley, 1980).

PERFORMING DATA ANALYSIS

Although data analysis occurs throughout data collection, the next two stages—discovering cultural themes and taking a cultural inventory—focus solely on data analysis.

Discovering Cultural Themes

The discovery of cultural themes requires ethnographers to carefully examine the data collected and identify recurrent patterns. Whether tacit or explicit, the patterns constitute the culture.

To complete the theme analysis, researchers must become immersed in the data, which requires focused concentration over an extended period. The purpose of immersion is to identify patterns that have not become apparent at the particular point in the study or to explore patterns that may have been generated previously to assure their soundness. Spradley (1980) has identified six universal themes that may be helpful during this stage of data analysis. These themes are not meant to explain all patterns, but they do provide a place to begin. The universal themes are (1) social conflict; (2) What types of conflicts are occurring between people in social situations? (cultural contradiction); (3) Is there information derived from the cultural group that appears contradictory? (informal techniques of social control); (4) Are there informal patterns of behavior that result in social control? (management of interpersonal relationships); (5) How do group members conduct their interpersonal relationships? (acquisition and maintenance of status); and (6) problem solving. Researchers then write an overview summary of the cultural scene to help identify themes they have not yet discovered.

Taking A Cultural Inventory

Completing a cultural inventory is the first stage in writing an ethnography. The inventory provides the opportunity to organize collected data. A cultural inventory involves listing cultural domains; listing analyzed domains; collecting sketch maps, which are drawings of places or activities; listing themes; completing an inventory of examples; identifying organizing domains; completing an index or table of contents; completing an inventory of miscellaneous data; and suggesting areas for future study (Spradley, 1980).

Interpreting the Findings

The purpose of an ethnographic study is to describe the culture. It is important to remember that no two researchers would likely describe a culture in the same way, because of issues within each researcher's culture, the period in which the study was conducted, and the information gathered by the researchers. Perhaps, some researchers would argue, these are reasons why qualitative methods and, in particular, ethnography can never be viewed as science. On the contrary, these are precisely the reasons why ethnography and other qualitative methods are science. What most qualitative methods of research seek to do is share a context-bound view of phenomena; in this case, the phenomenon is the culture of a group. Because culture is ever-changing and dynamic, the discoveries of today are applicable within context. These discoveries bring important insights but do not pretend to bring forward *the* truth but, rather, *a* truth. So, as ethnographers begin to write the study findings, they must remember that, if they used appropriate rigorous methods to collect and analyze data, then the product is one view of a truth.

"In the course of the final analysis, comparisons with existing ethnographies and other midrange theories are made. Existing theories may be supported or refuted and new midrange theories, in addition to the descriptive and explanatory theory of culture (the ethnography) may be induced" (Germain, 2001, p. 297). Once researchers have completed the inventory, interpreted the findings, and compared their work to that in the literature, they are ready to write the ethnography.

Writing the Ethnography

The purpose of writing an ethnography is to share with people what the researcher has learned and to attempt to make sense out of the cultural patterns that present themselves. To do so, an ethnographer must ask, For whom am I writing? Based on the answer to this question, the document will look different. If writing for a scholarly community, details will be important. If writing for the popular press, insights with exemplars will be most useful. If writing for an organization in the form of a formal report, the researcher must pay attention to those details that reflect the concerns that directed the inquiry.

One of the best ways to know what to write is to look for examples of what has been written. Ethnographers may choose to report natural history organized chronologically or spatially, or they may choose to organize information based on significant themes (Omery, 1988). A review of published texts that chronicle macro-ethnographies or scholarly journals that have published focused or micro-ethnographies will provide good examples of how to organize the final ethnographic report. Every detail or idea may not be collapsible into one journal article or one book. Focusing on aspects of the research for several books or articles may be the only feasible way to report the findings of an ethnographic study.

Researchers may write several drafts until the document reflects the study. They may recruit colleagues to critique the work. Colleagues can help neophyte researchers discover whether the researchers have appropriately covered the topic.

ETHICAL CONSIDERATIONS

The protection of study participants is important regardless of the research paradigm, whether a qualitative or quantitative approach, phenomenology, grounded theory, ethnography, action, or historic. Because ethics is covered broadly in Chapter 16, this section shares unique ethical issues specific to ethnography.

When conducting ethnographic research, researchers by virtue of their roles as participant-observers are in a unique position to fit in. Researchers live among the people and therefore have the ability to be invisible at times in the researcher capacity. The invisible nature of researchers has significant value in data collection but can present potential dilemmas from an ethical standpoint. The important elements in conducting any type of research study are to inform participants fully about the matter to which they are consenting, inform participants they can withdraw from the study at any time for any reason, reduce all unnecessary risks, ensure that the benefits of the study outweigh the risks, and ensure that the researchers who will be conducting the study have appropriate qualifications (Lipson, 1994).

Informed consent is an ethical principle that requires researchers to obtain voluntary consent, including description of the potential risks and benefits of participation. Munhall (1988) has recommended "process consent" (p. 156) rather than the traditional consent signed in the beginning of most studies and not revisited unless participants question their obligations related to the study. *Process consent* or "consensual decision-making" (Ramos, 1989, p. 61) means that researchers renegotiate the consent as unforeseen events or consequences arise (Munhall, 1988; Ramos, 1989). By providing the opportunity to renegotiate the consent and be part of the decision making as the study develops, ethnographers afford participants the chance to withdraw or modify that to which they initially agreed.

Lipson (1994) has suggested that consent in the field becomes somewhat more difficult. For instance, the researcher secures consent before formal fieldwork begins. Some time passes and the researcher is in the field at the time an unexpected event occurs, such as the birth of a child. Although it is important that the researcher inform the group that he or she is chronicling this event for research purposes, it would be intrusive to address consent at that point. One way to handle this situation would be for the researcher to inform participants at a later time that the birth experience gave him or her insight into cultural values. If objections were to arise, it is obvious that the researcher could never erase the memory of the event; however, to protect the informants, it is imperative that he or she not formally include those data in the study. Covert participation in all research is regarded as a violation of individuals' rights. Therefore, ethnographers should always be forthright with their objectives.

Risk is another major concern. Researchers should never put a participant group in danger to collect data. For example, the researcher in the field discovers that some young men are staging a gang fight in which they plan to use weapons. Believing that it would be important to learn more about conflict and how the group handles it, the researcher plans to go as an observer. In this situation, the risk to the people involved far outweighs the goal to observe how the group handles conflict. Intervention is necessary. How the researcher intervenes should be determined by a number of factors. A research mentor is invaluable in helping the researcher sort out when and how to intervene. Too many variables are involved to offer a simple answer. The important principle is that the researcher does not engage in data collection to achieve his or her own goals when significant risk to research participants is involved.

Another principle described by Lipson (1994) is the researcher's qualifications. Usually, institutional review boards will assess the researcher's qualifications based on review of the submitted research proposal. An unqualified researcher can do substantial damage to a culture. It is essential that, even as a neophyte ethnographer, one clearly understands what it is he or she is doing and the potential risks in conducting a study without adequate sensitivity and knowledge.

Roper and Shapira (2000) also suggest that researchers adopt specific strategies to address ethical dilemmas. The ones recommended are to

> deliberately evaluate their own effects on the research process by consciously identifying biases brought to the field and also emotional responses resulting from their experiences.
>
> Next,...come up with an explicit description of their role during data collection. Finally,...establish mechanisms that guarantee honest and trustworthy research relationships. (p. 114)

It is essential that all qualitative researchers—but, in particular, ethnographers—be aware of and knowledgeable about their responsibilities to research participants. Specifically, because of the intimate nature of the relationships that develop when ethnographers live among study participants, these researchers have a important duty to inform and protect informants.

SUMMARY

This chapter discussed the ethnographic approach to research and presented issues related to selection of the method, interpretations of the approach, application of the approach, and interpretation of the findings. A thorough explanation of how to conduct ethnographic research has been shared to provide a framework from which to conduct the first ethnographic inquiry.

Ethnography offers a significant research approach to individuals interested in learning about culture, willing and able to report data in narrative format, comfortable with ambiguity, able to build trusting relationships, and comfortable working alone (Germain, 1986). The study of culture, whether in a well-known nursing unit or in a country whose health practices are unknown, offers exciting discovery opportunities. Nurse–researchers who choose to use this approach will find that the focus of the study will become an intimate part of their daily existence until they have fully explored, described, and interpreted that focus.

Chapter 10 provides a review of research that uses the ethnographic approach. It is hoped that the review will further assist those individuals interested in the approach to understand the method and will provide concrete criteria from which to judge the merits of published reports.

REFERENCES

Agar, M. H. (1982). Toward an ethnographic language. *American Anthropologist, 8*(4), 779.795.
Agar, M. H. (1986). *Speaking of ethnography*. Newbury Park, CA: Sage.
Anderson, J. M. (1991). Reflexivity in fieldwork: Toward a feminist epistemology. *Image, 23*(2), 115–118.

Atkinson, P. (1999). Ethnography: Post, past, and present. *Journal of Contemporary Ethnography, 28*(5), p. 460–470.

Atkinson, P., & Hammersley, M. (1994). Ethnography and participant observation. In N. K. Denzin & Y. S. Lincoln (Eds.), *Handbook of qualitative research* (pp. 248–261). Thousand Oaks, CA: Sage.

Benedict, R. (1934). *Patterns of culture*. New York: Houghton Mifflin.

Boas, F. (1948). *Race, language and culture*. New York: Macmillan.

Boyle, J. S. (1994). Styles of ethnography. In J. M. Morse (Ed.), *Critical issues in qualitative research methods* (pp. 159.185). Thousand Oaks, CA: Sage.

Chase-Ziolek, M. (1999). The meaning and experience of health ministry within the culture of a congregation with a parish nurse. *Journal of Transcultural Nursing, 10*(1), 46–55.

Fontana, A., & Frey, J. H. (1994). Interviewing: The art of science. In N. K. Denzin & Y. S. Lincoln (Eds.), *Handbook of qualitative research* (pp. 361–376). Thousand Oaks, CA: Sage.

Geertz, C. (1973). *The interpretations of culture*. New York: Basic Books.

Germain, C. P. (1986). Ethnography: The method. In P. L. Munhall & C. J. Oiler (Eds.), *Nursing research: A qualitative perspective* (pp. 147–162). Norwalk, CT: Appleton-Century-Crofts.

Germain, C. P. (2001). Ethnography: The method. In P.L. Munhall (Ed.), *Nursing research: A qualitative perspective* (3rd ed). Sudbury, MA: National League for Nursing.

Goetz, J. P., & LeCompte, M. D. (1984). *Ethnography and qualitative design in educational research*. Orlando, FL: Academic Press.

Goodenough, W. (1970). *Description and comparison in cultural anthropology*. Chicago: Aldine.

Goodenough, W. (1971). *Culture, language and society*. Reading, MA: Addison-Wesley.

Graff, C., Roberts, K., & Thornton, K. (1999). An ethnographic study of differentiated practice in an operating room. *Journal of Professional Nursing, 15*(6), 364–371.

Grant, L., & Fine, G. A. (1992). Sociology unleashed: Creative directions in classical ethnography. In M. D. LeCompte, W. L. Millroy, & J. Preissle (Eds.), *The handbook of qualitative research in education* (pp. 405–446). San Diego, CA: Academic Press.

Haglund, K. (2000). Parenting a second time around: An ethnography of African American grandmothers parenting grandchildren due to parental cocaine abuse. *Journal of Family Nursing, 6*(2), 120–136.

Hammersley, M., & Atkinson, P. (1983). *Ethnography: Principles in practice*. London: Tavistock.

Hughes, C. C. (1992). "Ethnography": What's in a word—Process? Product? Promise? *Qualitative Health Research, 2*(4), 439–450.

Leininger, M. (1970). *Nursing and anthropology: Two worlds to blend*. New York: Wiley.

Leininger, M. (1978). *Transcultural nursing: Concepts, theories and practices*. New York: Wiley.

Leininger, M. (1985). Ethnography and ethnonursing: Models and modes of qualitative data analysis. In M. Leininger (Ed.), *Qualitative research methods in nursing* (pp. 33–71). Orlando, FL: Grune & Stratton.

Lipson, J. G. (1994). Ethical issues in ethnography. In J. M. Morse (Ed.), *Critical issues in qualitative research methods* (pp. 333–355). Thousand Oaks, CA: Sage.

Lipson, J. G. (2001). We are the canaries: Self-care in multiple chemical sensitivity sufferers. *Qualitative Health Research, 11*(1), 103–116.

Lundberg, P. C. (1999). Meanings and practices of health among married Thai immigrant women in Sweden. *Journal of Transcultural Nursing, 10*(1), 31–36.

Magilvy, J. K., & Congdon, J. G. (2000). The crisis nature of health care transitions of rural older adults. *Public Health Nursing, 17*(5), 336–345.

Malinowski, B. (1922). *Argonauts of the Western Pacific*. London: Routledge & Kegan Paul.

Malinowski, B. (1961). *Argonauts of the Western Pacific*. New York: Dutton.

Manias, E., & Street, A. (2001). Rethinking ethnography: Reconstructing nursing relationships. *Journal of Advanced Nursing, 33*(2), 234–242.

Mead, M. (1949). *Coming of age in Samoa*. New York: New American Library, Mentor Books.

Morin, K. H., Patterson, B. J., Kurtz, B., & Brzowski, B. (1999). Mothers' responses to care given by male nursing students during and after birth. *Image: Journal of Nursing Scholarship, 31*(1), 83–87.

Morse, J. M., & Field, P. A. (1995). *Qualitative research methods for health professionals*. Thousand Oaks, CA: Sage.

Muecke, M. A. (1994). On the evaluation of ethnographies. In J. M. Morse (Ed.), *Critical issues in qualitative research methods* (pp. 187–209). Thousand Oaks, CA: Sage.

Munhall, P. L. (1988). Ethical considerations in qualitative research. *Western Journal of Nursing Research, 10*(2), 150–162.

Omery, A. (1988). Ethnography. In B. Sarter (Ed.), *Paths to knowledge: Innovative research methods for nursing* (pp. 17–31). New York: National League for Nursing.

Radcliffe-Brown, A. R. (1952). *Structure and function in primitive society*. London: Oxford University Press.

Ragucci, A. T. (1972). The ethnographic approach and nursing research. *Nursing Research, 21*(6), 485–490.

Ramos, M. C. (1989). Some ethical implications in qualitative research. *Research in Nursing and Health, 12, 57–63.*

Roper, J. M., & Shapira, J. (2000). *Ethnography in nursing research*. Thousand Oaks, CA: Sage.

Rowe, J. H. (1965). The Renaissance foundation in anthropology. *American Anthropologist, 67,* 1–20.

Sanday, P. R. (1983). The ethnographic paradigm(s). In J. Van Maanen (Ed.), *Qualitative methodology* (pp. 19–36). Beverly Hills, CA: Sage.

Savage, H. (2000). Ethnography and health care. *British Medical Journal, 321*(7273), 1400–1403.

Schulte, J. (2000). Finding ways to create connections among communities: Partial results of an ethnography of urban public health nurses. *Public Health Nursing, 17*(1), 3–10.

Spradley, J. P. (1980). *Participant observation*. New York: Holt, Rinehart & Winston.

Spradley, J. P., & McCurdy, D. W. (1972). *The cultural experience: Ethnography in complex society*. Prospect Heights, IL: Waveland Press.

van Maanen, J. (1983). The fact of fiction in organizational ethnography. In J. van Maanen (Ed.), *Qualitative methodology* (pp. 36–55). Beverly Hills, CA: Sage.

Wanta, B. A. (1998). Planning for death and dying while healthy: Lessons for the Gulf War mobilization. *Holistic Nursing Practice, 13*(1), 22–31

Wolf, Z. R. (1988). *Nurses' work, the sacred and the profane*. Philadelphia: University of Pennsylvania Press.

Woods, P. (1992). Symbolic interactionism: Theory and method. In M. D. LeCompte, W. L. Millroy, & J. Preissle (Eds.), *The handbook of qualitative research in education*. San Diego, CA: Academic Press.

10

Ethnography in Practice, Education, and Administration

A s a means of studying nursing and the cultural practices imbedded within it, ethnography creates unlimited prospects for nurses interested in using this approach. The study of patterns within a culture provides an excellent opportunity to describe the practices of the people for whom nurses care, to understand the health-related phenomena of people within various cultures, and to examine nursing's own unique culture. Ethnography provides a chance to explore both the clinical aspects of nursing and its administrative and educative patterns and lifeways.

This chapter provides an overview of ethnographic studies that have explored cultures of interest to nursing. In addition, it critiques *focused* ethnographic studies that reflect clinical nursing practice, nursing education, and nursing administration to provide readers with examples of published works and the contributions these works have made to the field. The ethnographic studies examined in this chapter have been critiqued using the guidelines in Box 10.1. The critiquing guidelines offer specific directives for determining the quality of the ethnographic works presented in this chapter and in the literature. The questions in Box 10.1 are specific to ethnographic research and reflect the most important aspects researchers must evaluate in an ethnographic report. A reprint of Haglund's (2000) article found at the end of this chapter assists readers in understanding the critiquing process. Table 10.1 summarizes a recent series of ethnographic studies representing the areas of nursing education, administration, and practice.

APPLICATION TO PRACTICE

Ethnographic research methodology offers an exceptional opportunity for nurses interested in examining clinical practice issues. Whether the interest is in studying hospice (Wright, 2001), public health (Schulte, 2000) or parish nursing (Tuck & Wallace, 2000), or the culture of grandmothers parenting their grandchildren (Haglund, 2000), ethnographic research provides the framework for exploring the richness of nursing and nursing-related phenomena. Haglund's (2000) study of African American grandmothers parenting grandchildren owing to parental cocaine abuse is the reference for critique in this section.

CRITERIA FOR CRITIQUING ETHNOGRAPHIC RESEARCH

Focus

1. What is the culture being studied?
2. What is the focus or scope of the study?
3. What is the purpose of the study?

Method

1. How does ethnography fulfill the purpose of the study?
2. Is the study conducted in the field?
3. What guidelines have been established for participant consent?
4. How has the researcher protected study participants' rights?

Sampling

1. Why is the group selected to inform the study appropriate?
2. Does the researcher discuss how key informants are selected and why?

Data Collection

1. What strategies were used to collect data?
2. How do the strategies selected fully inform the study?
3. What was the researcher's role in the study?
4. How has triangulation of data sources (observation, interview, collection of artifacts) enhanced credibility of findings?
5. Is time in the field adequate to meet the purpose of the study?

Data Analysis

1. What strategies were used to analyze data? Were they consistent with the method?
2. How is the cyclic nature of data collection or data analysis reported?
3. Based on the report, can another researcher follow the logic of the researcher's conclusions?

Rigor

1. How has the researcher maintained his or her "objectivity"?
2. How has the researcher documented the authenticity of the data?
3. What role do the informants play in validating the researcher's findings?

Findings

1. Do the findings make clear a description of the culture studied?
2. In what context are the findings presented?

(continues)

Box 10.1

Criteria for Critiquing Ethnographic Research (Continued)

3. Are findings presented in a rich narrative format providing readers with a "feel" for the culture?
4. Do the findings go beyond the description to explain why particular aspects of the culture are as they are?
5. Are the findings reported in a systematic way, such as by themes?

Conclusions

1. How do the conclusions relate to the findings of the study?
2. What is the relevance of the findings to nursing and how can they be used in practice?
3. What future directions for research are offered?

It is important to point out that it is not unusual for ethnographic researchers who publish ethnography in a research journal to focus on only one facet of a larger study. Because of the significant amount of information generated in a long-term cultural study, many ethnographies are published as books. When researchers choose to publish their ethnographic work in a journal, the scope of the report must meet the page guidelines of the selected journal. In the case of Haglund's (2000) study, although not reported as such, the study is a focused ethnography. Focused ethnography has as its focal point a distinct problem that is studied within a single context with a limited number of individuals.

Haglund's (2000) study clearly identifies the culture studied. The author reported that she was interested in describing "a group of six African American grandmothers parenting their grandchildren secondary to cocaine abuse on the part of the parents" (p. 1). The focus or scope of the study is a group of six African American grandmothers. The limited number of informants is to be expected in a focused ethnography. If the study were traditional in its focus, the scope would be larger, looking at, for example, the culture of African American families caring for grandchildren. In the case of the traditional ethnography, a variety of reasons for grandparenting grandchildren might become apparent. In this case, the researcher reports that the focus is on grandmothers and particularly those caring for grandchildren whose parents are cocaine abusers.

The purpose of the study is to "examine the phenomenon of parenting grandchildren from the grandmothers' perspectives and to specifically investigate how parenting grandchildren affected the grandmothers' health" (Haglund, 2000, p. 2). The method used to conduct the inquiry is appropriate. Because of the researcher's reported intent to look specifically at the impact parenting had on the *health* of the grandmothers, ethnography is particularly valuable. If the purpose of this study was to describe the experience of grandmothers who parent grandchildren whose

TABLE 10.1 SELECTIVE SAMPLING OF MICRO-ETHNOGRAPHIC AND FOCUSED ETHNOGRAPNIC STUDIES

Author	Domain	Culture
Chase-Ziolek (1999)	Practice/ administration	Urban United Methodist Congregation
Graft, Roberts, & Thornton (1999)	Administration	Operating room at the University of Kansas Hospital
Haglund (2000)	Practice	African-American grandmothers
Higginbottom (2000)	Practice	Years 7 and 10 secondary school children of African and African-Caribbean descent
Higgins & Learn (1999)	Practice	Hispanic women aged 20-40 living in urban New Mexico County
Holland (1999)	Education	English College of Nursing students in a new model of education
Lipson (2001)	Practice	Individuals living with multiple chemical sensitivity
Lundberg (1999)	Practice	Thai immigrant women living in Sweden with Swedish husbands
Magilvy & Congdon (2000)	Practice	Thirteen counties in two rural areas of Colorado
Morin, Patterson, Kurtz, & Brzowski (1999)	Education	Women who delivered children in a 14-bed maternal and infant unit in a community hospital in the mid-Atlantic region of the United States
Neal, Brown, & Rojjanasrirat (1999)	Administration	Inpatient psychiatric unit at the University of Kansas Hospital
Pulsford, Rushford, & Connor (2000)	Practice	Individuals who were treated with Woodlands therapy for dementia

Focus	Data Collection Strategies	Data Analysis
Health ministry	Participant observation Interview Review of documents	Spradley (1979)
Differentiated practice	Participant observation Interviews	Document analysis Analyzed for common categories and themes

Parenting grandchildren
  of cocaine-abusing
  parents
	Participant observation
	Interviews
	Supplementary data sources
		Spradley (1979)

Heart health-associated
  health beliefs
  and behaviors
	Focus groups	Atlas/ti

Health practices	Interview	Analyzed for themes and categories

Becoming a nursing
  student
	Participant and nonparticipant
	  observations
	Interview
		Thematic analysis

The experience of living
  with multiple chemical
  sensitivities
	Participant observation
	Semistructured interview
		Coded for themes and
		  categories

Meanings and practices
  of health
	Participant observation
	Interview
		"Identification of
		  descriptors, structural
		  analysis to eventual
		  theme formulation"
		  (p. 33)

Nature of health care
  transitions for rural
  older adults
	Minimally structured interviews
	Participant observation
	Photographs
	Review of cultural artifacts
		Ethnographic analysis
		  (Spradley, 1979; Rubin
		  & Rubin, 1995;
		  Fetterman, 1998)

Mothers' responses to
  care given by male
  nursing students
	Semistructured interview	NUD*IST

Implementation of case
  coordinator role
	Nonparticipant and participant
	  observation
	Interview
		Theme identification

Responses of dementia
  patients treated with
  Woodlands therapy
	Videotape
	Reflective discussions
		Discourse analysis

(continues)

TABLE 10.1	SELECTIVE SAMPLING OF MICRO-ETHNOGRAPHIC AND FOCUSED ETHNOGRAPNIC STUDIES (CONTINUED)	
Author	**Domain**	**Culture**
Schulte (2000)	Practice/ administration	Public health nurses in a large, Midwestern urban health department
Smyer (1999)	Practice	Consumers of respite care in a 24-bed hospital-based skilled nursing facility in Western United States
Tuck & Wallace (2000)	Practice/ administration	Parish nursing program in Southeastern U.S. city
Wright (2001)	Practice/ administration	Community-based hospice agency in the Pacific Northwest

parents are cocaine abusers, phenomenology would have been a more appropriate choice.

Clearly, the study is conducted in the field. The researcher reported that she carried out participant observation of the families in their home environments. Also, Haglund (2000) observed support group meetings in which the grandmothers were involved.

Haglund (2000) reports that pseudonyms are used in the report. The assumption is that this is done to protect the identity of informants. There is no reference to formal institutional review board (IRB) approval of this study. It is important to share with research consumers the procedures used to protect the informants. Most researchers would agree that reporting IRB approval demonstrates the most appropriate way to make evident human subjects' protection. Further, in light of the close relationship ethnographers develop with their participants, it is critical to report how participants are protected.

The sample for the study is somewhat confusing as reported. Haglund (2000) shares in the first sentence of the article that six African American grandmothers comprise the sample. However, later in the study, the researcher tells the reader that four women were the primary informants. She then goes on to say that those who were not grandmothers but "were in similar situations (such as a great grandmother and a great-aunt) or others who were intimate with the grandmothers" (p. 3) helped to understand the culture. The confusion stems from the

Focus	Data Collection Strategies	Data Analysis
Description of the culture	Participant observation Interview Document examination	Not reported
Development of a typology of respite care users and a description of the process of adaptation to its use	Participant observation Interview Review of artifacts	Constant comparative analysis
Parish nursing as a nursing specialty	Interview Participant observation Document analysis	Spradley (1979)
Perception of knowledge and skill base essential to practice of hospice nursing	Observation Interview Examination of agency manuals, records, and literature	Not reported

reference to six grandmothers, then a later reference to four primary informants who the reader can assume were grandmothers, with additional reference to two who were in similar situations. It is totally appropriate in ethnography to interview and observe others who are familiar with the culture under study. What makes the report of the sample confounding is the description of other than grandmothers who appear to be considered part of the primary group of informants. This conclusion has to be drawn based on the reference to six grandmothers early in the report. It is important to note that the researcher clearly identifies how she selected primary informants. She states "primary informants were African American grandmothers who had parented their grandchildren for at least 1 year because of cocaine addiction of the children's mothers. All the informants had legal custody of the children" (p. 3).

Haglund (2000) reports that three types of data collection were used: participant observation, interviewing, and review of supplementary data. Participant observation provides the researcher with the opportunity needed *in the field* to most effectively observe the culture with the intention of improving his or her understanding of it.

Interviewing can help the researcher to determine where to begin observations, or following observations can help to clarify and examine more carefully what has been observed. In Haglund's (2000) study, she gives the reader specific information about the primary informants from whom she collected data. The information shared provides a context in which to view the culture and hopefully leads to understanding of the cultural experience.

Supplementary data sources such as observation of support group meetings for grandmothers parenting their grandchildren, personal documents of the informants, newspaper articles, and a TV special on grandparents parenting their grandchildren were also included in data collection and analysis. Use of supplementary data helps to understand the culture but also corroborates other types of data collected during the course of the study.

In addition to participant-observation, interviews, and use of supplementary data sources, Haglund (2000) kept a fieldwork journal. A journal is a valuable tool for ethnographers. The journal can serve as a "reality check" of a researcher's motivation for and role in participating in the culture's activities (Werner & Schoepfle, 1987). In this study, the researcher reports that the journal was used to keep a record of field experiences, reactions and ideas about them, and logistics of the fieldwork.

The use of multiple types of data is an excellent way to enhance credibility of the findings. The term used to describe use of multiple data sources in a study is called data triangulation. More about data triangulation can be found in Chapter 15. In Haglund's (2000) study, it is clear that she uses multiple types of data collection, leading her to a cultural understanding with greater depth.

Time in the field is another way to enhance the credibility of the findings. It is difficult to ascertain the total amount of time spent in the field as reported in this study. The researcher reports that 37 hours was spent in direct observation and that there were 12 1-hour interviews with the primary informants. It would be helpful to know whether this study was conducted in a week, a month, or over a year. Time in the field is one of the criteria usually used to determine the credibility of the findings. Based on Haglund's (2000) report that credibility was achieved through "participant observation, prolonged engagement, and a search for clarification and confirmation" (p. 4), the reader can conclude that adequate time was spent in the field.

Haglund (2000) does an excellent job of explaining how she analyzed her data. She reports that she used the methods described by Spradley (1979). In accordance with Spradley's method, she conducted domain and taxonomic analyses. Based on these analyses, cultural themes are offered for the reader. Additionally important is her reporting of the cyclic nature of data collection and analysis. The process of engaging in data collection followed by data analysis with a subsequent return to data collection is a hallmark of ethnographic research.

It is easy, based on reading the subjective comments offered by Haglund (2000), to get a sense of the lives of the individual women. It is more difficult, however, to get a sense of whether the comments shared fit into the cultural themes offered or whether the cultural themes emerged from the data collected. Because the study is reported as a focused ethnography, the audience can conclude that what the researcher presents is *focused* on the health impacts resulting from assuming parenting responsibilities of the grandchildren; however, health effects is only one of the four cultural themes reported. The other three, parenting a second time around, sacrifice, and God's presence in daily lives seem reflective of the larger cultural experience and not just that of their health. The researcher does report that the informants spent very little time talking about their health and were anxious to move onto other topics. Therefore, focusing on the health of these women might be important to the nursing community but appears to be less important to the culture being studied.

Several times in the study, Haglund (2000) refers to the use of a reflective journal. The use of a reflective journal is one of several ways that objectivity is practiced. In addition to the journal, the researcher includes peer review, consultation with experts, and confirmation by the informants to reduce her bias. Authenticity of the data is documented through the use of excerpts of interviews with the informants. The study participants confirm data analysis, which is essential in assuring rigor.

Reading the cultural theme sections of this report gives the reader a view of what life is like for the grandmothers. Although limited, the richness of the data is found in the comments offered. Using narrative comments to engage readers is important in helping them get a good sense of the culture. In addition to reporting the comments offered by the informants, Haglund (2000) offers some insightful statements reflecting analysis of what she has seen and heard. Sharing insights based on the analysis helps to place the study in the context of what is already known. This ultimately helps the reader place the findings in a context that will be useful. In this case, Haglund tells us what the value is of this study for the practice of nursing. Finally, based on conclusions and implications, the researcher offers directions for future research.

APPLICATION TO EDUCATION

Nursing education presents another context in which nurse–researchers can conduct ethnographic studies. The teaching-learning environment, connecting students, faculty, and in clinical settings clients and health care providers, creates its own culture. Few published studies have specifically illustrated the lifeways of students and faculty. The limited number of studies in nursing education since the publication of the second edition of this text clearly illustrates this. No published ethnographic research studies focusing on students and faculty could be found after 1999. Clearly, ethnographic research has a role in the teaching-learning process and offers the qualitative education researcher rich opportunities. The article "Mothers' Responses to Care Given by Male Nursing Students During and After Birth" (Morin, Patterson, Kurtz, & Brzowski, 1999) serves as the reference for critique in this section. It was selected because it demonstrates the use of ethnography in studying a student clinical learning situation.

In the article, Morin et al. (1999) clearly identify that the purpose of the study is to describe "the rationale maternity patients use in determining whether to accept care by a male student nurse" (p. 83). The focus is also clear. The authors are interested in looking at how mothers make decisions about whether to accept a male nursing student for delivery and postpartum care. What is not as clear is the identification of the culture. The reader has to make some assumptions that may not be accurate. Is the culture the clinical learning environment created between male nursing students and maternity patients? Since the women are interviewed based on their presumed response to a male nursing student's care, this seems unlikely. Is it the culture of women who deliver babies in the institution described? This may well be the case since Morin et al. describe in great deal the demographic features of the women interviewed. Since the study is an ethnography, it is vitally important to clearly state the culture being studied. This is as important in a focused ethnography as it is in a traditional or classical ethnography. In a focused ethnography, the focus may be on a distinct problem, and the researcher may collect data from a smaller group of people; however, the purpose of all ethnography is the description of behavioral patterns of individuals and groups within a specific culture (Agar, 1986; Bernard, 1994; Roper, & Shapira, 2000).

The authors are able to collect the information they are interested in and are able to draw some conclusions based on the study; however, it is unclear why ethnography was selected to conduct the study. The reason for conducting the study is reported very clearly. Morin et al. (1999) tell the reader that the data regarding pregnant women's opinions and attitudes about being cared for by male students are inconsistent. The real question from a methodological perspective remains: Why ethnography? What will this method bring to light that other methods have failed to do?

As would be expected, the study is conducted in the field. All interviews and observations were conducted on the maternal and infant unit described. The authors share that prior to data collection, "the study was approved by an institutional review board for the study of human subjects" (Morin et al., 1999, p. 84).

There is no reported distinction between key informants and others who are interviewed. The researchers report that 32 women were interviewed as part of a purposive sample. Based on the information presented, the reader must assume that all 32 women were key informants. Morin et al. (1999) offer a description of who the women were and the criteria for exclusion from the study. There are statements reflecting that if husbands were in the room during the interview that their comments were included in data analysis.

Interviewing was the primary method of data collection. Researchers did record information about people in the room during the interview, personal items in the room, and any technical problems encountered during the interview. In addition, observations of male nursing students on the unit were made. Roper and Shapira (2000) state:

> Focused ethnographies share with classical ethnographies a commitment to conducting intensive participant observation activities within the naturalistic setting, asking questions to learn what is happening, and using other available sources of information to gain as complete an understanding as possible of people, places and events of interest (p. 7).

A view of the informants' feelings was offered in the report. The primary reporting focus is on what the mothers perceived. Although this was the purpose of the study, there is limited opportunity to gain an in-depth understanding of the culture. This situation exists because of the difficulty in clearly identifying the culture under study. The research team collected and analyzed the data. There is reference to observations of male nursing students on the unit lending "additional support" (Morin et al., 1999, p. 85) to one or more of the themes identified by the women. The authors do not report the length of time in the field so it is impossible to determine if the time in the field was adequate. The authors do report staying in the field until saturation was achieved. An assumption that might be drawn is that if interviews were conducted until data were saturated that the time spent in the field was ample.

Data were managed using the computer program NUD*IST. No one philosophical or methodological procedure was offered for data analysis. Instead, the researchers share linear steps for data analysis. Morin et al. (1999) report that analysis was ongoing throughout the study. It is reported that data analysis was ongoing during data collection. No specific examples are offered of the cyclic nature of data collection and analysis. Based on what is reported, the reader would be able to follow the data shared and come up with similar conclusions.

Researcher subjectivity was managed through the use of reflective journal. The reader is unable to determine from what is reported whether there was one journal or whether each member of the team kept her own journal. The authenticity of the data is offered through the use of quotes made by informants. There is no reference leading the reader to conclude that data were returned to the participants for validation.

The findings reported do share a perspective offered by the women interviewed on their opinions about being cared for by male nursing students during the delivery and postpartum period. However, this perspective is mostly based on what the women think, not on what they actually experience. The findings don't represent their patterns of behavior. Rather, the study offers results based on what might be the case if they were placed in the position of being cared for by male nursing students.

Morin et al. (1999) clearly reiterate that their findings relate only to the study situation. The narrative presented does let you hear the thoughts of the women and men who were interviewed. The report does not overstate the implications of the study. Themes are reported based on personal and contextual factors. Increased use of quotes made by informants could have provided a greater depth to the reader's understanding.

The conclusions focus on the student and what responsibility nursing educators have to male nursing students and patients in maternity settings. Also, the researchers share some ideas about what male nursing students should know before entering the maternity setting. Finally, Morin et al. offer suggestions for future research.

This study offers valuable insights into decision making by postpartum women with regard to their choice to have a male nursing student care for them during delivery and the postpartum period and for that, the study makes a substantial contribution. What is less clear from this report is why ethnography was selected, particularly since those studied do not seem to have shared an experience of being cared for by a male nursing student, leaving the reader with a sense that the study is more about perceived actions rather than actual patterns of behavior within a culture.

APPLICATION TO ADMINISTRATION

In previous editions of this text, it was extremely difficult to find ethnographic studies that reflected the area of nursing service administration. Again, this is the case. There is a paucity of qualitative studies in the area of nursing service administration, making it an extremely fertile research area for qualitative researchers. By broadening the definition of administration to include the culture of specific types of nursing practice, a more recent ethnographic research article is available for critique. Wright's (2001) published report of her ethnographic research on hospice nursing as a specialty will be the focus of the critique. As you will note in Table 10–1, research studies that are based on the culture of specific types of nursing practice have been identified as both practice and administrative reports.

Wright (2001) shares that the culture she is interested in studying is that of "the hospice nurse in the culture of hospice care" (p. 21). The focus of the study is the same as the purpose in this study. The purpose of studying the culture of the nurses in this organization is twofold. First Wright wants to "identify and delineate what experienced hospice nurses perceive as the knowledge and skills base essential to their practice" (p. 20). Secondly, she wants "to determine the methods hospice nurses use for knowledge and skills acquisition" (p. 20). Instead of studying a more general culture such as hospice nursing, Wright specifies what it is she wants to focus on, making the study a focused ethnography.

The researcher reports that the reason for selecting ethnography is because she wants "to examine hospice nurses in the context of their own community-based agency" (p. 21). Wright's (2001) explanation justifies why she chose ethnography. She wants to study hospice nurses within the culture of hospice nursing. The field nature of the work and the interest in the patterns of behavior meet two of the major criteria for conducting ethnography. One of the shortcomings in this report is the lack of specific information on consent or human subjects' protection. It is essential when evaluating any type of qualitative or quantitative research that the reader be able to ascertain that human subjects were protected. As stated earlier, the easiest way to assure the reader that the participants have been protected is to report that the study was reviewed by an institutional review board.

The informants for this study included hospice nurses and other agency personnel including board members, social workers, nursing assistants, volunteers, and clerical staff. In addition, hospice patients' family members provided data. Wright (2001) reports that the key informants were experienced hospice nurses whom she defines very specifically. Since she is interested in knowing about hospice nursing, it is appropriate that she identify her key informants as experienced hospice nurses.

Wright (2001) uses a variety of data collection strategies including participant observation, interviews, review of records, and analysis of key events. The use of multiple data sources assists in strengthening the findings by allowing the researcher to cross-validate information. It is clear that Wright is the researcher; however, what specific role she played within the culture is unclear.

She shares that data analysis and data collection occurred continuously. Although not specifically stated, one can assume from this that there was cyclic collection of data, analysis, and collection of more data with further analysis. The cyclic nature of data collection is another hallmark of ethnographic research. Based on the data presented, one can follow the researcher's line of reasoning. Wright (2001) reports that she spent 20 hours a week for 8 weeks in the field. She conducted over 45 interviews. When her data analysis was complete, she returned to the key informants for verification and validation. The activity is essential in assuring the credibility of the findings.

Data analysis was not reported based on any one methodological or philo-sophical approach. Wright (2001) reports that she coded data, organized it into categories, and then returned her findings to participants. It is preferable to use one set of methodological procedures; however, it is not unusual for ethnographers to report strategies similar to those reported here. Since she validated her conclu-sion with the participants, it is safe to assume that her analysis strategies were pro-ductive in attaining the results. After reading the 11 categories that emerged from the study, the reader is able to follow the logic and conclusions offered.

Wright (2001) does not report how she maintained her objectivity. The most common way for an ethnographer to reduce personal bias is to keep a reflective journal. If she did keep one, it is not reported. The quotes shared contribute to the authenticity of her findings. And as stated earlier, she increases the credibility of the findings by returning her analysis to the informants for "verification and clar-ification" (p. 22).

The findings of this study demonstrate the knowledge and skills needed by hospice nurses to do their jobs. Further, it is clear from the information offered how they attained the knowledge and skills needed. These statements are true for the nurses in this study. Wright (2001) shares the findings within the context of what is already known on the topic she explored. As stated earlier, the subjective comments offered give you a feel for the patterns recognized to be important by hospice nurses.

The findings of this study are presented as categories of data. This type of reporting is typical of ethnographic research. Wright (2001) does make some rather far-reaching suggestions on how to use the data, specifically as it relates to educational programming. Suggestions about distance education are beyond the reported findings. The author indicates that her study needs to be repeated to demonstrate its utility to larger groups.

Overall, Wright (2001) has contributed significantly to the body of nursing research in general but specifically to the literature on hospice nursing. In addition, her use of ethnographic research methodology contributes to the growing body of ethnographic nursing research

SUMMARY

This chapter reviewed samples of published ethnographic research in the areas of nursing practice, education, and administration. Each critique presents the strengths and limitations of reporting ethnographic research. The reviewed authors have contributed to the literature and provided readers with an opportunity to become part of the culture or subculture they studied.

Ethnographic research and the studies that use ethnography as a method add to the richness and diversity of the human experience by allowing readers to share in the lives of the people studied. As nurse–researchers become more comfortable with multiple ways of knowing and multiple realities, they will benefit by participating in the creation and dissemination of the knowledge imbedded in the cultural realities that are a person's life.

REFERENCES

Agar, M. H. (1986). *Speaking of ethnography*. Newbury Park, CA: Sage.
Bernard, H. R. (1994). *Research methods in anthropology: Qualitative and quantitative approaches* (2nd ed.). Thousand Oaks, CA: Sage.
Chase-Ziolek, M. (1999). The meaning and experience of health ministry within the culture of a congregation with a parish nurse. *Journal of Transcultural Nursing, 10*(1), 46–55.
Fetterman, D. M. (1998). *Ethnography step by step* (2nd ed.). Thousand Oaks, CA: Sage.
Graff, C., Roberts, K., & Thornton, K. (1999). An ethnographic study of differentiated practice in an operating room. *Journal of Professional Nursing, 15*(6), 364–371.
Haglund, K. (2000). Parenting a second time around: An ethnography of African American grandmothers parenting grandchildren due to parental cocaine abuse. *Journal of Family Nursing, 6*(2), 120–136.
Higginbottom, G. M. A. (2000). Heart health-associated health beliefs and behaviours of adolescents of African and African Caribbean descent in two cities in the United Kingdom. *Journal of Advanced Nursing, 32*(5), 1234–1242.
Higgins, P. G., & Learn, C. D. (1999). Health practices of adult Hispanic women. *Journal of Advanced Nursing, 29*(5), 1105–1112.
Holland, K. (1999). A journey to becoming: The student nurse in transition. *Journal of Advanced Nursing, 29*(1), 229–236.
Lipson, J. G. (2001). We are the canaries: Self-care in multiple chemical sensitivity sufferers. *Qualitative Health Research, 11*(1), 103–116.
Lundberg, P. C. (1999). Meanings and practices of health among married Thai immigrant women in Sweden. *Journal of Transcultural Nursing, 10*(1), 31–36.
Magilvy, J. K., & Congdon, J. G. (2000). The crisis nature of health care transitions for rural older adults. *Public Health Nursing, 17*(5), 336–345.
Morin, K. H., Patterson, B. J., Kurtz, B., & Brzowski, B. (1999). Mothers' responses to care given by a male nursing student during and after birth. *Image: Journal of Nursing Scholarship, 31*(1), 83–87.
Neal, J., Brown, T., & Rojjanasrirat, W. (1999). Implementation of a case coordinator role: A focused ethnographic study. *Journal of Professional Nursing, 15*(6), 349–355.

Pulsford, D., Rushforth, D., & Conner, I. (2000). Woodland therapy: An ethnographic analysis of a small-group therapeutic activity for people with moderate or severe dementia. *Journal of Advanced Nursing, 32*(3), 650–657.

Roper, J. M., & Shapira, J. (2000). *Ethnography in nursing research.* Thousand Oaks, CA: Sage.

Schulte, J. (2000). Finding ways to create connections among communities: Partial results of an ethnography of urban public health nurses. *Public Health Nursing, 17*(1), 3–10.

Smyer, T. (1999). A typology of consumers of institutional respite care. *Clinical Nursing Research, 8*(1), 26–51.

Spradley, J. P. (1979). *The ethnographic interview.* Fort Worth, TX: Harcourt Brace Jovanovich College.

Tuck, I., & Wallace, D. (2000). Exploring parish nursing from an ethnographic perspective. *Journal of Transcultural Nursing, 11*(4), 290–299.

Werner, O., & Schoepfle, G. M. (1987). *Foundations of ethnography and interviewing* (Vol. 1). Newbury Park, CA: Sage.

Wright, D. J. (2001). Hospice nursing: A specialty. *Cancer Nursing, 24*(1), 20–27.

RESEARCH ARTICLE

Parenting a Second Time Around: An Ethnography of African American Grandmothers Parenting Grandchildren due to Parental Cocaine Abuse

Kristin Haglund

This study describes a group of six African American grandmothers parenting their grandchildren secondary to cocaine abuse on the part of the parents. It explores the manner in which such parenting affected the grandmothers' health. Data for this ethnography design were collected through participant observation, field notes, taped interviews, and supplementary data sources. The identification of cultural themes evolved from domain and taxonomic analyses. The themes—parenting a second time around, sacrifice, and God's presence in daily life—expressed aspects of the grandmothers' culture. The effects on health varied from none to exacerbation of chronic illnesses. The study results, and its picture of life from the grandmothers' perspectives, suggest areas of nursing assessment and intervention that otherwise might be left unexplored.

African American grandmothers are often portrayed in literature and popular culture as matriarchs, central stabilizing figures that hold a family together (Burton, 1992; Franklin, 1997). It often is assumed that a grandmother will naturally accept the role of parenting her grandchildren. However, this assumption represents a limited picture of the African American grandmother (Burton & Dilworth-Anderson, 1991); urbanization, individualistic values, and changes in childbearing patterns and family structures might have rendered the grandmothers less willing to assume this role (Burton & Bengston, 1985). Today, many African American grandmothers desire a relationship with their grandchildren that still allows time for their own interests and self-development (Burton, 1992; Minkler & Roe, 1993; Shore & Hayslip, 1994); as a result, taking on the role of parenting grandchildren may be physically, emotionally, and economically exhausting. It may also elicit ambivalent feelings, especially if the role is assumed out of necessity, as often is the case when the grandchild's parent is abusing cocaine.

Parenting grandchildren in the wake of a parent's cocaine abuse may be a different experience than parenting as a result of parental unemployment, divorce, or teen parenthood. These grandmothers have the difficult task of caring for children who may

Kristin Haglund, RN, MSN, Program Administrator, Milwaukee Adolescent Health Program, Medical College of Wisconsin, Department of Pediatrics, Milwaukee; PhD Candidate, University of Wisconsin-Milwaukee.

have been prenatally exposed to drugs and to dysfunctional parenting, neglect, or abuse. As noted by several authors (Besharov, 1989; Koppleman & Jones, 1989; O'Reilly & Morrison, 1993), such children subsequently may have emotional, behavioral, or physical problems and special needs that present significant parenting challenges.

Additional challenges for these grandparents may include dealing with hostile, abusive persons who steal money or property to obtain drugs (Chychula & Okore, 1990). The family members of the cocaine-abusing person witness the deterioration of their loved one and suffer the loss of this person. Thus, although the experience of parenting a grandchild may have positive aspects, it might also be a source of stress and distress in a grandmother's life. When parenting a grandchild is coupled with the parenthood of a cocaine abuser, the likelihood of stress and distress is increased (Turpin, 1993).

EFFECTS ON HEALTH WHILE PARENTING GRANDCHILDREN

Studies on parenting grandparents, most of whom were grandmothers, have found positive and negative effects on the health of grandparents. Negative effects included complications of diabetes and arthritis, perceptions of decreased health, increased psychological distress, and increased health risk behaviors such as alcohol and cigarette use (Burton, 1992; Kelly & Damato, 1995; Minkler & Roe, 1993). Grandparents parenting grandchildren have reported feelings of depression and anxiety (Burton, 1992) and exhaustion (Minkler & Roe, 1993). They also reported feelings of anger and helplessness amid their inability to help their children become responsible parents (O'Reilly & Morrison, 1993) and resentment toward their children for not accepting parental responsibilities (Robinson, 1989; Shore & Hayslip, 1994). Furthermore, some of these grandparents reported significantly decreased satisfaction with grandparenting and decreased overall well-being (Shore & Hayslip, 1994).

The effects on these grandparents' health were attributed to a number of stressors, including financial drain, overwhelming responsibilities, lack of time to attend to personal needs, social isolation, lack of child care, and observation of the cocaine-abusing child's deterioration (Burton, 1992; Kelly & Damato, 1995; Minkler & Roe, 1993). Finally, grandparents felt stress because of fears that their own health would suffer and result in death or an incapacitating illness and subsequent inability to care for the grandchildren (Kelly, 1993; Shore & Hayslip, 1994). Some grandparents in these studies may have downplayed the negative effects of surrogate parenting on their health for fear of losing custody of the children (Minkler & Roe, 1993).

Alternatively, fear of losing the grandchildren led some grandparents to improve their health by quitting smoking, losing weight, and getting medical care (Minkler & Roe, 1993). Other positive effects were feelings of purpose and usefulness, self-satisfaction, and the experience of love from the children (Burton, 1992; Kelly & Damato, 1995). Finally, some grandparents reported improved health amid reduced contact with their cocaine-abusing child, knowledge that the grandchildren were safe, increased activity with less time to worry, and coming to terms with the drug abuse of their child (Minkler & Roe, 1993).

The phenomenon of parenting of a grandchild holds many complexities. Many grandparents would rather not assume parental responsibility for their grandchildren, yet when the children must be removed from parental custody because of drug abuse, most grandparents accept the children. Although parenting grandchildren may lead to adverse effects on health, some of its aspects may lead to improvements. This study was done to examine the phenomenon of parenting grandchildren from the grandmothers' perspectives and to specifically investigate how parenting grandchildren affected the grandmothers' health.

METHOD

Sample

This ethnographic study included families recruited from the caseloads of public health nurses in a large midwestern city. The sample was chosen according to who provided the richest data (Germain, 1993) and who was representative of the culture (Leininger, 1985). The primary informants were African American grandmothers who had parented their grandchildren for at least 1 year because of cocaine addiction of the children's mothers. All of the informants had legal custody of the children. All of the names used in this report are pseudonyms. Four women were primary informants.

Three to seven visits were made with all the primary informants except Ms. Lewis, whose lack of time permitted only one visit. Each visit was an average of 1.5 hours; the visits lasted from 15 minutes to 5 hours.

Ophelia Johnson was 44, married, and parenting three grandchildren, ages 4, 5, and 7 years. Ms. Johnson had custody of these children for 5 years. Martha Brown, 56 and divorced, was parenting 5 grandchildren, ages 1, 2, 6, 7, and 11 years. She had custody of these children for 11 years. Angela Jones, also 56, was a widow, parenting 4 grandchildren ages 3 months, 1, 3, and 16 years. She had custody of these children for 9 years. Finally, Nancy Lewis was 41, divorced, parenting two grandchildren ages 1 and 7 years in addition to her own three minor children and also providing care for her chronically ill father. Ms. Lewis had custody of the children for 7 years. Except for Ms. Lewis, all the women had at least two chronic illnesses, including asthma, arthritis, scoliosis, degenerative joint disease, obesity, sarcoidosis, hypertension, or diabetes.

Those who were not grandmothers parenting grandchildren but were in a similar situation (such as a great-grandmother and a great-aunt), or others who were intimate with the grandmothers and whose experiences were necessary to develop an understanding of the culture (Schulte, 1992), were included as supplementary informants.

One home visit was conducted with Abigail Adams, a 57-year-old widow who suffered from chronic headaches. She had parented her great-grandchildren, ages 4 months and 4 years, for the past 4 years. One home visit and interview was conducted with Lavonda Wilson, a 60-year-old widow with hypertension. Ms. Wilson was helping her daughter, who had legal custody, parent her great-niece. In addition, informal interactions occurred during home visits between the researcher and many of the grandchildren, some of the cocaine-abusing mothers, the grandmothers' other adult children, and family friends.

DESIGN

This study was designed as a small-scale ethnography with a specific focus (Leininger, 1985). An ethnography uses at least three types of data collection: participant-observation, in-depth interviewing, and supplementary data sources (Germain, 1993). Participant-observation involved observation of the grandmothers and their families within their home environments. Field experiences ranged from 15 minutes to 5 hours, with a total of 37 hours spent in direct observation.

The home interviews were conducted through a repertoire of query strategies (Agar, 1980). As cultural understanding grew, more specific questions were asked. When the situation was appropriate, interviews were taped, although Ms. Lewis and Ms. Adams refused to be audiotaped. During other visits, the researcher simply stayed beside the grandmother, her grandchildren, and a variety of other people, but taping was precluded as the grandmother divided her attentions between the needs of her family and the researcher. Some field notes were taken; then, immediately following the field experiences, complete notes, including verbatim quotations, were generated. Twelve 1-hour interviews with four informants were taped and transcribed.

Supplementary data sources included observations during a support group meeting for parenting grandmothers; personal documents shared by the informants, including letters, photographs, and writings; newspaper articles; and a television special on grandparents parenting grandchildren. A fieldwork journal contained a record of field experiences, researchers' responses and ideas, and a logistics log. The journal was used to identify personal biases as part of the audit trail (Lincoln & Guba, 1985).

Data Analysis

Data analysis occurred concurrently with data collection. Transcribed interviews, field notes, supplementary data, and the fieldwork journal were analyzed by domain and taxonomic analyses (Spradley, 1979). A domain is a symbolic, limited category of knowledge that includes phrases and words, semantically related to a cover term. The data were searched for repeated phrases, ideas, or experiences, grouped into domains, and labeled with a cover term. In this analysis, 15 domains were identified: setting, characteristics of grandmothers, characteristics of mothers, characteristics of grandchildren, health promotion practices, chronic illnesses, sources of illness, effects on health secondary to parenting, events leading up to placement, ways to help mom get treatment, reasons for taking the children, personal sacrifice, sources of support, love, and faith in God.

The taxonomic analysis involved categorizing the items in a domain to identify subsets of cultural knowledge. Taxonomies were developed in seven of the identified domains. For example, the domain called effects on health was categorized into negative and positive effects. Finally, the identification of cultural themes evolved out of the domain and taxonomic analyses, repeated reading of the field journal and transcripts, and relistening to the audiotapes. A cultural theme is a cognitive principle, assumed or explicit, that recurs in more than one domain and connects different subsystems of a culture (Spradley, 1979). The identified domains were divided into four themes: health effects, parenting a second time around, sacrifice, and God's presence in daily life. Identified themes were tested in the field and confirmed by informant agreement. Characteristics of the grandchildren were not reported in this article.

Rigor

Rigor in qualitative designs can be measured in terms of credibility, transferability, dependability, and confirmability (Lincoln & Guba, 1985).

Credibility is the faithful depiction of the informant's lived experiences that would be recognizable to themselves, as opposed to the verification of a preconception of those events. Credibility was achieved through participant observation, prolonged engagement, and a search for clarification and confirmation from informants.

Transferability is the capacity to transfer the conclusions to another setting. Thick descriptions and verbatim quotations were presented so that a person using the research could judge the appropriateness of transferring the study findings to another group.

Dependability is achieved when a different researcher is able to reach similar conclusions using the researcher's perspective, raw data, and analytical documents.

Finally, confirmability refers to the maintenance of neutrality and the prevention of personal bias influence on the research. Bias was controlled through the use of a reflexive journal, peer review, consultation with expert researchers, and confirmation from informants.

RESULTS

The effects on the grandmothers' health were varied, but in general, the informants spent little time discussing their own health. They often made comments such as "doing pretty good" and then approached a different topic.

Health Effects

The women had a variety of chronic illnesses, including hypertension, arthritis, scoliosis, sarcoidosis, asthma, obesity, diabetes, degenerative joint disease, and headaches. The reported parenting effects on these problems ranged from none to persistent aggravation.

Ophelia Johnson, who had scoliosis and arthritis and needed hip replacement surgery, said,

> It's hard, because by me being disabled, I have back problems and leg problems. Sometimes I can hardly get up to take care of them, but regardless of how much pain I be in...I got to get up. But I got to have an operation for an artificial hip to replace that cup [sic]. That's another thing. I want to take the operation so I can better my leg. But I can't take it because I talked to my doctor. He's talking about 6 to 7 weeks, maybe a couple of months of not being able to walk. Who's going to take care of the kids? I don't have anybody who can take care of my grandkids.

Parenting of grandchildren had a definite effect on Mrs. Johnson's health, as it caused her to postpone her surgery. Other participants denied that specific health problems or exacerbation of chronic diseases were related to the children, yet later, they did report health complaints. Angela Jones denied that caring for the children had any negative effects on her diabetes or arthritis. However, she said that her blood sugar had been running high because of concern that her daughter would be killed by the drug-abusing people with whom she associated. Other grandmothers also reported that they worried about the safety of their drug-abusing child.

Exhaustion and stress were the most often cited health problems. Abigail Adams was fatigued from sleepless nights with her 4-month-old great-granddaughter Andrea and from chasing her 4-year-old great-granddaughter Annie during the day. The infant was on an apnea monitor, which required someone familiar with the equipment and competent in infant CPR to be with her at all times. This limited child care to family members only.

Andrea cried at night until she was picked up, then fell asleep in her great-grandmother's arms. Because she awoke when returned to the crib, Abigail slept in a chair holding the baby. Abigail sometimes napped during the day but regretted it "because then things get away from me." In response to the question of effects on her health, she stated that she did not have much time to think about the subject. Yet, she reported feeling very tired and said, "I'm too old to have these little kids. Pretty soon I will need someone to take care of me."

To manage their chronic illnesses and to maintain their health, the grandmothers practiced a variety of behaviors, including dietary measures such as decreases in salt intake, consumption of fruit, vitamins and herbs, and fasting; abstinence from cigarette and alcohol use; relaxation in a hot bath or reading; exercise through play with the grandchildren and through walking; consumption of prescription medication and maintenance of preventive health care such as mammograms, checkups, and Pap tests; searches for support from people with similar problems; viewership of talk shows; and finally, through personal activities such as singing, praying, and maintaining interests outside the home.

Some grandmothers did report positive benefits on their emotional health due to parenting their grandchildren. They reported that they experienced positive well-being from feeling and expressing love. They stated that they enjoyed time with their grandchildren and that they were happy to get to know them intimately. Finally, they reported that the knowledge that the children were in a safe, stable environment, rather than with their mothers or in foster care, provided relief.

Parenting a Second Time Around

The women in this study described themselves as hardworking. They had raised their own children largely as single parents due to divorce, spousal alcoholism or drug abuse, death, or abandonment. All the women worked outside the home while raising their children. Lavonda Wilson said,

> I raised five children by myself because my husband died young. I raised my children up, and I just raised them, I guess. I'd get up, take my kids to school and my grandchildren. Drop them off, everybody, and go on to my job. If you know you got a family to raise, there's no husband around, you're going to raise [the children] if you want to do it. You can do anything that you want to do, all you got to do is make up your mind that you want to do it and you can do it.

Each of the informants had similar experiences leading to the placements of their grandchildren. The natural mothers had custody of their children at birth, but the parenting situation deteriorated because of the mothers' drug use. For a period of time, the grandmothers and other family members tried to help their daughters abstain from drugs and resume appropriate parenting of their children. Some families rented the mother an apartment, allowed her to live with family members in town, or sent her out of town to another relative's home. Some practiced tough love, talking, or confrontation, whereas others provided food or money to help support the children. They left the children with the cocaine-abusing mothers for a period of time, hoping that the responsibilities of motherhood would preclude the drug abuse. They also attempted to put the cocaine-abusing women out of the house, letting them hit rock bottom, and they threatened to take away parental rights.

In the end, the families' attempts failed. The women continued to use drugs, and the caretaking of their children deteriorated. Child abuse and neglect, such as leaving the children home alone unsupervised, not providing food for the children, spending the family's money on drugs, leaving the children at the homes of relatives and failing to return to get them, and incarceration led to the placement of the children with their grandmothers. Ophelia Johnson explained how her grandchildren came to live with her:

> My oldest daughter started using cocaine, and she started abusing the children. She was living with my mother in an upstairs apartment, but she kept leaving the children on my mother. She'd just leave them and tell my mother that she's going to the store, and she wouldn't come back. She did this repeatedly. We had been warning her about it; she just kept on, kept on doing it. She'd beat her kids. She wouldn't take care of the kids. She'd go off and come back and wouldn't have any money. So the last time she did it, she had went off like 5 days and then came back. So after the third day, my mother called me and she told me. She says, "Ophelia you're going to have to come and get the kids. We're going to have to do something." I told her, I said, Where's Vicki at, where's the kids at?" She said, "Vicki been gone; I just didn't want to tell you she been gone for days." And so I went over there and got them. When I went over there and got them, I said, well, I'm going to do her the same way that other people do. I love her, but I want to do this for her health, and called social services. They came in that day and they talked to my mother and they talked to me, and we told them that, you know, I love my daughter but it's not fair to the children. So the social service stepped in, and then that's how I ended up with the kids. I've had them like for 5 years now.

After a period of time, Child Protective Services and the court system were involved with all the families, and the grandmothers received legal custody of the children. The grandmothers stated that although they loved their daughters, they ultimately chose to protect their grandchildren. As Angela Jones said, "I still love her. I stand by her as much as I can. I can't abide by her mistreating the kids, because they didn't ask to be born and somebody's got to take care of them." The grandmothers ultimately accepted parental responsibility for the children because of love for the children and for their daughters, a sense of family responsibility, an aversion toward foster care, and to protect the children.

Acceptance of the grandchildren began the experience of parenting a second time around. Parenting the grandchildren was a long-term commitment, vastly different than a child's visit to grandma's house. These children were with their grandmothers for years, many since infancy. Over time, some came to think of their grandmothers as their mothers and their birth mothers as a friend or playmate. This phenomenon was evident during a home visit with Angela Jones. As Angela's 1-year-old grandson's nose ran, she handed him some tissue and said, "Go by your mama and get your nose cleaned." The child walked back and forth from Kim, his mother, to Angela, finally stopping by Angela. Kim said, "He thinks that she's his mother. I have a hard time getting him to come by me." This experience was echoed by Ophelia Johnson, who said, "When she's [the children's mother] got her head together, she'll run and play with them. That's what they like about being around her, it's like being with another kid." Thus, the experience of parenting a second time represented a commitment to the grandchildren.

Sacrifice

The theme of personal sacrifice, integral to parenting, was evident in the lives of the informants. "Eighteen years of sacrifice, then you want to enjoy yourself, but here comes the grandbaby," a participant at a support group for parenting grandparents said. A common sacrifice involved the grandmothers' abandoning or postponing long-term plans, activities, and dreams. They expressed the feeling that they should have time to pursue their own interests after their own children were grown.

Ophelia Johnson had plans to go to school and to spend more time with her recently retired husband. She said,

> I've asked God why. I know you are not supposed to question, but I just have to ask...I was going to school for secretary work when I got the grandchildren. I had to stop then because I couldn't concentrate with them being so little. I was getting ready to start into LPN, but that got cut out, and I'm taking care of kids again. I imagine a lot of other grandmas feel the same way; you just can't get your life together...You think at this time in my life, I'm still young enough to enjoy life, can't go when I want to go, I got to get up to be sending kids to school, taking them to the doctors and washing clothes.

Ms. Johnson made sacrifices in her education and in her relationship with her husband, and other participants experienced sacrifices in personal relationships. For example, Martha Brown wanted to spend more time with her elderly mother in Mississippi but was not able to see her as often or as long as she felt was needed because of obligations to the grandchildren.

The women also reported anger and resentment in response to the sacrifices. They reported anger with their daughters for rejecting their parental responsibilities and that their grandchildren were not experiencing true parent-child relationships. Angela Jones explained,

> Children are supposed to be with their mothers. Grandmothers love them and see after them, but the place of the kids is with their mothers. Kids shouldn't grow up without knowing their mother and father, doesn't matter if their mother and father are not together.

They were also angry with the paternal families for not being involved with the children emotionally or financially. Nancy Lewis explained,

> I do resent the mother and the father and the father's family for not taking care of the baby. They only want to see the kids on their birthdays to give them gifts or to see them and say how big they are, but do not want to make any contributions to their life.

For the most part, the grandmothers were solely responsible for the majority of work and expense involved in taking care of their grandchildren.

God's Presence in Daily Lives

The women expressed the conviction that God existed and was active in their daily lives. They frequently made spontaneous remarks about their relationship with God. God's presence in daily life represented a cultural theme because it appeared to permeate the grandmothers' lives. Martha Brown said it simply: "I am a very spiritually minded lady, and I believe highly in God. I believe this is how God has my life fated so I won't be alone."

God's presence also appeared to be a source of strength and support for the women to persevere in spite of difficulties. Nancy Lewis stated that she "would not have made it without faith." Ophelia Johnson said, "Sometimes I just want to give up; I have to pray and ask God to give me strength." Martha Brown identified a lack of social support that was filled by assistance from God. She said,

> Well, my children, I talk to them, but sometimes I be having problems and I be wanting to talk to them and [they say] "ah Mama, we ain't got time." "I don't want to hear that right now." Well, see then, I don't have nowhere to go and turn to. With God in my life, I can lock my door and I can talk to God about it. I never hear it again, and it's worked out and don't nobody know it but me and God.

Most informants were active in their churches in a variety of ways, including ushering, teaching Sunday school, participating in the church choir, sending the grandchildren to Sunday school, and regularly attending services.

DISCUSSION

This study captures only a small portion of a rich culture, yet it provides a picture of life from the grandmothers' perspectives. Although the findings may not be accurate for all African American grandmothers parenting their grandchildren, they do suggest areas for assessment that could yield important information about a woman's health, lifestyle, and family.

Ethnographic studies reflect the phenomenon as it was experienced during a period of time and under certain conditions. The results of this study might not be replicated as women's experiences and perceptions change. Nonetheless, thick descriptions of the women's experiences created an opportunity for the reader to determine the application of the findings.

Limited time was spent in the field, and a White female nurse, who was 13 years the junior of the youngest informant, conducted the study. Although a concerted effort was made to present a faithful account of the informants' experiences, this report may be biased by the researcher's interpretations. Observations and themes were verified by the informants during the study, thus increasing the credibility of this account.

Many people feel it is a grandmother's duty to take responsibility for her grandchildren when the parents no longer provide adequate care. It is not unusual for children to live with their grandparents; in fact, in the last census, approximately 3.2 million children lived with their grandparents or other relatives (U.S. Bureau of the Census, 1991). Thus, because it is not unusual, a woman may not volunteer that she is parenting her grandchildren. She also may be reticent to divulge this information because she is parenting amid her child's substance abuse.

Nurses must be sensitive to the possibility that their clients are parenting grandchildren. It is important for them to ask the women who lives with them and for whom they provide care. As reported, some grandmothers deny that their parenting responsibilities adversely affect their health. They may attribute suspicious blood sugars or high blood pressure to age or ascribe exacerbated respiratory conditions to the weather. Nurses working with parenting grandmothers may help them by exploring the effects on their health. This process may help the grandmothers achieve insights into their health and may facilitate discovery of methods to ameliorate negative effects.

Alternatively, exploring the effects of parenting grandchildren can identify benefits that might help develop health promotion practices and interventions. Knowledge of positive effects from the situation might aid the grandmothers in stressful times. Also, women in this study reported a key coping mechanism: the knowledge that others shared their life situation. Accordingly, nurses working with these families might help them by informing them that they are not alone.

In addition, some grandmothers may appreciate referrals to a sensitive mental health care provider or to a local support group for parenting grandmothers, for parents of cocaine-affected children or children with special needs, or for relatives of substance abusers.

Further research is needed to identify ways to support grandparents who are compelled to parent their grandchildren. Future studies also should investigate the grandchildren's experiences when their grandparents assume parental responsibility for them.

Parenting grandchildren is not unusual and may become more common as states institute welfare reform. A recent article in The New York Times (DeParle, 1999) reported that in the welfare reform state of Wisconsin, increasing numbers of children are being placed with their grandmothers amid their mother's substance abuse problems, work schedules, or lack of money.

As identified in this study, parenting grandchildren is not easy and is not always desired by grandparents. Yet, for many children in need of placement outside their parents' custody, grandparents often are the best alternative. Without grandparents, many of these children would be placed in foster care or in institutions or would fend for themselves. The men and women who take in their grandchildren provide an opportunity for the grandchildren to thrive within the comfort of their own families. They also relieve the community of the responsibility and expense for care in institutions or in foster settings.

Current welfare reform programs require recipients to work as a condition of receiving benefits. Grandmothers who assume parental responsibility for their grandchildren and who require assistance should be exempt from these work requirements. Public policy should guarantee parenting grandparents financial assistance for basic living expenses such as health care, food, clothing, personal care items, and day care. These assistance programs must be publicized and readily accessible: "Welfare policy reforms should be undertaken to ensure that grandparent caregivers are supported, rather than penalized, for the critical role they are playing in raising some of the nation's most vulnerable children" (Minkler & Fuller-Thomson, 1999, p. 1388).

Grandparents require and deserve support for maintenance of their own, and their grandchildren's, health and well-being. Supporting grandparents in these efforts is a worthwhile investment for the community and the children.

Research article taken from: Haglund, K. (2000). Parenting a Second Time Around: An Ethnography of African American Grandmothers Parenting Grandchildren due to Parental Cocaine Abuse. *Journal of Family Nursing, 6*(2), 120–136. (Reprinted with permission.)

References

Agar, M. (1980). The professional stranger. San Diego, CA: Academic.
Besharov, D. (1989). The children of crack. Public Welfare, 47, 6–11.
Burton, L. M. (1992). Black grandparents rearing children of drug-addicted parents: Stressors, outcomes, and social service needs. The Gerontologist, 32(6), 744–751.
Burton, L., & Bengtson, V. L. (1985). Black grandmothers: Issues of timing and continuity of roles. In V. I. Bengtson & J. E. Robertson (Eds.), Grandparenthood (pp. 61–77). Beverly Hills, CA: Sage.
Burton, L., & Dilworth-Anderson, P. (1991). The intergenerational family roles of aged black Americans. Marriage and Family Review, 16(3/4), 311–330.
Chychula, N., & Okore, C. (1990). The cocaine epidemic: A comprehensive review of use abuse and dependence. Nurse Practitioner, 15(7), 31–39.
DeParle, J. (1999, February 21). As welfare rolls shrink, load on relatives grows. The New York Times, pp. 1, 20.
Franklin, D. (1997). Ensuring inequality: The structural transformation of the African American family. New York: Oxford University Press.
Germain, C. (1993). Ethnography: The method. In P. Munhall & C. Oiler Boyd (Eds.), Nursing research: A qualitative perspective (pp. 237–268). New York: National League for Nursing.
Kelley, S. (1993). Caregiver stress in grandparents raising grandchildren. Image, 25(4), 331–337.
Kelley, S., & Damato, E. (1995). Grandparents as primary caregivers. American Journal of Maternal Child Nursing, 20(6), 326–332.
Koppleman, J., & Jones, J. M. (1989). Crack: It's destroying fragile low-income families. Public Welfare, 47, 13–15.
Leininger, M. (1985). Ethnography and ethnonursing: Models and modes of qualitative data analysis. In M. Leininger (Ed.), Qualitative research methods in nursing (pp. 33–71). Orlando, FL: Grune & Stratton.
Lincoln, Y., & Guba, E. (1985). Naturalistic inquiry. Beverly Hills, CA: Sage.
Minkler, M., & Fuller-Thomson, E. (1999). The health of grandparents raising grandchildren: Results of a national study. American Journal of Public Health, 89(9), 1384–1389.
Minkler, M., & Roe, K. (1993). Grandmothers who care. Newbury Park, CA: Sage.
O'Reilly, E., & Morrison, M. (1993). Grandparent-headed families: New therapeutic challenges. Child Psychiatry and Human Development, 23(3), 147–159.
Robinson, L. (1989). Grandparenting: Intergenerational love and hate. Journal of American Academy of Psychoanalysis, 17(3), 483–491.
Schulte, J. (1992). Finding ways to create connections among communities: Ethnography of urban public health nurses. Doctoral dissertation, University of Colorado.
Shore, R., & Hayslip, B. (1994). Custodial grandparenting: Implications for children's development. In A. Gottfried & A. Gottfried (Eds.), Redefining families implications for children's development (pp. 171–218). New York: Plenum.
Spradley, J. (1979). The ethnographic interview. New York: Holt, Rinehart & Winston.
Turpin, S. (1993). Moral support for grandparents who care. American Journal of Nursing, 93, 52–56.
U.S. Bureau of the Census (1991). Current population reports: Marital status and living arrangements, March 1990 (Series P-20 No. 450). Washington, DC: Author.

Historical Research Method

Nursing care for clients includes acquiring a nursing history. If nurses did not collect background data, they would—through ignorance—greatly jeopardize decisions regarding a client's current health care needs and future chance of achieving a higher level of wellness. A historical understanding is crucial to providing nursing care because of nursing's essential holistic nature. Looking at the whole person requires recognition of multiple factors that influence the person. Similarly, decisions related to the nursing profession today, such as unionization, risk failure and inadequacy of response if the profession ignores history.

All knowledge has a historical dimension; conversely, historiography provides individuals with a way of knowing. Tholfsen (1977) explained that "the past is present in every person and in the cultural and institutional world that surrounds [them]" (p. 248). This means, Tholfsen continued, that historians must know the historical conditions of the period they are studying. Knowledge of the past helps to inform most other research designs that include explanatory background that establishes an understanding of the phenomenon under study. Selecting a historical research design as the methodology requires that researchers have an understanding of what history is; a knowledge of various social, political, and economic factors that affect events, ideas, and people; an interest in the subject; and creativity in approach (Christy, 1978; Rines & Kershner, 1979).

HISTORICAL RESEARCH DEFINED

Many definitions and explanations exist related to the meaning and nature of history. Austin (1958) defined *history* as "an integrated, written record of past events, based on the results of a search for the truth" (p. 4). Kruman (1985) explained history as "facts (ideas, events, social, and cultural processes) filtered through human intelligence" (p. 111). Kruman referred to an *objective relativism* that permits the objective reality of one historian to coexist with different historical interpretations of others, thus promoting change in ideas and advances in historical inquiry. Matejski (1986) conceived of history "as a past event, a record, or account of something that has happened" (p. 175). Furthermore, Matejski explained history as a field of study with its own set of criteria and methods that enables researchers to collect data and interpret findings. Having its own method that has often borrowed from other disciplines, historical inquiry examines the interactions of people, activities, and "multiple variables" (Matejski, 1986, p. 177) that affect human thought and activity. The narrative that results from a historian's findings must creatively weave the many factors into a readable and interesting story.

Historical research opens windows into the past, creating new ideas and reshaping human thinking and understanding. Ashley (1978) explained the crucial role historical research plays in the foundation of nursing scholarship by defining history as "the study of creative activity in human behavior [that] gives one the courage to create and respond to what is new without fear of losing one's identity with the whole of humanity" (p. 28). As Lynaugh (1996) suggested, history becomes "our source of identity...it helps us gain identity and personal meaning in our work, improves our comprehension and our planning, and validates social criticism" (p. 1).

Like nursing, history is an art and science. The discipline of history requires the use of scientific principles to study the interrelationship of social, economic, political, and psychological factors that influence ideas, events, institutions, and people. Yet, to explain the findings of historical inquiry while balancing the rigors of scientific inquiry and the understanding of human behavior, historical researchers must revert to the "art of contemplation, speculation, and of interpretation" (Newton, 1965, p. 24).

Researchers who choose historical methods must exhibit more than just a curiosity about the past. Researchers formulate a thesis about the relationship among ideas, events, institutions, or people in the past. Chronologically ordering events over time does not explain the established links and ties. Probing for explanations between historical antecedents requires questioning, reasoning, and interpreting. Christy (1978) explained that "healthy skepticism becomes a way of life for the serious historiographer" (p. 6). Historiographers seeking to discover meanings in the past must sift through data and examine each piece closely for clues.

D'Antonio (1999) speaks of the use of cross-disciplinary interpretation in the writing and rewriting of nursing history. This "'two-way street' between the historical traditions of nursing and those of the liberal arts" (D'Antonio, 1999, p. 268) has led to significant change in the understanding of nurses' work. Most nursing historiograpies in the late twentieth century will usually include some kind of reference to issues relating to gender, class, race, and politics of professionalism (D'Antonio, 1999). Yuginovich (2000) states "history is probably a stronger force than language in moulding our social consciousness" (p. 70). Examining nurses' role as caregivers, leaders, administrators, educators, and practitioners in light of a multidisciplinary framework provides the historiographer with a variety of useful sources, broad interpretations, and necessary tools with which to examine the data.

When studying the past, historical researchers use a variety of sources such as private letters, personal journals, books, magazines, professional journals, and newspapers. Researchers travel in time and explore these materials, seeking a relationship among ideas, events, institutions, or people. The purpose of such a study is not to predict but, rather, to understand the past in order to explain present or future relationships. From historical documents, historiographers derive insight from past lived experiences that they can adapt to generate new ideas (Barzun & Graff, 1985).

Researchers use a historical design if they believe something from the past will explain something in the present or the future. Conflict between what the researcher thinks and what he or she may have read about a particular topic also influences the decision to do historical research. For example, a misconception regarding nurses' participation in the late nineteenth-century women's movement led Lewenson (1990, 1996) to study the relationship between the women's suffrage movement and the four nursing organizations that had formed in America between 1893 and 1920. Lewenson (1990, 1996) conducted a historical inquiry to dispel the tension resulting from a contemporary understanding of the past, also called a present-mindedness, that omitted nursing's political response to the events of the late nineteenth and early twentieth centuries. *Present-mindedness* refers to using a contemporary perspective when analyzing data collected from an earlier period. Such data analysis is stigmatized as unhistorical and leads to inaccurate conclusions when ideas and lived experiences of people in the past are compared with later events (Tholfsen, 1977). Although Tholfsen has warned historians to be careful of absolutes and the dangers of present-mindedness, he has argued that "the best history is rooted in a lively interest in the present" (p. 247). Nevertheless, history refers to constant change, and it is this change that "produces the endless diversity characteristic of the historical world" (p. 248). Researchers must study each period within the context of its age to avoid judging or interpreting the past without respect to changes made over time. Hence, difference found in every age must "be understood in its own terms" (p. 248).

Nurses and history make a good match. Nurses come from rich, diverse backgrounds with many contacts they may use to better understand and explain human behavior. Nurses, who are adept at studying human behavior, are well suited to historical inquiry in which they study human behavior in the context of an event, a place, a person, an institution, or an idea in the past. Like historians, nurses identify and interpret patterns of behavior that occur over time.

HISTORICAL RESEARCH TRADITIONS

Morse and Field (1995) have identified two traditions or schools of thought in historical research: the positivistic or neo-positivistic and the idealist schools. In the *neo-positivistic school*, historians take a more quantitative posture. The focus is on "reducing history to universal laws" (p. 33). Historians use data analysis to verify or categorize information. "There is a strong effort to show cause-effect relationships" (p. 33).

In the *idealist school*, historians are most concerned with getting inside an event and trying to understand the thoughts of individuals involved in the event while considering the time, place, and situations (Fitzpatrick, 2001; Morse & Field, 1995). The idealist school represents more closely the values of qualitative research as shared in the present text.

Regardless of the tradition observed by historical researchers, the intent is always the "interpretation and narration of past events" (Morse & Field, 1995, p. 33). Historical researchers must clearly identify the focus of the study and then make a commitment to a philosophic position.

FUNDAMENTAL CHARACTERISTICS OF HISTORICAL RESEARCH

Although no single historical method exists, Lynaugh and Reverby (1987) have pointed out essential guideposts and rules of evidence to ensure the credibility and usefulness of the historian's findings. Lusk (1997) has identified several methodological stages: selecting "a topic and an appropriate theoretical framework, finding and accessing the resources, and analyzing, synthesizing, interpreting, and reporting the data" (p. 355). In search of an approach, Barzun and Graff (1985) wrote that, "without form in every sense, the facts of the past, like the jumbled visions of a sleeper in a dream, elude us" (p. 271). The next section offers beginning researchers a guide on how to develop a historical design. As in any process, researchers must allow fluidity between the steps of the guide, that is, they must easily move from one step to another, in both directions. For example, the data collected may direct the literature review and the literature review, in turn, may determine the thesis.

SELECTION OF HISTORIOGRAPHY AS METHOD

To understand the wholeness of the past, nurse–historians select a framework to guide the study. However, as Lynaugh and Reverby (1987) have warned, no one formula or specific method exists for doing historical research. Tholfsen (1977) has contended that "history lacks a coherent theoretical and conceptual structure" (p. 246). No one theoretical framework exists for the study of history. Although there is no "set methodology...some methodological consensus exists" (Lusk, 1997, p. 355). History is a discipline with many structures that Cramer (1992) has described as "permanent or semipermanent relations of elements that determine the character of the whole" (p. 6). Superimposed structure enables researchers to organize the data. For example, when using geography to frame a study, the researcher may write a regional history, or when using a particular topic to organize a study, the researcher may focus on women's work (Cramer, 1992).

Society asks historians to analyze an experience and use that experience to explain and prepare society for similar events in the future. For example, historians study the records of war so that society will learn what may help in future wars (Hofstadter, 1959). Writing for a specific function creates further tension between the dual nature that exists within the historian's role: the writing of a historical narrative and the writing of a historical monograph. According to Hofstadter, the historical narrative tells a story but often is disappointing in the analysis, and the historical monograph approximates a scientific inquiry but lacks literary style and frequently offers insufficient analytic data. However, both functions are enriched by interrelating social sciences and historical inquiry. Hofstadter believed that a combination of social sciences and historical research produces fresh ideas and new insights into human behavior.

Historians look at other disciplines to help inform and structure their work. To understand the development of nursing education in North America and to provide a theoretical framework, historians might use research from women's and educational history in the United States. Knowledge of U.S. labor history, which is important to nursing history because of nurses' apprenticeship role in hospitals, would also be a useful framework for historiographers to conceptually organize the data. To study history using a variety of approaches, such as philosophical, national, psychohistorical, or economic, allows researchers to explore a point in time with a conceptual guide from a particular discipline (Ashley, 1978; Matejski, 1986).

Nurse–historians ponder different theoretical frameworks that structure historical research. They may select from theoretical approaches such as biographic, social, and intellectual histories. A *biographical history*, the study of an individual, opens a wide vista to an entire period (Brown, D'Antonio, & Davis, 1991). Biography uses the story of a person's life to understand "the values, expectations, tensions and the conflicts of the time and culture within which he or she lived" (Brown et al., 1991). Interpretation requires historians to familiarize themselves with a period so that they may derive meanings from within the particular time frame rather than superimpose them from a later, contemporary distance. For example, to understand the life of the early twentieth-century nurse and birth control activist Margaret Sanger, it is essential to understand society's beliefs about woman's roles and beliefs about procreation.

Social history explores a particular period and attempts to understand the prevailing values and beliefs by examining the everyday events of that period. Historian Vern Bullough described a strategy for doing a social history: Use specific quantitative data to understand the life experiences of "'ordinary' men and women" (Brown et al., 1991, p. 3). An analysis of census data, court records, and municipal surveys, for example, assists historians to go beyond the boundaries of class, ethnicity, economics, and race, hence enabling them to gain a broader understanding of the study subject.

Intellectual history, in which "*thinking* is the event under analysis," lends itself to several approaches (Brown et al., 1991, p. 2). Historians may explore the ideas of an individual considered to be an intellectual thinker of a period; for example, they might study the ideas of public health nurse Lillian Wald. Or historians may explore the history of ideas over time, such as nursing leaders' ideas that influenced the development of U.S. nursing education. Another approach may be to explore the attitudes and ideas of people who are not considered intellectual thinkers of the period, such as the ideas of practicing nurses (Hamilton, 1991). However, historians must be aware that conflict may arise between the ideas and the contextual backgrounds that gave rise to them (Hamilton, 1993).

Historical researchers must be ready to "live in permanent struggle with conceptual ambiguities, missing evidence and conflicting viewpoints" (Lynaugh &

Reverby, 1987, p. 4). Historians continually face a methodological polarity whereby tension exists between the "general and the unique, [and] between the particular and the universal" (Tholfsen, 1977, p. 249). However, these tensions and ambiguities are essential to history because they mirror human experience with all of life's contradictions and ambiguities (Tholfsen, 1977). When approaching historical research, researchers must expect ambiguity of design as well as data. Researchers must decide on a particular theoretical framework and understand the conflicting views and ideas regarding the approach. Keeping this information in mind, historians can then begin to construct a creative design that addresses their research interest.

DATA GENERATION

Developing a Focus

To apply a historical design, researchers must first define the study topic and prepare a statement of the subject (Kruman, 1985). A clear, concise statement tells readers what researchers will be studying and their reasons for selecting the subject. Researchers must explain their interest in the topic and justify its relationship with other topics. In addition, researchers establish the purpose and significance to nursing and nursing research in the statement (Rines & Kershner, 1979). According to Lusk (1997), topics "should be significant, with the potential to illuminate or place a new perspective on current questions" (p. 355).

When selecting a topic, Austin (1958) has suggested that the subject be "part of a larger whole, and one which can be isolated" (p. 5). Isolating a part of the topic makes the study more manageable. For example, it may be easier to study the curriculum of three nurse training schools in 1897 than to tackle all of nursing education in the late nineteenth century.

Because historical study does not predict outcomes, there is no hypothesis. A researcher's interest and hunches about the topic guide the study and move the research toward a particular field or discipline. Researchers base their ideas on background information they have obtained. Patterns that emerge in the initial fact-finding and knowledge-building step aid in the creative formation of a thesis. For example, instead of predicting the effect of apprenticeship training on the development of nursing education, historians might identify themes or ideas about nursing education and use those themes to convey their ideas on the subject. An example is the Hanson (1989) study on the emergence of liberal education in nursing education.

To accomplish this important step, researchers must gather information regarding the period to be studied. They must have a working knowledge of the social, cultural, economic, and political climate that prevailed and how these factors influenced the subject. This knowledge helps researchers establish patterns and identify relevant points regarding the subject and justifies the selection of the historical method. Moreover, when selecting a topic, researchers need to be aware of the accessibility of the sources, the relevance of the topic to the audience, and its potential to enhance understanding (Lusk, 1997).

Selecting a Title

Once historians have identified the focus of the study, it is helpful to delimit the project by titling it. The title tells readers what to expect from the study and narrows the topic for the historian. Typically, the title includes the time frame and purpose, for example, A Review of Critical Thinking in Nursing, 1990–2000.

Although the title appears first in a completed study and concisely describes the research topic, it may be the researcher's final step. The advantage of titling a study early in the project is to assist in focusing the work. Historians can always modify the title as the project develops and should be open to change based on data they uncover. A well-focused and delimited study will assist researchers in making the literature search effective and meaningful. It is essential, though, that historians do not prematurely close the literature search because the materials discovered are outside of the predetermined time frame. Rather, historians should continue their review of materials until they are comfortable that they have fully examined the thesis. It is easier to adjust the title than to risk having a poorly developed study.

Conducting a Literature Review

A good starting point for a literature review is to identify major works published on the selected topic. If historians want to study the history of critical thinking, then they must assess what has been written on the subject and identify the themes and ambiguities related to critical thinking that exist in the literature. Part of the review includes identifying the problems connected with the topic, for example, the ambiguities that have arisen over time in defining and evaluating critical thinking. The anticipation of problems that may arise with methodology or with the interpretation of data allows historical researchers time to plan problem resolution. A search of the literature for references from several periods allows for a greater understanding of the subject. Various computer databases provide a means by which researchers may obtain some data needed in the literature review.

A literature review helps researchers formulate questions they need to address, delineate a time frame for the study, and decide on a theoretical framework. In addition, the review affords researchers an opportunity to learn what types of materials are available. For example, a researcher learns whether he or she can obtain primary sources or firsthand accounts of an event, such as the letters written by an individual living during the period of study. The researcher also learns of secondary sources or secondhand accounts of an event, such as histories or newspapers that have already been written on the particular study subject.

Based on the literature review, historians formulate questions regarding events that influenced the chosen subject. To elucidate the subject, researchers ask questions beginning with How, Why, Who, and What in light of the ideas, events, and institutions that existed and individuals who existed. If, for example, a researcher narrows a topic such as U.S. public health nursing to the study of public health nurses living at the Henry Street Settlement, then questions such as the following may guide the direction of the literature search: How did the Henry Street Settlement begin? Who began the Henry Street Settlement? What is a settlement house? Why was Henry Street the location? These questions may prompt the researcher to examine biographies of people who participated in the settlement house movement during the late nineteenth and early twentieth centuries. Or to better understand life at that time, the historian might read city records regarding population statistics or examine published materials to understand another historian's perception of women's roles, education, work, and life during the study period. Newspaper accounts, written histories, proceedings of minutes, photographs, biographies, letters, diaries, and films may help historians seeking a greater understanding of a particular subject.

During the literature review, historians must develop an organizing strategy that will help them analyze the data. Some facts they had obtained may seem trivial in the beginning of the project, but may become crucial to explaining or connecting events learned later in the study. Thus, careful documentation using an index card filing system or a directory in a word processing program will help researchers retrieve the information at a later time (Austin, 1958; Barzun & Graff, 1985). The bibliographic entry should include the author, title, abstract, place of publication, date, and particular archive or library where the researcher found the information. Researchers must include any pertinent information in the notes so that, during data analysis, they will be able to easily retrieve important information or go back to the original source, if necessary.

During this phase of the project, historians begin to develop a bibliography. Using historical source materials from libraries, archives, bibliographies, newspapers, reviews, journals, associations, and the Internet, researchers begin to comprehend the extent of the subject under investigation (Matejski, 1986). To accomplish this important step, historians use collections in libraries and archives. Libraries and archives contain different types of reference materials that require different methods of storage and classification. To enable researchers to use each method appropriately, it is necessary they be familiar with both.

Libraries contain published materials that researchers often use as secondary materials. To locate materials, researchers use a card catalog, computerized catalog system, or computerized database that allows them to locate works. A call number, usually given in the catalog, designates the unique location of each volume in the library; volumes are usually arranged by subject. Libraries have purchased many of the books and thus permit them to circulate (Termine, 1992), whereas archival materials remain on-site.

Archives differ from libraries in their holdings, cataloging, and circulation policies. Archives contain unpublished materials that are considered primary source materials, such as the "official records of an organization or persons...[that]

are preserved because of the value of the information they contain" (Termine, 1992). Instead of using a card catalog to find a book, researchers use a *finding aid*, a published book or catalog that lists what is in the archive or repository. The finding aid identifies a collection using a record group, a series, and a subseries. However, instead of being stored according to these designations, collections are stored haphazardly within aisles, shelves, and box numbers. Libraries contain a discrete number of volumes, whereas archives contain linear (cubic) feet of records. Archives acquire their material by collections. For example, many organizations cannot store or maintain their records and transfer this task to archives.

Unlike libraries, where books are circulated, archives require that researchers use the materials on-site. In most archives, researchers may only use pencil and paper to collect data; other archives permit the use of a laptop computer. Newer technologic advances have enabled researchers to use handheld scanners in conjunction with their laptop computers. Scanners provide a safe method for copying materials (Lusk, 1997). Archives usually require that researchers make appointments to discuss their project with an archivist. Besides offering researchers primary source references needed in historical research, archives provide materials and memorabilia researchers may use in exhibitions such as the history of an organization or a person. Because some of the primary source materials are fragile, archivists will only permit scholars engaged in historical research to use the collections (Termine, 1992).

Archivists and librarians assist researchers to access materials, thus rendering an important informational service. However, because of the differences between libraries and archives, the work of professional archivists and librarians varies. Whereas archivists work with the records, papers, manuscripts, and nonprinted materials found in the collections, librarians manage the books and publications (Termine, 1992). Table 11.1 summarizes the differences between libraries and archives.

DATA TREATMENT

Identifying Sources

Historic researchers must find some way to understand what actually occurred during an earlier period. To research historical antecedents, researchers must identify sources from the period. Primary sources give firsthand accounts of a person's experience, an institution, or of an event, and may lack critical analysis. However, primary sources such as personal letters or diaries may contain the author's interpretation of an event or hearsay. Thus, researchers must analyze and interpret the meaning of the primary sources.

Ulrich (1990) wrote about Martha Ballard, an eighteenth-century midwife from Hallowell, Maine. Using Ballard's diary as a primary source, Ulrich wrote a rich biographic account of Ballard as well as a historical rendering of everyday life

TABLE 11.1   DIFFERENCES BETWEEN LIBRARIES AND ARCHIVES

	Libraries	Archives
Holdings	Published materials	Unpublished materials: records, manuscripts, papers
Locators	Card catalog Call number Unique location by subject	Finding aid Record group, series, subseries Haphazard location of "boxes" by aisle, shelf, box number
Stored	Volumes (titles)	Linear (cubic) feet
Acquired	Purchased by volume or issue	Donated or purchased collections
Use of materials	Circulation	Noncirculation; use of paper and pencil only or laptop computer to collect data

From Termine, J. (1992, March). Paper presented at the State University of New York, Health Science Center at Brooklyn, College of Nursing, Brooklyn, NY. Adapted with permission.

during this period. Ballard's diary, which she kept daily for more than 27 years, connected "several prominent themes in the social history of the early Republic" (p. 27). More important, Ulrich explained, "It [the diary] transforms the nature of the evidence upon [which] much of the history of the period has been written" (p. 27). Earlier historians did not consider the potential the diary had for uncovering historical data about this period in the United States. Rather, they perceived Ballard's daily record as trivial and too filled with daily life to be of any importance because she documented the deliveries with which she assisted, the travel she endured to reach laboring women, the stories she wrote about other people, and the accounts of her own family. However, on viewing the same diary, Ulrich believed that it reached directly to the "marrow of eighteenth century life" (p. 33). The "trivia that so annoyed earlier readers provides a consistent, daily record of the operation of a female-managed economy" (p. 33).

Unlike primary sources that are written by people directly involved in an event, secondary sources are materials that cite opinions and present interpretations. Newspaper accounts, journal articles, and textbooks from the period being studied are secondary sources that place researchers within the context of a period. For example, newspaper accounts of the 1893 Columbian World Exposition held in Chicago added authenticity to the story about the founding of the American Society of Superintendents of Training Schools for Nurses (known today as the National League for Nursing). However, researchers may use secondary sources as primary sources, depending on the researchers' questions or the purpose of the study (Austin, 1958). For example, although newspaper articles from the late nineteenth century gave secondary accounts of what happened, they also offered insight into what was considered important during that period. Thus, if researchers are studying the insights of individuals present at a particular point in history, then they may use newspaper accounts as primary as well as secondary sources. Chaney and Folk (1993), for example, used cartoons found in the American Medical Association journal *American Medical News* as a primary source in the study "A Profession in Caricature: The Changing Attitudes Towards Nursing in the *American Medical News*, 1960–1989."

Confirming Source Genuineness and Authenticity

When selecting primary sources, the genuineness and authenticity of those sources become important issues. Barzun and Graff (1985) have explained that historians are responsible for verifying documents to assure they are genuine and authentic. *Genuine* means that a document is not forged; *authentic* means that the document provides the truthful reporting of a subject (Barzun & Graff, 1985). Authenticating sources requires several operations, none of which is fixed in a specific technique. Researchers rely on "attention to detail, on common-sense reasoning, on a 'developed' field for history and chronology, on familiarity with human behavior, and on ever-enlarging stores of information" (p. 112). Authenticity of letters or journals becomes even more important when researchers find them in a nursing school attic or closet. More than likely, primary sources within archival collections have already been found to be genuine and have been authenticated by the institution in which they are housed. Nevertheless, researchers are responsible for the final authenticity of a document. A careful reading of the document, an examination of the type of paper and the condition of the material, and an extensive knowledge of the period can help researchers verify the document as authentic.

The validity of historical research relies on measures that address matters concerning external and internal criticism. *External criticism* questions the genuineness of primary sources and assures that the document is what it claims. *Internal criticism* of the data is concerned with content authenticity or truthfulness. Kerlinger (1986) has suggested that internal criticism "seeks the 'true' meaning and value of the content of sources of data" (p. 621). Researchers must ask, Does the content accurately reflect the period in which it indicates it is written? Do the facts conflict with historical dates, meanings of words, and social mores?

Spieseke (1953) has emphasized that, when determining the reliability of the contents, researchers must evaluate when authors of primary sources wrote their account—whether it was close to the event or 20 years later. Other questions researchers must ask are, Did a trained historian or an observer write the story? Were facts suppressed? If so, why? To ensure the accuracy of the writer, Spieseke has suggested that researchers check for corroborating evidence, look for another independent primary source that supports the data, and identify any disagreements between sources. Ulrich (1990), for example, authenticated Ballard's diary by corroborating some of Ballard's entries regarding feed bills with other sources from the town in which she lived.

What data researchers can validate externally as genuine, however, may be inconsistent when researchers examine the data contents. For example, an individual may have written letters in the nineteenth century, but the content may conflict with known facts of that period and pose serious questions regarding the truth of the content (Kerlinger, 1986). Nevertheless, external criticism "ultimately...leads to content analysis or internal criticism and is indispensable when assessing evidence" (Matejski, 1986, p. 189). Austin (1958) illustrated this point by explaining that learning the date of a source (external criticism) helps researchers determine if the content reflects the period in which it was written (internal criticism), and vice versa.

In historical studies where the story can be enhanced or explained by someone who is still alive and who has lived through a period of time, then an oral history provides a useful data source. Collecting oral histories provides an important primary source for many historical studies and adds to the understanding of the history of nursing. The collection of stories told by nurses who have experienced changes in the hospital or the way we care for the terminally ill provides depth and richness to the historical tapestry. "Over the past 20 years, research using oral history method has played a significant role in retrieving and recording historical experiences of 'non-elite' nurses and their patients who have no record of their lives or historical documents" (Biedermann, 2001, p. 61).

To do an oral history, the historiographer uses many of the same steps used in doing a historiography. One of the key differences in collecting oral histories is that live subjects are used and thus require consideration afforded to all research using human subjects. The Oral History Association (2000) web page provides detailed explanation of the responsibilities of the interviewer, the interviewee, the organization sponsoring the oral histories, archives, and transcribers. Readers interested in using an oral history method in their study are referred to other sources such as the Oral History Association for a more comprehensive understanding of this method.

DATA ANALYSIS

Data analysis relies on the statement of the subject including the questions raised, purpose, and conceptual framework of the study. The themes developed by researchers direct the data analysis. Researchers frame the findings according to research questions generated by the thesis. According to Spieseke (1953), the purpose of the study often directs the data analysis. If researchers want to teach a lesson, answer a question, or support an idea, then they organize the selection of relevant data accordingly. How researchers analyze the material depends, in part, on the thematic organization of conceptual frameworks used in the study. Use of social, political, economic, or feminist theory will structure the data and enable researchers to concentrate on particular areas.

In data analysis, researchers must deal with the tension between the conflicting truths so that they may find interpretations or an understanding regarding the subject. In some way, researchers must strike a "balance between conflict" (Tholfsen, 1977, p. 246). They need to ask questions such as, Is the content found in the primary and secondary sources congruent with each other or are there conflicting stories? If a conflict does exist, is there supporting evidence to justify either side of the argument?

Another important aspect of analysis is researcher bias about the subject and the influence of that bias on data interpretation. Awareness of their bias helps researchers identify a particular frame of reference that may limit or direct their data interpretation. Self-awareness promotes a researcher's honesty in finding the truth and decreases the influence of bias on data interpretation (Austin, 1958; Barzun & Graff, 1985).

Through data analysis, researchers should develop new material and new ideas based on supporting evidence rather than just rehash ideas (Matejski, 1986). Researchers seek to discover new truths from the assembled facts. However, given the same data, individuals will analyze the data differently and thus contribute to the tentative nature of interpretation (Austin, 1958). To interpret the findings and get at a truth, historians must be conscious of the role ideology plays in analysis. Researchers must question how ideology, or any set of ideas, influences the analysis of a particular event. For example, a paternalistic ideologic view of the nurse's role in the health care system may starkly contrast with an interpretation of the same data using a feminist lens. Awareness of ideologic influence forces researchers to study the full effect ideas have on an event and to avoid accepting ideas on face value. Tholfsen (1977) argued that history will suffer if taught from any one ideologic stance; instead, its aim should be the "commitment to the disinterested pursuit of truth, accompanied by an openness to continuing debate and discussion" (p. 255). With this understanding, researchers analyze and sort out data and try to find new truths that the evidence produced by the data can support.

Analysis occurs throughout the process of data collection. Historians look for evidence to explain events or ideas. By interpreting primary and secondary documents, researchers form a picture of historical antecedents. However, these documents become part of history only when "they have been subjected to historiography that bridges the gap between lived occurrences and records" (Matejski, 1986, p. 180).

In their search of true meanings and in their attempts to bridge the gap, researchers must not only be aware of their own bias and that of ideology but also bias from the sources themselves that may impede interpretation. For example, in biographic research, the use of both informants through interviews and materials found in archival collections raises issues regarding the accuracy and validity of the data. Historians doing a biographic study need to be cautious of interviews that often present a biased or one-sided view of the individual being studied. Researchers may also suspect bias in archival holdings of an individual's papers, because the individual may have determined what to include in the collection (Brown et al., 1991).

ETHICAL CONSIDERATIONS

An ethical concern regarding the use of an institution's or individual's private papers is the right to privacy versus the right to know. Although discussion of this concern is beyond the scope of this chapter, it is important for historical researchers to be aware of this dilemma. Researchers must have a clear idea of the kinds of information they need to obtain from data. If they find the source in an archive, then the archivist is responsible for seeing that "policy, regulations, and rules—governing his action do exist and are effective" (Rosenthal, 1982, p. 4). However, scholars are ultimately responsible for using the data appropriately. If historiographers have as a goal to further the understanding of social, political, or economic relationships among individuals, institutions, events, or ideas, then they must question what purpose is served if they expose exploitative or embarrassing details. Historians who misuse data and generate sensationalism by "[presenting] conclusions regarding motives and behavior that transcend the evidence...[and] turn an ordinary book into a best seller" (Graebner, 1982, p. 23) are discouraging future access and preservation of primary sources. If this misuse involves the past, then only a historical reputation is damaged; however, if it involves people who are still living or their immediate ancestors, then it places at risk the right to access future contributions of papers from other families or institutions. When determining how to use data, Graebner (1982) has suggested that "decisions, events, and activities which affect the public welfare or embrace qualities of major human interest—and thus add legitimately to the richness of the historical record—set the acceptable boundaries of historical search and analysis" (p. 23).

The confidentiality of source material has become more of an ethical concern for historians as researchers have placed greater emphasis on the lives of ordinary people (Lusk, 1997). Several professional organizations such as the American Historical Association (1987), American Association for the History of Medicine (1991), and Oral History Association (2000) have developed ethical guidelines for historical research. Nurse–historians Birnbach, Brown, and Hiestand (1991), members of the American Association of the History of Nursing, have published ethical guidelines as well as professional standards for doing historical inquiry in nursing.

INTERPRETATION OF THE FINDINGS

The historical narrative is the final stage in the historical research process. During this stage, researchers tell the story that interprets the data and engages readers in the historical debate. Synthesis occurs and findings are connected, supported, and molded "into a related whole" (Austin, 1958, p. 9). Decisions regarding what to include and what to emphasize become important. In historical exposition, researchers explain not only what happened but how and why it happened. They explore relationships among events, ideas, people, organizations, and institutions and interpret them within the context of the period being studied. The political, social, and economic factors set a stage or backdrop from which to compare and contrast the historical data collected. Historical judgments, based on historical evidence, must pass through the filter of "human understanding of human experience" (Cramer, 1992, p. 7). To accomplish this task, researchers must be sensitive to the material; must show genuine engagement in the subject; and must balance the forces of self-interest, societal interest, and historical interest. Along with these attributes, researchers need creativity to achieve a coherent, convincing, and meaningful account (Ashley, 1978; Spieseke, 1953).

When writing the narrative, researchers are charged with creatively rendering the events, explaining the findings, and supporting the ideas. Researchers must possess discipline, organization, and imagination to accomplish this Herculean task. Historiographers must set aside time to write daily, find a quiet place to concentrate and contemplate the data, use a detailed outline to direct the writing of the manuscript, plan the story using the thematic framework established earlier in the study, and use time and place as landmarks to give balance and direct the flow of the story while critically interpreting the findings (Austin, 1958).

Historians weave together historical facts, research findings, and interpretations influenced by the conceptual framework into a coherent story. To guide them in the writing process, researchers may divide the narrative into chronologic periods. Or, they may use geographic places such as regional areas in the United States, thematic relationships, research questions, or political, social, cultural, or economic issues to organize the narrative. These ad hoc inventions are determined by each researcher and thus are subject to the researcher's interest, bias, and understanding of the historical method (Cramer, 1992; Fondiller, 1978).

Writers of history who want readers to hear the words spoken during the period studied may use direct quotations. Direct quotations also provide corroboration of and credibility to a researcher's interpretation. However, although authentic quotes are a useful narrative tool, researchers must avoid using too many direct quotations. It is better to paraphrase and use limited direct quotes to give the narrative the flavor of a person.

Historiography displays a researcher's creativity and imagination as the story unfolds. Creativity connects thoughts, quotes, and events into a readable story and gives birth to new ideas (Christy, 1978). The interpretations and response to the themes and questions rely on historians' ability to go beyond the known facts and develop new ideas and new meanings. No two historians who view the same data will respond in exactly the same way. The human filter through which all information passes will alter researchers' responses to the data and will provide the catalyst for the creation of new ideas (Barzun & Graff, 1985; Christy, 1978).

SUMMARY

The nursing profession needs the infusion of new ideas, new meanings, and new interpretations of its past to explain its place in history and its future direction. Ashley (1978) confirmed that connection when she wrote, "With creativity as our base, and with strong historical knowledge and awareness, nurses can become pioneers in developing new types of inquiry and turn inward toward self-knowledge and self-understanding" (p. 36). The historical method gives qualitative researchers tools to explore the past. Using certain guideposts along the way, historiographers formulate ideas, collect data, validate the genuineness and authenticity of those data, and narrate the story. However, to make the research meaningful, historians must relate the research questions and the findings to the present.

REFERENCES

American Association for the History of Medicine. (1991). Report of the committee on ethical codes. *Bulletin of the History of Medicine, 65*(4), 565–570.

American Historical Association. (1987). Statement on standards of professional conduct. *History Teacher, 21*(1), 105–109.

Ashley, J. (1978). Foundations for scholarship: Historical research in nursing. *Advances in Nursing Science, 1*(1), 25–36.

Austin, A. (1958). The historical method. *Nursing Research, 7*(1), 4–10.

Barzun, J., & Graff, H. F. (1985). *The modern researcher* (4th ed.). San Diego, CA: Harcourt Brace Jovanovich.

Biedermann, N. (2001). The voices of days gone by: Advocating the use of oral history in nursing. *Nursing Inquiry, 8,* 61–62.

Birnbach, N., Brown, J., & Hiestand, W. (1991). *Ethical guidelines for the nurse historian, and standards of professional conduct for historical inquiry into nursing.* Paper Presentation.

Brown, J., D'Antonio, P., & Davis, S. (1991, April). *Report on the Fourth Invitational Nursing History Conference.* Unpublished manuscript.

Chaney, J. A., & Folk, P. (1993). A profession in caricature: The changing attitudes towards nursing in the *American Medical News*, 1960–1989. *Nursing History Review, 1,* 181–201.

Christy, T. (1978). The hope of history. In M. L. Fitzpatrick (Ed.), *Historical studies in nursing* (pp. 3–11). New York: Teachers College Press.

Cramer, S. (1992). The nature of history: Meditations on Clio's craft. *Nursing Research, 41*(1), 4–7.

D'Antonio, P. (1999). Rewriting and rethinking the rewriting of nursing history. *Bulletin of the History of Medicine, 73,* 268–290.

Fitzpatrick, M. L. (2001). Historical research: The method. In P. L. Munhall (Ed.), *Nursing research: A qualitative perspective* (3rd ed., pp. 403–414). Sudbury, MA: Jones and Bartlett.

Fondiller, S. (1978). Writing the report. In M. L. Fitzpatrick (Ed.), *Historical studies in nursing* (pp. 25–27). New York: Teachers College Press.

Graebner, N. A. (1982). History, society, and the right to privacy. In *The scholar's right to know versus the individual's right to privacy: Proceedings of the first Rockefeller Archive Center Conference, December 5, 1975* (pp. 20–24). Pocantico Hills, NY: Rockefeller Archive Center Publication.

Hamilton, D. (1991, April). *Intellectual history.* Paper presented at the meeting of Fourth Invitational Conference on Nursing History: Critical Issues Affecting Research and Researchers, Philadelphia, PA.

Hamilton, D. B. (1993). The idea of history and the history of ideas. *Image, 25*(1), 45–50.

Hanson, K. S. (1989). The emergence of liberal education in nursing education, 1893 to 1923. *Journal of Professional Nursing, 5*(2), 83–91.

Hofstadter, R. (1959). History and the social sciences. In F. Stern (Ed.), *The varieties of history* (pp. 359–370). New York: Meridan.

Kerlinger, F. N. (1986). *Foundations of behavioral research* (3rd ed.). New York: Holt, Rinehart & Winston.

Kruman, M. (1985). Historical method: Implications for nursing research. In M. M. Leininger (Ed.), *Qualitative research methods in nursing* (pp. 109–118). Orlando, FL: Grune & Stratton.

Lewenson, S. B. (1990). The woman's nursing and suffrage movement, 1893–1920. In V. Bullough, B. Bullough, & M. Stanton (Eds.), *Florence Nightingale and her era: A collection of new scholarship* (pp. 117–118). New York: Garland.

Lewenson, S. B. (1996). *Taking charge: Nursing, suffrage and feminism, 1873–1920.* New York: NLN Press.

Lusk, B. (1997). Historical methodology for nursing research. *Image, 29*(4), 355–359.

Lynaugh, J. (1996). [Editorial]. *Nursing History Review, 4,* 1.

Lynaugh, J., & Reverby, S. (1987). Thoughts on the nature of history. *Nursing Research, 36*(1), 4–69.

Matejski, M. (1986). Historical research: The method. In P. L. Munhall & C. J. Oiler (Eds.), *Nursing research: A qualitative perspective* (pp. 175–193). Norwalk, CT: Appleton-Century-Crofts.

Morse, J. M., & Field, P. A. (1995). *Qualitative research methods for health professionals* (2nd ed.). Thousand Oaks, CA: Sage.

Newton, M. (1965). The case for historical research. *Nursing Research, 14*(1), 20–26.

Oral History Association. (2000). *Oral history evaluation guidelines* (Pamphlet No. 3) [On-line]. Available: www.dickinson.edu/oha/EvaluationGuidelines.html.

Rines, A., & Kershner, F. (1979). *Information concerning historical studies.* Unpublished manuscript. New York: Teachers College, Columbia University, Department of Nursing.

Rosenthal, R. (1982). Who will be responsible for private papers of private people? Some considerations from the view of the private depository. In *The scholar's right to know versus the individual's right to privacy: Proceedings of the first Rockefeller Archive Center Conference, December 5, 1975* (pp. 3–6). Pocantico Hills, NY: Rockefeller Archive Center Publication.

Spieseke, A. W. (1953). What is the historical method of research? *Nursing Research, 2*(1), 36–37.

Termine, J. (1992, March). *A talk about archives.* Paper presented at the State University of New York, Health Science Center at Brooklyn, College of Nursing, Brooklyn, NY.

Tholfsen, T. R. (1977). The ambiguous virtues of the study of history. *Teachers College Record, 79*(2), 245–257.

Ulrich, L. T. (1990). *A midwife's tale: The life of Martha Ballard based on her diary, 1785–1812.* New York: Vintage Books.

Yuginovich, T. (2000). More than time and place: Using historical comparative research as a tool for nursing. *International Journal of Nursing Practice, 6,* 70–75.

12

Historical Research in Practice, Education, and Administration

U sing a historical method to study nursing practice, education, and administration provides a better understanding of relationships and allows us to view the world from a broader perspective. Lynaugh (1996) explained "history yields self-knowledge by structuring a mind capable of imagining life beyond one's own life-span" (p. 1). Applying a historical methodology creates a synergy among the past, present, and future.

This chapter highlights how researchers in nursing practice, education, and administration apply historical methodology to understand patterns of our past and interpret those patterns to gain a better understanding of the current and future world. Included in the chapter are three critiques of historical research articles in the areas of practice, education, and administration. Based on criteria developed from the material discussed in Chapter 11, guidelines were created for critiquing historical research (Box 12.1). A reprint of the Brush and Capezuti (2001) article, "Historical Analysis of Siderail Use in American Hospitals" appears at the end of the chapter to help readers understand the critiquing process. Table 12.1 offers a sampling of selected historical research publications.

CRITIQUE GUIDELINES

To critique historical research, historiographers need to understand what is expected in the process. This section reviews the essential components of doing historical research and suggests questions researchers might ask when using this design. Researchers may use these same questions—which have been applied to the three critiques in this chapter—to evaluate historical research.

Historiographers search for facts and evidence that will unveil the nature and relationships regarding historic events, ideas, institutions, or people. To accurately assess historical meanings, researchers must assure readers of external validity that confirms that the source is what it claims. Simultaneously, researchers must establish the internal validity of the source, verifying the consistency between the genuineness of the primary source and the authenticity of the data. Historiographers may use a framework that helps to organize ideas and makes connections and, simultaneously, acknowledges personal and ideologic bias. To interpret the mate-

Box 12.1	GUIDELINES FOR CRITIQUING HISTORICAL RESEARCH

DATA GENERATION

Title

1. How does it concisely reflect the purpose of the study?
2. How does it clearly tell readers what the study is about?
3. How does it delineate the time frame for the study?

Statement of the Subject

1. Is the subject easily researched?
2. What themes and theses are studied?
3. What are the research questions?

Literature Review

1. What are the main works written on the subject?
2. What time period does the literature review cover?
3. What are some of the problems that may arise when studying this subject?
4. What primary sources can be identified?
5. How was the subject narrowed during the literature review?
6. What research questions were raised during the literature review?

DATA TREATMENT

Primary Sources

1. How were primary sources used?
2. Were they genuine and authentic?
3. How was external validity determined?
4. How was internal validity determined?
5. Were there inconsistencies between the external validity and internal validity?
6. Does the content accurately reflect the period of concern?
7. Do the facts conflict with historical dates, meanings of words, and social mores?
8. When did the primary author write the account?
9. Did a trained historian or an observer write the source?
10. Were facts suppressed, and, if so, why?
11. Is there corroborating evidence?
12. Identify any disagreements between sources.

(continued)

Box 12.1   GUIDELINES FOR CRITIQUING HISTORICAL RESEARCH (CONTINUED)

Secondary Sources

1. What were the secondary sources used?
2. How were secondary sources used?
3. Do they corroborate the primary source?
4. Can you identify any disagreements between sources?

DATA ANALYSIS

Organization

1. What conceptual frameworks were used in the study?
2. How would the study be classified: e.g., intellectual, feminist, social, political, biographic?
3. Were the research questions answered?
4. Was the purpose of the study accomplished?
5. If conflict exists within the findings, was there supporting evidence to justify either side of the argument?

Bias

1. Was the researcher's bias identified?
2. Was analysis influenced by a present-mindedness?
3. What were the ideologic biases?
4. How did bias affect data analysis?

Ethical Issues

1. Was there any infringement on a historical reputation?
2. Was there a conflict between the right to privacy versus the right to know?
3. Did the research show that decisions, events, and activities of an individual or organization affected the public welfare or embraced qualities of major human interest?

INTERPRETING THE FINDINGS

Narrative

1. Does the story describe what happened, including how and why it happened?
2. Were relationships among events, ideas, people, organizations, and institutions explained, interpreted, and placed within a contextual framework?
3. How were direct quotations used? (Too limited or too long?)
4. Was the narrative clear, concise, and interesting to read?
5. Was the significance to nursing explicit?

rial and to make sense of the data as the story unfolds, researchers must possess clear narrative and explanatory skills.

Accuracy is extremely important to historiographers. The systems that researchers develop will help them maintain accuracy. How researchers collect data, organize the bibliography, and number the different drafts of the narrative assists in the accurate accounting of the story. Historiographers must organize the data and tell the story in a logical fashion. Furthermore, researchers must honestly address questions that arise from the data, trying to understand and explain what the data are describing. Researchers must be prepared to answer questions such as, Did an event noted in a source actually happen? Could it have happened as it was noted in the primary source? Throughout the study, historiographers must be true to the data, allowing them to unfold and bring a better understanding of the subject. This process requires researchers to be aware of their own bias and degree of honesty in relationship to the findings. Does their own bias hinder discovery of new meanings that may be revealed? Essential to the historical method is imagination. Imagination lets researchers make connections in the data and create a story that assists in learning more of the truth (Barzun & Graff, 1985).

According to Spieseke (1953), historical researchers must be able to locate and collect data, analyze the reliability of the data, organize and arrange the data into a pattern, and express "it [the data] in meaningful and effective language" (p. 37). The narrative should show the successful attainment of these important skills, thus providing a method to evaluate the process. The narrative not only tells the story but also allows researchers (and others) to critique the study.

Box 12.1 organizes the data presented in Chapter 11 and suggests criteria to use when critiquing historical research. The criteria were used to critique published studies in the areas of nursing practice, education, and administration; these studies are presented later in the chapter. However, because published historical research should read as an interesting narrative, analysis using a specific instrument such as Box 12.1 might be inhibiting. Reviewers need to know that such an instrument is just a guide—not an absolute rule. Headings in a published article may not clearly delineate primary or secondary sources or personal bias (as perhaps they might in a historical dissertation or in other forms of reported research). Nevertheless, used as a guide, Box 12.1 highlights important features of historical research and helps consumers critique its worth more effectively.

An answer to the question, What comes first: The chicken or the egg?, epitomizes the dilemma in deciding whether to use the historical method first or to let the area of interest guide the decision regarding choice of method. Why select historical method in nursing practice, education, or administration when so many other methods are available to researchers? The research questions or conflicts that need historical explication determine the selection of method. Armed with the appropriate tools, historical researchers venture into these areas and formulate specific questions. Following the selection of the subject, researchers must narrow the topic to enable them to study the area in depth. To build a body of knowledge requires teamwork or the linkage of several historical studies that eventually will fill gaps and offer a fuller understanding of history (Bloch, 1964). Historians probe historical antecedents in broad areas of nursing such as practice, education, and administration to explain relationships, ideas, or events that influenced nursing's professional development. A review of previous studies helps researchers determine their own course of study and stimulates imagination. Table 12.1 offers a sampling of historical research studies.

APPLICATION TO PRACTICE

During the early modern nursing movement, nursing education and nursing practice were so closely related that studying one often meant studying the other. During the late 19th century and well into the 20th century, hospitals relied heavily on student nurses to provide patient care. Changes in the traditional, apprenticeship educational model and the move to university-based educational settings dramatically and economically altered the delivery of care in hospitals and nursing practice. Before these changes, graduate nurses, on completing their training, were rarely hired to staff hospitals and were forced to look elsewhere for jobs. They worked outside of hospitals as private duty and public health nurses.

In 1928, Wolf (1991) addressed the National League of Nursing Education (now known as the National League for Nursing [NLN]) regarding the transition of graduate nurses employed by hospitals. Wolf explained how graduate nurses who provided client care—as opposed to student nurses—would be advantageous to hospital administrators, nursing educators, and to the graduate nurses. Aside from stabilizing nursing service, providing an excellent service, and profiting the employer and employee, Wolf argued that hiring graduate nurses would improve the value society placed on nursing service. Wolf believed that graduate nurses faced undue criticism from hospital administrators, who believed that student nurses were more "buoyant, resilient, and enthusiastic" (Wolf, 1991, p. 140) than graduates. Yet, Wolf argued that "the graduate nurse sees more to be done for a patient than a student, she knows better what to do" (p. 140).

Wolf's (1991) speech provides historians with a perspective of someone personally involved in the changes in nursing practice history that had profound effects on the shape of things to come. Historical research in the development of nursing practice might examine nursing practice in hospitals, private duty, or public health. External factors such as wars, economic depressions, and advances in medicine and science affected the development of the nursing profession and created an infinite number of ways to approach the study of nursing practice. Researchers can find primary and secondary sources in published nursing textbooks, hospital manuals, speeches presented at various professional meetings, minutes of professional meetings, and graduation addresses. Archives of hospitals, schools of nursing, and visiting nurse services contain data that tell the story of nursing practice.

Discussions in the literature that have defined nurses' roles, specialization, and society's value of care find their origins in history. Bullough (1992) explained that "clinical specialization started in the early 20th century as nurses with advanced

TABLE 12.1	SELECTIVE SAMPLING OF HISTORICAL RESEARCH STUDIES	
Author/Date	**Title**	**Findings**
Biedermann, Usher, Williams, & Hayes (2001)	The wartime experience of Australian Army nurses in Vietnam, 1967–1971	Most of the Australian nurses sent to Vietnam had no idea of the work that they were to do or the conditions under which they would do it. They were clinically unprepared for what they had to do. The expectation was that because they were nurses, they could do the work. The study revealed that the nurses did adapt professionally and are affected by their memories of the work they did there.
Brown, Nolan, & Crawford (2000)	Men in nursing: Ambivalence in care, gender, and masculinity	Men in nursing have experienced the outcomes of a profession that was "feminized" during the nineteenth century. As a result of Florence Nightingale's strong influence on nursing, the mid-nineteenth century saw nursing undergo a change. Nursing, once a masculine endeavor, changed to being seen as solely female. Nursing in the United States followed Nightingale's model and became more feminized and controlled by women. The authors use an oral history approach to study the issue of how two men between the 1940s and 1970s describe their experiences in nursing. Both men identified changes in nursing from moving away from "institutional hierarchies towards a more patient-centered model."
Carter (2001)	Trumpets of attack: Collaborative efforts between nursing and philanthropies to care for children crippled with polio 1930 to 1959	Strong community support for nurses' work with polio led to them being able to attract foundations' support of the care of child polio victims. The support they received resulted in increased employment and educational opportunities "primarily for white nurses." "Middle and upper class fear of polio enabled the development of powerful and successful private organizations to supplement the available government services" (p. 253).

TABLE 12.1	SELECTIVE SAMPLING OF HISTORICAL RESEARCH STUDIES (CONTINUED)	
Author/Date	**Title**	**Findings**
D'Antonio (2001)	Founding friends: Families and institution building in early 19th century Philadelphia	This study examines the historical roots of the relationship between families, clinicians, and health care institutions, specifically the Friends Asylum in Philadelphia. Families "presented clinicians not just with dilemmas, but with solutions that carried substantial cultural weight" (p. 260). The study suggests that "theoretical innovations in healthcare might draw from the transformations in normative rules about domestic, work, and social rules" (p. 260).
Fairman (2000)	Economically practical and critically necessary?	Fairman examines the opening in 1954 of the intensive care unit at Chestnut Hill Hospital, a small community hospital in Pennsylvania. The paper examines the context in which the intensive care unit developed and the interplay among the many factors that led to its opening. The hospital chose this strategy among several others to care for the critically ill patient. The analysis provides the reader with "a glimpse of the foundation of contemporary dilemmas surrounding this most expensive form of hospital care, as the meaning and substance of intensive care changed over time for its multiple participants" (p. 81).
Fairman & Mahon (2001)	Oral history of Florence Downs	This study looks specifically at one individual, Florence Downs, and her career. "Several strands emerged that defined Downs' extended career, including the importance of developing a community of scholars both in and outside of nursing, the dangers of parochialism, and the necessity of a perspective on life that melded a keen sense of humor." Factors that affected Downs' style and choice, especially her mother, and her educational experiences, were revealed.

(continued)

TABLE 12.1	SELECTIVE SAMPLING OF HISTORICAL RESEARCH STUDIES (CONTINUED)	
Author/Date	**Title**	**Findings**
Robbins (2001)	The tuberculosis nurses' debate	This study presents the debate about the nursing care and treatment of people with tuberculosis between 1908 and 1914. The debate addressed familiar issues to the public health worker today such as "defining goals, evaluating success and failure, weighing the needs and rights of individual patients against those of the public at risk" (p. 36).
Rosenfeld (2001)	From the Lower East Side to the Upper Galilee: The pioneering experiences of Sara Bodek Paltiel, 1909–1993	Rosenfeld examines the unique experiences of Sara Bodek Paltiel, considered the first American to graduate from the Hadassah School of Nursing in Israel. Raised in a middle-class Jewish family, Paltiel studied nursing in Israel between 1933 and 1936. She remained in Israel and became one of the pioneering nurses working in the developing country. Rosenfeld writes that "Paltiel's pioneering spirit was equaled by her devotion to nursing, health care, and social justice" (p. 156). She concludes by noting that "one is struck by the singular track Paltiel follows. At every fork in the road of life, she chooses the less traveled road. Confident in her belief in Zion and armed with her nursing skills, she chose to stay 'behind the scenes' and actively worked to transform her idealism to the reality we now share" (p. 157).
Ryder (2000)	Nursing reorganization in occupied Japan, 1945–1951	This study describes the reorganization of professional nursing in occupied Japan following World War II. The change in nursing education and practice initiated by the American government took place within a 6-year time period. As a result of the Japanese "social, economic, and cultural climate," nursing in Japan prior to World War II did not share in the educational and service developments with nursing in the United States. The successful introduction of the ideas about nursing education and service led to the growth of nursing schools and better practice, but it also

TABLE 12.1	SELECTIVE SAMPLING OF HISTORICAL RESEARCH STUDIES (CONTINUED)	
Author/Date	**Title**	**Findings**
		served as the foundation for contemporary nursing concerns in Japan: Nursing remains more a vocation than a profession because nurses are mostly educated in certificate programs rather than university programs; and the remains of the rigid and bureaucratic systems established during the American occupation have led to the inefficient "handling of problems" in nursing.
Wall (2001)	Definite lines of influence	Wall tells the story of how Catholic sisters adapted their approach to nursing to bring it in line with societal expectations for training both religious and lay women. "This legitimized their nursing practice and enhanced their influence with students, physicians and hospital groups" (p. 314). As the sisters admitted lay women, they moved toward professional standards and placed their mark on their distinct understanding of nursing in a secular society.

knowledge and training were needed to care for groups of patients with special needs" (p. 254). Specialties emerged in nursing such as nurse-anesthetist, nurse-midwifery, public health nursing, and critical care nursing that demanded additional education, practical experience, and, in some instances, certification. Unanswered questions about the development of different specialties and the needed qualifications for each lend themselves to historical inquiry.

Critique of a Study in Practice

In this well-written historical study, Brush and Capezuti (2001) examine the evolution of the use of bed siderails in hospitals in their work titled, "Historical Analysis of Siderail Use in American Hospitals." The title clearly reflects the purpose of the study but does not give the reader a timeframe. Instead, Brush and Capezuti inform the reader immediately in the statement of the subject that the use of siderails during the 20th century will be reviewed. In the opening of the paper, the authors explain the relevance of analyzing the use of siderails in American hospitals. Given that raising of bed siderails "remains the most frequently used intervention to prevent bed-related falls and injuries" (Brush & Capezuti, 2001, p. 381), it is necessary to understand the evolution of this intervention in order to appreciate why new practice models are not readily adopted even when data support their validity. The authors present their argument that the use of siderails in practice has been "based more on a gradual consensus between law and medicine than on empirical evidence for nursing practice" (p. 381). This gives the reader the researcher's rationale for undertaking this historical inquiry into nursing practice and provides the framework for exploration of the factors that influenced the use of this nursing intervention.

Brush and Capezuti (2001) used a "social historical research method" (p. 381) to analyze data. A *social historical* method guided the historical investigation toward the examination of the patterns of siderail use as well as the perceived value of this safety intervention. The treatment of data was presented in the opening part of the paper to help the reader understand the authors' bias, framework, and organization of the material. A variety of primary sources were used including "medical trade catalogs, hospital procedure manuals, newsletters, photographs, and other archival materials" (p. 381). The authors identified three different archives from which data were obtained as well as included a list of other source material. Materials about bed design, such as journal articles, government documents, published histories, and textbooks in nursing and medicine, provided additional documentation. Secondary sources were not specifically reported; however, some of the sources identified could have been used as both primary and secondary sources. Assurances of the authenticity and the genuineness of data were not provided by the authors, nor is it usually addressed in published research articles. However, the wide variety of resources allows the reader to assume the external validity criterion was established. The varying types of data studied, including textbooks, manuals, and photographs, reflected the period represented in the study.

Brush and Capezuti (2001) begin their paper with Isabel Adams Hampton in 1893, thus leading the reader to consider nursing just prior to the beginning of the 20th century. An individual not familiar with the modern nursing movement or with the social history of nursing at that time becomes quickly acquainted with the meaning of caring for patients and the use of beds on a hospital unit in the 1890s. This lets the reader understand that period of time (1890s) in perspective and avoids the interpretation of the use of beds from a present-minded point of view.

The authors organized the paper using distinct headings to delineate different sections. The social historical method provided a way to look at the material that was identified in the heading titles. For example, the title "Rendering the Obstinate Docile" (Brush & Capezuti, 2001, p. 382) demonstrated the role nurses played in hospital safety and what the standard of "good" nursing practice included. This allows the reader to better understand the data and their subsequent relevance in the analysis presented in the final section, "Implications for Current Practice" (p. 382)

In the telling of the historical narrative, the authors also used a chronologic approach. The 1890s ideal bed and its dimensions set the stage for later adaptations because of changes in the way hospitals viewed patient safety and comfort, changes in staffing numbers, institutional liability, and legal issues pertaining to safety. Use of medical and nursing textbooks, medical studies, and legal cases throughout the 20th century provided the data that supported the narrative. Ethical issues did not present themselves in the use of the data, and thus were not addressed. The researchers avoided a present-mindedness when they interpreted the data by framing their findings within the context of the period they described. In the 1950s when the authors noted that the use of siderails became linked to the issue of institutional liability, they explained this finding using social, political, and legal influences from that same time period. Factors that influenced the use of siderails included changes in state laws, resulting in modification of the charitable hospital liability, a post-World War II nursing shortage that created an inability to observe patients as closely as in earlier times, as well as changes in bed manufacturers' interest in patient safety.

The narrative highlights connections between research from the different periods and social, political, and legal factors. Brush and Capezuti (2001) noted, for example, how in the 1980s and 1990s, the use of siderails continued even when the research showed the positive relationships between patient mobility and healing. Analysis of the data allowed the authors to provide the readers with some important implications regarding this issue in nursing practice. By using studies from the 1990s and 2000s, especially the guidelines issued by the Health Care Finance Administration (HCFA) that were designed to "deter health care providers from routinely using siderails" (Brush & Capezuti, 2001, p. 384), the authors contrasted the long-held belief about siderail use with the idea that other interventions, such as patient assessment, might be more appropriate in practice.

The historical analysis allowed the authors to observe how beliefs about siderails came into use, how they changed over time, and how the need for more research in the area of siderail use is essential to make changes in patient care. The final words of the authors calling for the use of "empirical outcomes rather than untested consensus" highlights the significance of the study to nursing and supports their beliefs (or bias) that research must guide nursing practice.

APPLICATION TO EDUCATION

Researchers interested in nursing education are concerned with varied aspects of this subject, such as an analysis of nursing texts (Davis, 1988b), the entry into practice dilemma (Leighow, 1996), the history of accreditation in Canada (Richardson, 1996), the development of university education in nursing (Baer, 1992), or the biography of an important figure in nursing education (Downer, 1989). Using historic frameworks, researchers may address topics in nursing education ranging from curriculum design to control of education. This approach not only provides background descriptive information but answers relevant questions regarding issues that concern nursing today.

Currently, topics such as adult learners, critical thinking, and cultural diversity concern nursing educators. However, historians may question whether the concept of adult learners is a new idea in nursing education and may attempt to understand this topic by studying nursing students of the past. Historians may examine past records of nurse training schools or professional studies of nursing. For example, the 1923 Goldmark (1923/1984) study *Nursing and Nursing Education in the United States* indicated that, in 1911, about 70% of the training schools required students to be aged 20 or 21 years old for admission; however, within 7 years, the age requirement had dropped to ages 18 or 19 years. Why did the admission age drop at that time and why did training schools initially believe older women would be better training school candidates? What teaching strategies worked better with older women than with younger ones? Both questions address the past and yet relate to current, pertinent issues related to adult learners.

Another contemporary issue, encouraging critical thinking among nursing students, has its roots in nursing's history. For example, in 1897, Superintendent of Bellevue Training School [Agnes] Brennan addressed the Superintendent's Society: "An uneducated woman may become a good nurse, but never an intelligent one; she can obey orders conscientiously and understand thoroughly a sick person's need, but should an emergency arise, where is she? She works through her feelings, and therefore lacks judgment" (Brennan, 1991, p. 23). Was Brennan referring to critical thinking when she reasoned that nurses needed to have the knowledge and theory regarding pathology to understand the appropriate care of sick people? Brennan suggested it was equally important for nurses to spend time in clinical practice learning the "character of the pulse in different patients or finding out just why some nurses can always see at a glance that this patient requires her pillow turned" (p. 24). She firmly believed that a trained nurse required both theoretical and practical knowledge and that, without both, something would be missing in the nursing care provided. As she pointed out, "Theory fortifies the practical, practice strengthens and retains the theoretical" (p. 25). Brennan discussed clearly her views on the theory-practice dichotomy that still baffles nursing educators today. However, Brennan firmly believed that nurses must be educated to think so they may practice.

Historiography has addressed the contemporary issue of cultural diversity by studying racial tensions in nursing and in society and offering researchers a better understanding of the inherent conflicts. Historians may question, Was there cultural diversity in nursing? From where did the nursing student at the beginning of the 19th century come? What socioeconomic-political background did the student bring to nursing? In the book *Black Women in White: Racial Conflict and Cooperation in the Nursing Profession, 1890–1950*, Hine (1989) described the opening of nurse training schools for African Americans who had been excluded from most of the existing U.S. nurse training schools. Of the schools that did not racially discriminate, many admitted African Americans using quotas. The very origin of the National Association of Colored Graduate Nurses (NACGN) in 1908 speaks to the early exclusion of African Americans from the first two national nursing organizations: American Society of Superintendents of Training Schools for Nurses (renamed the National League of Nursing Education in 1912) and the Associated Alumnae of the United States and Canada (renamed the American Nurses Association [ANA] in 1911). Historians need to look at what was, as well as what was not, to better understand historic events. For example, How did nursing handle cultural diversity? When did the profession welcome people of a different race, color, and creed into the profession? Who were the advocates of an integrated society?

Historians who search for answers may learn that nursing political activist Lavinia Dock spoke out against prejudicial treatment of any professional nurse. Dock (1910) cited the need for nursing to demonstrate practical ethics and ardently hoped that the nursing association (ANA) would not ever "get to the point where it draws the color line against our negro sister nurses" (p. 902). She believed that the nursing association was one place in the United States where color boundaries were not drawn. However, as the ANA expanded, Dock witnessed evidences that made her remark "that this cruel and unchristian and unethical prejudice might creep in here in our association" (p. 902). Dock said that under no circumstances should nurses emulate the cruel prejudices displayed by "men" and urged nurses to treat each nurse of color "as we would like to be treated ourselves" (p. 902). She supported black nursing leader Adah Thomas, who became president of the NACGN and a politically active nursing leader who, in 1929, wrote the history of African American nurses in the book *The Pathfinders* (Davis, 1988a).

Questions that arose from conflicting ideas in the data and the omission of information in the narrative suggest new areas for historic inquiry. An example is Mosley's (1992) historical doctoral dissertation "A History of Black Leaders in Nursing: The Influence of Four Black Community Nurses on the Establishment, Growth, and Practice of Public Health Nursing in New York City, 1900–1930." Mosley included a section specifically addressing institutional racism as it existed in nursing during the first 30 years of the 20th century. To understand the prejudice experienced by African American nurses, Mosley focused on the lives and contributions of four leaders in public health nursing: Jessie Sleet Scales, Mabel Staupers, Elizabeth W. Tyler, and Edith M. Carter.

Critique of a Study in Education

In "An Experiment in Leadership: The Rise of Student Government at Philadelphia General Hospital Training School, 1920–1930," Egenes (1998) examines the successful initiation of a student government at the Philadelphia General Hospital Training School (PGH) between 1920 and 1930. The title clearly informs readers of the time frame and subject. Although the researcher has not specifically identified primary and secondary sources in the article, Egenes does use and clearly reference them throughout the text. For example, some of the primary sources include periodicals of the period such as *The National Hospital Record* and *The American Journal of Nursing*; reports such as the *Annual Report of the Bureau of Charities of the City of Philadelphia for the Year Ending December 31, 1919*, located in the Center for the Study of the History of Nursing; and archival material from the PGH collection and minutes of PGH Student Government Association student council meetings. Secondary sources that support the narrative include historiographies by researchers such as Kalisch and Kalisch (1986), Rosenberg (1992), and Reverby (1987). Egenes uses the historians' work to provide the contextual setting for the article, and references them appropriately. For example, Reverby's (1987) work explained how women in the 1920s had more opportunities available to them other than nursing. Jobs with considerably shorter working hours, less of the perceived drudgery, and more independence competed with careers in nursing. Egenes uses Reverby's account to explain the social context of the 1920s and its effect on recruitment of educated middle-class women into nursing. Egenes examines the establishment of self-government at PGH as a way of inducting new recruits into the profession.

The opening paragraph of Egenes's (1998) study clearly presents the purpose of the study. Despite the perceived notion that the period under study was "considered a time of little progress in nursing education" (p. 71), an experiment in reforming the authoritarian nature of training schools was under way. Egenes explains that nursing schools were under public scrutiny for the poor care of students' health. In 1906, the *Ladies Home Journal* published an account of how training schools failed to adequately nourish their nurses. Letters from nurse graduates of training schools who had undergone some of the hardships of training supported these allegations. Other articles also deplored the strict, authoritative, and militaristic-type training. Nursing leaders acknowledged and recognized this criticism as barriers to recruiting intelligent middle-class women into the ranks of the nursing profession. Egenes uses the important Rockefeller Foundation's Goldmark (1923/1984) report published in 1923 to support the need to reform nurse training. The researcher explains that the Committee for the Study of Nursing Education-the authors of the Goldmark report-called for the introduction of student government to "broaden the educational experience of training school students" (p. 72).

Egenes (1998) analyzes the data in the context of the prevailing social, political, and economic climate of the 1920s. To attract college-educated women into nursing during World War I, nursing leadership had initiated the Vassar Training Camp. The Vassar Training camp recruited college-educated women into nursing; the nurses received their preliminary training in 1918 at Vassar and their clinical experience at various hospital-based programs. By 1921, following the armistice, Vassar Training Camp students who had remained to complete their training met to discuss how to improve nurse training and attract other women like themselves into the profession. Egenes intersperses interesting comments from the graduates who identified the need for student government. Those women viewed student government as a means to improve morale, allow for self-expression, and recruit better students into nursing.

In addition to pointing out the nursing leadership who supported the notion of student government, Egenes (1998) also includes the ideas of opponents. Egenes explains that detractors of student government believed that "student input on nursing service issues was deemed inappropriate" (p. 74). Egenes introduces PGH by identifying the excellent reputation it held in the 1920s. PGH was considered a reputable and progressive training school: The Vassar Training Camp and the Army School of Nursing selected PGH to offer clinical courses and the Committee for the Study of Nursing Education selected PGH to serve as part of the sample for its study. PGH proved to be an excellent place to carry out an experiment in student government. In addition, the leadership of PGH under nursing leader S. Lillian Clayton furthered the chance for the successful implementation of a student government. Clayton argued for students' personal rights on several occasions and was not averse to identifying the poor living conditions and ways to improve them.

Egenes (1998) clearly sets the background for the experiment in student government at PGH. The story slowly unfolds and Egenes narrates it articulately. The researcher presents and appropriately documents several examples of student government outcomes. From the PGH Student Government Association student council meeting minutes, Egenes weaves a story that supports the success of such an association. Initially, the idea of such an association was considered "revolutionary and frightening" (p. 77); however, it eventually became part of the fabric of the school and served as a model for other schools. Committees were formed that addressed some of the problems students confronted at PGH, such as wearing collars that were too high on uniforms, or gaining access to late passes, or receiving "gentlemen callers." Activities increased over time to include students' varied concerns and interests, such as glee clubs, book review clubs, and basketball teams. In the 1930s, according to Egenes, the activities of PGH shifted from student government toward the organization of student activities.

The conclusion of the report contains several succinct comments that support PGH's move toward creating a more progressive environment for nursing education between 1920 and 1930. Having a viable student government at a nurse training school meant that students would have increased opportunities for learning; be able to develop leadership skills; be responsible for enforcing rules of the nurses' home (which would free administrators from that task); create an empowered student body; facilitate cooperation between faculty and students; and serve as an excellent place to learn organizational skills that the students could apply to their work in professional organizations. The school and its administrative leadership created the right environment for the experiment in student government. In contrast to the commonly held belief that most schools of nursing were considered to be "too insular and impermeable" (Egenes, 1998, p. 82) to outside forces, PGH stood as an excellent example of change brought on by progressive nursing education administrators. Egenes suggests that the experiment had a substantial effect on the development of nursing education, supporting this comment with the National League of Nursing Education 1937 publication of a revised curriculum, which encouraged nursing schools to form a student organization. The final sentence in Egenes's study, "The noble experiment of PGH promoted student development and fostered a more humane environment in hospital training schools" (p. 82), remains an important idea today. Schools of nursing, especially in the 1990s, could benefit from the promotion of student development and the fostering of a more humane educational environment.

APPLICATION TO ADMINISTRATION

By now, it should be clear to readers that doing historical research requires creativity. Researchers may select a topic of interest and study it using different approaches. Studying the history of nursing organizations founded by nursing leaders provides researchers with a fertile field of study. An example of a nursing administration research study is one on the beginnings of the NLN, an organization that epitomizes the efforts of nurse-administrators to organize and control nursing education and practice (Birnbach & Lewenson, 1991). The NLN began in 1893 when a group of nursing superintendents in charge of nurse training schools met in Chicago at the Canada and Columbian Exposition. Superintendents throughout the United States met and founded the American Society of Superintendents of Training Schools for Nurses. In 1912, this organization became the National League of Nursing Education, and, in 1952, became the NLN. Superintendents started this organization so they could collectively address the issues confronting the developing profession. They advocated reforms such as improving educational standards, developing uniform training school curricula, decreasing working hours, and increasing the number of years of training. Through their efforts, the organization developed needed educational reforms in nursing and fostered the control of practice.

To study nursing administration, researchers might use biographies of nursing leaders. A biography offers insight into the characteristics of people as well as their role. Biographies of leaders before the modern nursing movement, such as the one done by Griffon (1998) on Mary Seacole, give a different perspective on women who contributed to establishing independent practice and setting the stage for future nurses. A biography need not be limited to one person but may compare and contrast the relationships among a group of leaders, such as the study by Poslusny (1989): "Feminist Friendship: Isabel Hampton Robb, Lavinia Lloyd Dock, and Mary Adelaide Nutting." The following section explores the reasons why nurses continued to work in hospitals following World War II (WWII) despite staffing shortages, long hours, low wages, and continued devaluing of their role. This study is used in this section because of the value it has for nurse administrators currently addressing the nursing shortage in health care in the twenty-first century.

Critique of a Study in Administration

In the paper, "A Hard Day's Work: Institutional Nursing in Post-World War II Era," Grando (2000) described the working conditions of nurses following WWII and their reaction to the conditions in which they worked. The title alerts the reader to the difficulty that nurses faced while working in hospitals and identifies the period following WWII as the focus of study. Grando narrows the time period further in the text where she refers to the years between the 1940s and 1950s as a period in which she studied nurses' responses to working conditions. Grando frames nurses' responses to working in institutions within the broader context of "women's lives and work patterns in the 1940s and 1950s" (p. 169). This helps the reader understand how the subject will be approached and understood in the period under review.

Rich in primary and secondary sources, Grando's study (2000) draws data from published articles and letters to the editor in nursing journals such as the *American Journal of Nursing* (AJN), United States census data, statistics from the Department of Labor, and nursing reports such as the Brown report to demonstrate the working conditions nurses found in hospitals following WWII. She culls the data for reactions nurses had to the overwork, underpay, and unfair labor practices. The context of the period is enriched by the data gathered from secondary sources such as Paul Starr's book *The Social Transformation of American Medicine* and Betty Friedan's *The Feminine Mystique*. Grando does not delineate the primary from secondary sources in the text, yet the reader can see in the list of references the wealth of sources that support the narrative.

Grando (2000) presents the study in an interesting style using direct quotes from many of the primary sources to provide the reader with vivid firsthand recollections of nurses' work and their individual responses to the conditions in which they practiced. The reader is privy to the feelings reflected by nurses in letters to the editor. Some of the letters noted the dismay they felt at the overwork expected of them, while others wrote about how they felt rewarded by a patient's recovery. The analysis of the data showed that, "nurses for the most part accepted the prevailing views of both the larger culture and the hospital culture" (p. 179). Nurses responded to the nursing shortage, worked regardless of the unpleasant working conditions, and "just like other women of the period, did what was expected of them" (p. 179). Grando also noted that while nurses continued to work in hospitals, they also organized to change the conditions in which they worked by establishing the American Nurses Association's Economic Security Program. Grando believed organizing this group was a very proactive when most women "did what was expected of them" (p. 179).

REFERENCES

Annual Report of the Bureau of Charities of the City of Philadelphia for the year ending December 1919. (1920). Philadelphia: City of Philadelphia 9–19. Center for the Study of the History of Nursing, School of Nursing. University of Pennsylvania (hereafter cited as CNHN) Accession #1993–14.

Baer, E. (1992). Aspirations unattained: The story of the Illinois Training School's search for university status. *Nursing Research, 41*(1), 43–48.

Baly, M. (1986). *Florence Nightingale and the nursing legacy*. London: Croom Helm.

Barzun, J., & Graff, H. F. (1985). *The modern researcher* (4th ed.). San Diego, CA: Harcourt Brace Jovanovich.

Biedermann, N., Usher, K., Williams, A. & Hayes, B. (2001). The wartime experiences of Australian Army nurses in Vietnam. *Journal of Advanced Nursing, 35*(4), 543–549.

Birnbach, N., & Lewenson, S. (Eds.). (1991). *First words: Selected addresses from the National League for Nursing 1894–1933*. New York: National League for Nursing Press.

Brennan, A. (1991). Comparative value of theory and practice in nursing. In N. Birnbach & S. Lewenson (Eds.), *First words: Selected addresses from the National League for Nursing 1894–1933* (pp. 23–25). New York: National League for Nursing Press. (Original speech presented in 1897.)

Bloch, M. (1964). *The historian's craft*. New York: Vantage Books.

Brown, B., Nolan, P., & Crawford, P. (2000). Men in nursing: Ambivalence in care, gender, and masculinity. *International History of Nursing Journal, 5*(3),4–13.

Brush, B. L., & Capezuti, E. (2001). Historical analysis of siderail use in American hospitals. *Journal of Nursing Scholarship, 33*(4), 381–385.

Bullough, B. (1992). Alternative models for specialty nursing practice. *Nursing and Health Care, 13*(5), 254–259.

Care, D., Gregory, D., English, J., & Venkatesh, P. (1996). A struggle for equality: Resistance to commissioning of male nurses in the Canadian military, 1952–1967. *Canadian Journal of Nursing Research, 28*(1), 103–117.

Carter, K. F. (2001). Trumpets of attack: Collaborative efforts between nursing and philanthropies to care for the child crippled with polio 1930–1959. *Public Health Nursing, 18*(4), 253–261.

D'Antonio, P. (2001). Founding Friends: Families and institution building in early 19th century Philadelphia. *Nursing Research, 50*(5), 260–266.

Davis, S. (1988a). Adah Belle Samuels Thomas. In V. Bullough, O. M. Church, & A. P. Stein (Eds.), *American nursing: A biographical dictionary* (pp. 313–316). New York: Garland.

Davis, S. (1988b). *Evolution of the American nursing history text: 1907–1983* (University Microfilm International Order No. PUZ8906485). New York: Columbia University, Teachers College.

Dock, L. (1910). Report of the thirteenth annual convention. *American Journal of Nursing, 10*(11), 902.

Downer, J. L. (1989). *Education for democracy: Isabel Stewart and her education, 1878–1963* (University Microfilm International Order No. PUZ9013541). New York: Columbia University, Teachers College.

Egenes, K. J. (1998). An experiment in leadership: The rise of student government at Philadelphia General Hospital Training School, 1920–1930. *Nursing History Review, 6*, 71–84.

Fairman, J. (2000). Economically practical and critically necessary? The development of intensive care at Chestnut Hill Hospital. *Bulletin of the History of Medicine, 74*, 80–106.

Fairman, J., & Mahon, M. M. (2001). Oral history of Florence Downs: The early years. *Nursing Research, 50*(5), 322–328.

Goldmark, J. (1984). *Nursing and nursing education in the United States.* New York: Garland. (Original work published 1923.)

Grando, V. (2000). A hard day's work: Institutional nursing in post WWII era. *Nursing History Review, 8*, 169–184.

Griffon, D. P. (1998). A somewhat duskier skin: Mary Seacole in the Crimea. *Nursing History Review, 6*, 115–127.

Hine, D. C. (1989). *Black women in white: Racial conflict and cooperation in the nursing profession, 1890–1950.* Bloomington: Indiana University Press.

Kalisch, P., & Kalisch, B. (1986). *The advance of American nursing* (2nd ed.). Boston: Little, Brown.

Leighow, S. R. (1996). Backrubs vs. Bach: Nursing and the entry-into-practice debate, 1946–1986. *Nursing History Review, 4*, 3–17.

Lynaugh, J. (1996). Editorial. *Nursing History Review, 4*, 1.

Mackintosh, C. (1997). A historical study of men in nursing. *Journal of Advanced Nursing, 26*, 232–236.

Mosley, M. O. P. (1992). A history of blacks in nursing: The influence of four black community health nurses on the establishment, growth, and practice of public health nursing in New York City, 1906–1930. (Doctoral dissertation, Columbia University, 1992).

Poslusny, S. (1989). Feminist friendship: Isabel Hampton Robb, Lavinia Lloyd Dock, and Mary Adelaide Nutting. *Image, 21*(2), 64–68.

Rendall, J. (1991). *Women in an industrializing society: England 1750–1880.* Oxford, England: Basil Blackwell.

Reverby, S. M. (1987). *Ordered to care: The dilemma of American nursing, 1850–1945.* New York: Cambridge University Press.

Richardson, S. (1996). The historical relationship of nursing program accreditation and public policy in Canada. *Nursing History Review, 4*, 19–41.

Robbins, J. M. (2001). The tuberculosis nurses' debate. *Nursing History Review, 9,* 35–50.

Rosenberg, C. (1992). *Explaining epidemics and other studies in the history of medicine.* New York: Cambridge University Press.

Rosenfeld, P. (2001). From the Lower East Side to the Upper Galilee: The pioneering experiences of Sara Bodek Paltiel, 1909–1993. *Nursing History Review, 9,* 141–158.

Ryder, R. S. (2000) Nursing reorganization in occupied Japan, 1945–1951. *Nursing History Review, 8,* 71–91.

Spieseke, A. W. (1953). What is the historical method of research? *Nursing Research, 2*(1), 36–37.

Wall, B. M. (2001). Definite lines of influence: Catholic sisters and nurse training schools. *Nursing Research, 50*(5), 314–321.

Wolf, A. (1991). How can general duty be made more attractive to graduate nurses? In N. Birnbach & S. Lewenson (Eds.), *First words: Selected addresses from the National League for Nursing, 1894–1933* (pp. 138–147). New York: National League for Nursing Press. (Original speech presented 1928.)

RESEARCH ARTICLE

Historical Analysis of Siderail Use in American Hospitals

Barbara L. Brush, Elizabeth Capezuti

Purpose: *To explore the social, economic, and legal influences on siderail use in 20th century American hospitals and how use of siderails became embedded in nursing practice.*
Design: *Social historical research.*
Methods: *Numerous primary and secondary sources were collected and interpreted to illustrate the pattern of siderail use, the value attached to siderails, and attitudes about using siderails.*
Findings: *The persistent use of siderails in American hospitals indicates a gradual consensus between law and medicine rather than an empirically driven nursing intervention. Use of siderails became embedded in nursing practice as nurses assumed increasing responsibility for their actions as institutional employees.*
Conclusions: *New federal guidelines, based on reports of adverse consequences associated with siderails, are limiting siderail use in hospitals and nursing homes across the United States. Lowering siderails and using alternatives will depend on new norms among health care providers, hospital administrators, bed manufacturers, insurers, attorneys, regulators, and patients and their families.*

Throughout most of the 20th century, the use of siderails as safeguards against patients' falls from hospital beds has spurred debate. Although researchers and practitioners have argued the merits and pitfalls of siderail use, few have explored how use of siderails evolved and gradually became embedded in nursing practice. Raising bed siderails remains the most frequently used intervention to prevent bed-related falls and injuries among hospitalized patients and institutionalized older adults (Capezuti, 2000; Capezuti & Braun, 2001).

Examining the social, economic, and legal influences on siderail use in 20th century American hospitals, we explored the centrality of the hospital bed to the mission and purpose of nursing and the shifting focus of bedside care from patient comfort to patient safety. We argue that use of siderails has been based more on a gradual consensus between law and medicine than on empirical evidence for nursing practice. Nevertheless, nurses, as hospital employees, adopted siderail use as part of their stan-

Barbara L. Brush, RN, PhD, CS, FAAN, Xi, Associate Professor, Boston College School of Nursing, Chestnut Hill, MA; Elizabeth Capezuti, RN, PhD, CS, FAAN, Xi, Associate Professor & Independence Foundation-Wesley Woods Chair of Gerontologic Nursing, Emory University School of Nursing, Atlanta, GA. This study was supported by a grant from the Xi Chapter of Sigma Theta Tau International. The authors thank Deborah J. Swedlow, MSS, MLSP, JD, Associate with Foley Hoag LLP in Boston, for assistance with obtaining and interpreting legal sources.

© 2001 Sigma Theta Tau International.

dard of bedside care (Barbee, 1957). Social historical research methods were used to collect and interpret data. Thus, the pattern of siderail use, the value attached to siderails as an example of benevolent care, and attitudes about raising siderails were examined as they evolved and shifted over time. Primary sources included medical trade catalogs, hospital procedure manuals, letters, photographs, and other archival materials from the New York Academy of Medicine, the College of Physicians in Philadelphia, and the Center for the Study of the History of Nursing at the University of Pennsylvania. Journal articles, government documents, published histories of hospital bed design, and nursing and medical texts provided additional sources of data.

THE HOSPITAL BED AS CENTRAL TO NURSING'S MISSION

In 1893, Isabel Adams Hampton made clear, in a chapter devoted entirely to hospital beds, that nurses were the overseers of beds and their occupants. As she put it, "A nurse who works over [beds] daily ought to be a fair judge of what is required in the way of a bed for the sick" (Hampton, 1893, p. 75). Hampton charged nurses to coordinate bed type to patient condition, maintain a neat and uniform bed appearance at all times, and ensure patient comfort during the period of recuperation.

In Hampton's day, the ideal bed was 6 feet 6 inches long, 37 inches wide, and 24–26 inches from the floor (Hampton, 1893). Although similar in length and width to standard twin beds in homes, hospital beds were approximately 6–8 inches higher to facilitate patient care and prevent unnecessary strain on nurses. Because beds were a fixed "nursing" height, stools were often used to accommodate patients as they transferred from bed.

Bed height, more than any other bed dimension, has consistently influenced bedside nursing care in American hospitals and long-term care facilities. Bed height and the outcomes of bed-related falls in hospitals have been the basic issues underlying numerous legislative and practice initiatives in the 20th century. Despite changes meant to remedy injurious outcomes from bed-related falls, however, patients falling from high beds are deemed at risk for increased morbidity and mortality (O'Keeffe, Jack, & Lye, 1996). Bed siderails, initially used as a temporary means to prevent confused, sedated, or elderly patients from falling from bed, are now permanent fixtures on most institutional beds (Braun & Capezuti, 2000; Capezuti & Braun, 2001). Their increased use in the latter half of the 20th century reflects a shifting emphasis from patient comfort to patient safety as hospitals, evolving from charitable institutions to modern medical centers, became increasingly subject to litigation (Stevens, 1989).

"Rendering the Obstinate Docile"

Bed siderails were rarely available on adult hospital beds until the 1930s. More common were cribs or children's beds equipped with full or partial crib sides, which, similar to siderails, were meant to protect infants and young children from falling from or leaving beds unattended. The primary intervention for agitated, confused, or other adults considered at risk of falling from bed was nurses' provision of "careful and continuous watchfulness" (Merck Manual, 1934, p. 36).

Haigh and Hayman's (1936) study of 116 "out of bed" incidents at the University Hospital of Cleveland, however, provided early evidence of siderail use to control adult patient behavior and prevent deleterious outcomes. The authors reported that in 31% of bed-related falls at the study institution, patients climbed over siderails, and an additional 7% removed a physical restraint and then proceeded over the rails before falling. Although siderails, as well as rails in combination with restraints, were ineffective in preventing falls or deterring patients from leaving beds unassisted, the nurse and physician authors concluded that siderails were a reasonable precautionary measure against falls from bed as well as necessary adjuncts in "rendering the obstinate docile" (Haigh & Hayman, 1936, p. 45).

When first used, siderails, also known as sideboards or side restraints, were not permanently fastened to hospital beds. Instead, they were accessories that nurses physically attached to beds when they deemed necessary or when prescribed by a physician (Tracy, 1942). Securing these devices was a time-consuming and cumbersome procedure that often required at least two people (Manley, 1944).

In the 1940s, siderail use on adult hospital beds gradually became the subject of legal action against personal injury and death. In 1941, for example, the parents of 21-year-old Edgar Pennington sued Morningside Hospital after their son fell from bed and sustained a fatal head injury (Morningside Hospital v. Pennington et al., 1941). When Mr. Pennington was initially hospitalized, his bed siderails were raised because of his irrational behavior. A few days later and presumably calmer, his side rails were removed and his left leg was chained to the bed instead. The plaintiffs argued that the nurses' failure to maintain side rails on their son's bed caused him to sustain his fatal fall. Whether his leg was still chained to the bed when he was found "with his bloody head on the concrete floor" was unsubstantiated. Ultimately, the case was dismissed.

A year earlier, the surviving husband of Jennie Brown Potter sued the Dr. W. H. Groves Latter-Day Saints Hospital for his wife's fall-related death, claiming that the hospital's failure to attach side boards to her bed constituted negligence. As in Morningside Hospital v. Pennington et al. (1941), the court ruled for the defendant, citing lack of evidence that standard of due care required the hospital to place sideboards on patients' beds (Potter et al. v. Dr. W.H. Groves, 1940).

The Nurse's Role in Hospital Safety

By the 1950s, siderail use became more visibly linked to institutional liability. Numerous factors contributed to this transition. First, many states adopted laws overturning charitable hospitals' immunity from the negligence of their employees, necessitating hospitals' purchase of expensive insurance policies (Hayt, Hayt, & Groeschel, 1952). Second, a severe post-war nursing shortage limited nurses' ability to provide previous levels of watchfulness over patients in their charge (Lynaugh & Brush, 1996). Finally, bed manufacturers expanded their focus in advertising to include patient safety along with patient comfort and rest. Consequently, institutional beds equipped with permanent full-length siderails became more readily available (Hospitals, 1954). Nurses raised siderails on patients' beds to reassure the public and hospital administrators that even if nurses were in short supply, at least patients were secure in their beds (Aberg, 1957; Barbee, 1957).

Ludham (1957) reinforced this notion in one of the first reported studies of hospital insurance claims involving bed incidents. In his study of 7,815 "out-of-bed" incidents in California hospitals, Ludham found that, although 63% (4,893) of reported incidents occurred when siderails were raised, claims paid by insurance companies increased ten fold when falls occurred in the absence of raised siderails. The imbalance in jury awards was largely attributed to the perception that raising siderails was a demonstrable effort, however unproved, to protect patients from falls and serious injury. With no supporting evidence, Ludham nonetheless echoed previous claims (Aston, 1955; Price, 1956) that out-of-bed incidents with raised siderails caused less severe injury because patients had something to grasp when falling. He recommended that hospitals establish standing orders or policies requiring siderail use with certain types of patients (e.g., sedated, confused, "older") as a national standard of hospital practice. Locally, the Council on Insurance of the California Hospital Association urged its hospitals to permanently attach siderails to every bed "as rapidly as possible" (Ludham, 1957, p. 47).

Professional journal articles and nursing texts also regularly encouraged nurses to use siderails as part of their therapeutic actions (Aberg, 1957; Harmer & Henderson, 1952; Price, 1954), especially because of the claim that "bedfalls, together with hot-water bottle burns account for more lawsuits involving nurses than all other risks combined" (Hayt, Hayt, Groeschel, & McMullan, 1958, p. 206). Although the standard hospital bed height was "not always comfortable to the patient (but) convenient for the nurse and the doctor" (Harmer & Henderson, 1952, p. 126), siderails, defined as restraints or restrictive devices, were advocated in the prevention of falls and injury from these high beds (Hayt, Hayt, & Groeschel, 1958; McCullough & Moffit, 1949; Price, 1954).

Meanwhile, bed manufacturers continued to sell to "safety-minded hospital administrators" (*Hospitals*, 1954, p. 197). The Hard Manufacturing Company's "Slida-Side" offered permanent siderails on every hospital bed, and the Inland Bed Company guaranteed portable siderails to "provide safety for your patients, protection for your hospital" (*Hospitals*, 1954, p. 197). Both the Hall Invalid Bed and the Simmons Vari-Hite bed could be manually lowered from the standard height of 27 inches to the "normal home bed height" of 18 inches (*Hospitals*, 1950). They were considered safer for two reasons: they eliminated the need for "slipping, tilting footstools" and they allowed patients to get up from a familiar bed height without calling for the nurse (*Hospitals*, 1950, pp. 87, 102). Thus, and most important, the Simmons Company reported, the Vari-Hite bed reduced "the likelihood of falling and serious injury" (*Hospitals*, 1950, p. 87).

The Hill-Rom Company also advertised its Hilow Beds as the pinnacle of modernization and fall prevention because the crank-operated bed could be lowered to 18 inches, making patients less likely to misjudge the distance to the floor, lose their balance, and fall (*Hospitals*, 1955). To make their point that lower beds eliminated the need for full siderails to prevent bed-related falls and injuries, advertisements depicted the Vari-Hite and Hall Invalid beds without siderails and the Hilow Bed with a half rail meant to assist patients to transfer independently.

Despite the availability of lower and variable height beds that eliminated the need for siderails, that were comfortable for patients, and increased nursing efficiency, fixed "nursing height" beds with permanent full-length siderails were used more regularly than were these new inventions (Smalley, 1956). The "common sense" notion that siderails were safety devices led to hospital-wide policies that standardized their use. Because nurses and hospital administrators failed to question siderail efficacy in preventing bedside falls, they also failed to use alternatives. Gradually, hospital-based nurses in the 1950s raised siderails to substitute for their physical presence at the bedside and to protect hospitals' legal interests.

The Standard of Good Nursing Practice

An escalating nurse shortage in the 1960s and 1970s, coupled with changes in hospital architecture from multi-patient wards to semiprivate and private patient rooms, prompted the continued use of siderails, as well as other physical restraints, as substitutes for nursing observation. By the 1980s, falls, especially from beds, were identified as a major hospital liability issue (Rubenstein, Miller, Postel, & Evans, 1983). In 1980 the National Association of Insurance Commissioners reported that falls represented 10% of all paid claims between 1975 and 1978; absence of siderails was identified as a principal justification. As a result, "routine use of bedrails" became "the standard of good nursing practice" (Rubenstein et al., 1983, p. 273).

As siderail use became common nursing practice, particularly to prevent falls among older patients, its scientific rationale was brought into question. Rubenstein and colleagues (1983) at Harvard Medical School labeled the continued use of siderails, in the absence of supporting data, an example of "defensive medicine" (p. 273). In other words, raising siderails was practice based on consensus rather than on scientific evidence. Based largely on legal action against hospitals and their personnel, siderail use became a means to promote patients' "right" to safety during hospitalization and nurses' "responsibility" to keep patients safe (Anonymous, 1984; Horty, 1973).

Shifting decisions about patient safety to nurses shifted liability from physicians to institutions. As a result, institutions took greater precautions to ensure that patients, especially the elderly, did not fall. Raising siderails for individuals deemed vulnerable to injury or death, in addition to using physical restraints for immobilization, reinforced the opinion that siderails and restraints were benevolent interventions (Cohen & Kruschwitz, 1997; Strumpf & Tomes, 1993). Although nurse attorney Jane Greenlaw found medication to be a major cause of negligence related to siderail use, she also noted the importance of a patient's mental state in determining liability. She noted, "Where it can be shown that a patient was senile, irrational, confused, or otherwise impaired, this can affect the hospital's duty to safeguard the patient" (Greenlaw, 1982, p. 125), and "Nursing responsibility to evaluate each person's safety and to act accordingly, regardless of whether the attending physician has done so" (Greenlaw, 1982, p. 127).

The nurse's duty to render independent judgment about siderail use was evident in the 1977 fall and injury case of John Wooten. Eighty-three-year-old Wooten suffered a severe head injury after falling at the Memphis, Tennessee Veterans Administration Hospital. During the evening, Wooten had risen from his bed unattended and walked a short distance before falling. Before the fall, Wooten's physician deemed him "stable" and gave an order for "bedrest with bedside commode and up in chair three times per day" (Anonymous, 1984, p. 4). Despite the physician's medical opinion, the U.S. District Court of Tennessee ruled that hospital personnel were negligent in caring for Wooten because his condition "mandated the use of siderails" (Anonymous, 1984, p. 4). The Court held that raised siderails was a reminder for patients to call nurses when they needed assistance to transfer from bed. Moreover, because Wooten was "older," he was at greater risk for confusion and disorientation. The Court awarded $80,000 in damages.

In 1981, 80-year-old Esther Polonsky was injured during her stay at Union Hospital in Lynn, Massachusetts, upon attempting to use the bathroom during the night. Several hours before the incident, the nurse had administered 15 milligrams of Dalmane to Polonsky to aid sleep. The Appeals Court of Massachusetts found that because the nurse failed to raise her bed siderails, a confused and disoriented Polonsky fell and fractured her right hip. She recovered $20,000 in damages (Regan, 1981).

While Polonsky's fall was directly linked to her medication, the case of Catherine Kadyszeski, like that of Wooten, illustrates the ageism often associated with siderail use (Tammelleo, 1995). Kadyszeski was 67 years old in 1985 when she fractured her left hip in a bathroom-related fall at New York's Ellis Hospital. Although heavily sedated with Demerol, Vistaril, and Phenobarbital, Kadyszeski did not win her claim on the basis of oversedation. Rather, the hospital was found negligent for failing to comply with its own rule that siderails be raised for all patients over age 65.

The continued use of siderails and restraints in the 1980s and 1990s sharply contrasted with new ideas about the importance of mobility during recuperation from acute illness or surgery (Allen, Glasziou, & Del Mar, 1999). The trend toward decreasing bedrest and increasing ambulation in hospitalized patients did not translate to the care of frail elders (Creditor, 1993; Sager et al., 1996). While younger patients' beds were equipped with half instead of full-length siderails to facilitate transfers, older patients continued to be immobilized in bed, in large part because nurses equated full siderail use with greater patient protection (Rubenstein et al., 1983). Even as negative consequences of immobilizing hospitalized elders, such as deconditioning, pressure ulcers, and pneumonia, were reported in the literature (Creditor, 1993; Hoenig & Rubenstein, 1991; Inouye et al., 1993; Sager et al., 1996), the use of siderails in this population did not abate.

IMPLICATIONS FOR CURRENT PRACTICE

Reports of siderail-related entrapment injuries and deaths over the past decade (Food and Drug Administration, 1995; Parker & Miles, 1997; Todd, Ruhl, & Gross, 1997) continue to challenge perceptions of siderails as safety devices. Many legal claims are now being won against hospitals for siderail misuse (Braun & Capezuti, 2000; Capezuti & Braun, 2001). The Health Care Finance Administration (HCFA) has issued surveyor guidelines redefining siderails as restraints when they impede the patient's desired movement or activity, such as getting out of bed (U.S. Department of Health & Human Services, 2000). The fundamental goal of these guidelines is to deter health care providers from routinely using siderails. Instead, they encourage a thorough assessment of patients' individualized needs and consideration of alternative interventions to siderail use (Capezuti et al., 1999; Capezuti, Talerico, Strumpf, & Evans, 1998). More broadly, the HCFA guidelines will likely influence siderail use by hospitals accredited through the Joint Commission on Accreditation of Healthcare Organizations (JCAHO). Because JCAHO must, at a minimum, meet applicable federal law and regulation, new standards, consistent with HCFA regulation, likely will be promulgated in the near future (Capezuti & Braun, 2001).

The acceptance and use of alternatives to siderails, however, will depend on a new consensus among health care providers, hospital administrators, bed manufacturers, insurers, attorneys, regulators, and patients and their families. To reach consensus, all parties need to understand how and why siderails became common practice in the first place and why, despite evidence to the contrary, they remain firmly entrenched as acceptable bedside care. Rethinking siderail use, especially with the elderly, will require new incentives for their discontinuation. The new guidelines by HCFA (U.S. Department of Health & Human Services, 2000) are a beginning step in this direction.

Bed manufacturers have also reintroduced adjustable low height beds, similar to the models first proposed in the 1950s. These "new" beds, as well as siderails with narrower rail gaps, will be on the market over the next few years. Financing the purchase of this equipment and retrofitting outdated bed systems will likely raise new concerns about siderail-related liability (Braun & Capezuti, 2000; Capezuti & Braun, 2001). Nurse researchers are in key positions to evaluate how legislative and manufacturing trends affect clinical outcomes.

Given the gradual evolution of siderail use in American hospitals, nurses can anticipate that attitudes and practices about use of siderails will not change quickly or easily. Changing views and practices of siderail use will require reinterpretation of nursing care standards and benevolent care. Given the evidence of these shifting ideas and practices now (Braun & Capezuti, 2000; Capezuti & Braun, 2001; Capezuti, 2000; Donius & Rader, 1994), new perceptions and habits will develop. Those changes should be based on empirical outcomes rather than on untested consensus.

Research article taken from: Brush, B.L., Capezuti, E. (2001). Historical analysis of siderail use in American hospitals. *Journal of Nursing Scholarship, 33*(4), 381–385. (Reprinted with permission.)

References

Aberg, H. L. (1957). The nurse's role in hospital safety. *Nursing Outlook, 5,* 160–162.
Allen, C., Glasziou, P., & Del Mar, C. (1999). Bed rest: A potentially harmful treatment needing more careful evaluation. *Lancet, 354,* 1229–1233.
Anonymous. (1984, February). Hospital policy re: "siderails" nurses' responsibility [Journal article]. *Regan Report on Nursing Law, 24,* 4.
Aston, C. S., Jr. (1955). Grasping bars means added safety. *Hospitals, 29,* 102–104.
Barbee, G. C. (1957). More about bedrails and the nurse. *American Journal of Nursing, 57,* 1441–1442.
Braun, J. A., & Capezuti, E. (2000). The legal and medical aspects of physical restraints and bed siderails and their relationship to falls and fall-related injuries in nursing homes. *DePaul Journal of Healthcare Law, 3,* 1–72.
Capezuti, E. (2000). Preventing falls and injuries while reducing siderail use. *Annals of Long-Term Care, 8*(6), 57–63.
Capezuti, E., Bourbonniere, M., Strumpf, N., & Maislin, G. (2000). Siderail use in a large urban medical center (Abstract). *The Gerontologist, 40*(Special Issue, 1), 117.
Capezuti, E., & Braun, J. A. (2001). Medicolegal aspects of hospital siderail use. *Ethics, Law, and Aging Review, 7,* 25–57.
Capezuti, E., Talerico, K. A., Cochran, I., Becker, H., Strumpf, N., & Evans, L. (1999). Individualized interventions to prevent bed-related falls and reduce siderail use. *Journal of Gerontological Nursing, 25,* 26–34.
Capezuti, E., Talerico, K. A., Strumpf, N., & Evans, L. (1998). Individualized assessment and intervention in bilateral siderail use. *Geriatric Nursing, 19*(6), 322–330.
Cohen, E. S., & Kruschwitz, A. L. (1997). Restraint reduction: Lessons from the asylum. *Journal of Ethics, Law, and Aging, 3,* 25–43.
Creditor, M. C. (1993). Hazards of hospitalization of the elderly. *Annals of Internal Medicine, 118,* 219–223.
Donius, M., & Rader, J. (1994). Use of siderails: Rethinking a standard of practice. *Journal of Gerontological Nursing, 20,* 23–27.
Food and Drug Administration. (1995, August 23). *FDA Safety Alert: Entrapment hazards with hospital bed side rails.* Rockville, MD: U.S. Dept. of Health and Human Services, Public Health Service, Center for Devices and Radiological Health.
Greenlaw, J. (1982, June). Failure to use siderails: When is it negligence? *Law, Medicine & Medicine,* 125–128.
Heigh, C., & Hayman, J. M., Jr. (1936). Why they fell out of bed. *The Modern Hospital, 47,* 45–46.
Hampton, I. A. (1893). *Nursing: Its principles and practice.* Philadelphia: WB Saunders.
Harmer, M., & Henderson, V. (1952). Textbook of the principles and practice of nursing. New York: Macmillan.
Hayt, E., Hayt, L. R., & Groeschel, A. H. (1952). *Law of hospital and nurse.* New York: Hospital Textbook Co.
Hayt, E., Hayt, L. R., Groeschel, A. H., & McMullan, D. (1958). *Law of hospital and nurse.* New York: Hospital Textbook Co.
Hoenig, H. M., & Rubenstein, L. Z. (1991). Hospital-associated deconditioning and dysfunction. *Journal of the American Geriatrics Society, 39,* 220–222.

Hospitals. (1950). Hall Invalid Bed; Simmons Vari-Hite [Advertisements]. *Hospitals, 24,* 86–87, 102.

Hospitals. (1954). Inland Bed Company; Hard Slida-Side [Advertisements]. *Hospitals, 28,* 19, 197.

Hospitals. (1955). Hill-Rom Hilow Beds [Advertisements]. *Hospitals, 29,* 161.

Horty, J. F. (1973). Hospital has duty to maintain premises, but employees have duty to be cautious. *Modern Hospital, 120,* 50.

Inouye, S. K., Wagner, D. R., Acampora, D., Horwitz, R. I., Cooney, L. M., Hurst, L. D., et al. (1993). A predictive index for functional decline in hospitalized elderly medical patients. *Journal of General Internal Medicine, 8,* 645–52.

Joint Commission on Healthcare Organizations (JCAHO). (1996). *Comprehensive accreditation manual for hospitals* (restraint and seclusion standards plus scoring: Standards TX7.1-TX7.1.3.3, 191–193). Oakbrook Terrace, IL: Author.

Ludham, J. E. (1957). Bedrails: Up or down? *Hospitals, 31,* 46–47.

Lynaugh, J. E., & Brush, B. L. (1996). *American nursing: From hospitals to health systems.* Cambridge, MA: Blackwell.

Manley, M. E., & The Committee on Nursing Standards, Division of Nursing, Department of Hospitals. (1944). Chapter VI: Preparation and care of beds. In *Standard Nursing Procedures of The Department of Hospitals City of New York* (pp. 109–125). New York: Macmillan.

Merck & Company (1934). *The Merck manual of therapeutics and materia medica* (6th edition.). Rahway, NJ: Author.

McCullough, W., & Moffit, M. (1949). *Illustrated handbook of simple nursing.* New York: McGraw-Hill.

Morningside Hospital & Training School for Nurses v. Pennington et al., 189 Okla. 170, 114P.2d943 (1941).

National Association of Insurance Commissioners. (1980). *Medical claims: Medical malpractice closed claims, July 1, 1975, through June 30, 1978* (Vol. 2). Brookfield, WI: Author.

O'Keeffe, S., Jack, C. I., & Lye, M. (1996). Use of restraints and bedrails in a British hospital. *Journal of the American Geriatrics Society, 44,* 1086–1088.

Parker, K., & Miles, S. H. (1997). Deaths caused by bedrails. *Journal of the American Geriatrics Society, 45,* 797–802.

Potter, et al. v. Dr. W.H. Groves Latter-Day Saints Hospital, 99 Utah 71, 103 P.2d 280 (1940).

Price, A. L. (1954). *The art, science and spirit of nursing.* Philadelphia: W.B. Saunders.

Price, A. L. (1956). Short side guards are safer. *Hospital Management, 82,* 86–89.

Regan, W. A. (1981). Legal case briefs for nurses. *Regan Reporting on Nursing Law, 21,* 3.

Rubenstein, H. S., Miller, F. H., Sholem, P., & Evans, H. B. (1983). Standards of medical care based on consensus rather than evidence: The case of routine bedrail use for the elderly. *Law, Medicine & Health Care, 11,* 271–76.

Sager, M. A., Franke, T., Inouye, S. K., Landefeld, C. S., Morgan, T. M., Rudberg, M. A., et al. (1996). Functional outcomes of acute medical illness and hospitalization in older persons. *Archives of Internal Medicine, 156,* 645–652.

Smalley, H. E. (1956). Variable height bed: A study in patient comfort and efficiency in care. *Hospital Management, 82,* 42–43.

Stevens, R. (1989). *In sickness and in wealth: American hospitals in the twentieth century.* New York: Basic Books.

Strumpf, N. E., & Tomes, N. (1993). Restraining the troublesome patient: A historical perspective on a contemporary debate. *Nursing History Review, 1,* 3–24.

Tammelleo, A. D. (1995). Siderails left down-patient falls from bed: "Ordinary negligence" or "malpractice"? *Regan Report on Nursing Law, 36,* 3.

Todd, J. F., Ruhl, C. E., & Gross, T. P. (1997). Injury and death associated with hospital bed side-rails: Reports to the U.S. Food and Drug Administration from 1985–1995. *American Journal of Public Health, 87,* 1675–1677.

Tracy, M. A. (1942). *Nursing: An art and a science.* St. Louis, MO: CV Mosby.

U.S. Department of Health & Human Services. (2000, June). *Health Care Financing Administration, guidance to surveyors.* Hospital conditions of participation for patients' rights (Rev. 17). Retrieved from http://www.hcfa.gov/quality/4b.htm.

13

Action Research Method

The hallmark of qualitative research is its focus on understanding human experience. Action research is a method that takes the intention of understanding human experience beyond the traditional researcher and participant dichotomy. Action researchers support a paradigm of liberation. Their goal is to democratize the research process. It is the interaction between researchers and participants that creates the action that is the hallmark of the action research process. According to Stringer (1999),

> The desire to give voice to people is derived not from an abstract ideological or theoretical imperative but from the pragmatic focus of action research. Its intent is to provide a place for the perspectives of people who have previously been marginalized from opportunities to develop and operate policies, programs, and services—perspectives often concealed by the products of a typical research process (p. 207).

Action research seeks to empower those who are part of the process to act on their own behalf to solve *real world problems*.

Nurses conducting research in the United States have not generally embraced action research. This is despite the fact that it is a research method that has demonstrated great success in the areas of social research. As Jenks (1999) states, "currently, English and Australian nurse–researchers most often engage in action research" (p. 251). It is the intention of this chapter to help the reader to understand the emancipatory process that is known as action research. The goal will be to share important insights about action research development, its fundamental roots, characteristics of the method, as well as information on how to generate, analyze and utilize the findings of an action research study. Once comfort with the method is achieved, it is hoped that it will be incorporated more often by nurse–researchers because of its significant utility in offering an action-based approach to problem solving for nurses and those they serve.

ACTION RESEARCH DEFINED

Action research has been known by various names, cooperative inquiry, action inquiry, participatory action research, community-based action research, collaborative research, and participative inquiry (Reason, 1994; Stringer, 1999; Tetley &

Hanson, 2001). The various terms make using one definition difficult. The definition of this approach may not be as important as its assumptions. It is the assumptions of the action research process that may better assist the neophyte in deciding whether action research represents a useful research approach.

Greenwood and Levin (1998) define action research as "social research carried out by a team encompassing a professional action researcher and members of an organization or community seeking to improve their situation" (p. 4). According to Winter and Munn-Giddings (2001), "it is a form of social research which involves people in a process of change, which is based on professional, organizational or community action" (p. 5). "Action research is first and foremost a group activity" (Bennett, 2000, p. 1). Some action researchers have suggested that rather than offering a single definition, action research should be seen as a continuum of methods with the ends of the continuum being both insider and outsider models (Badger, 2000; Rolfe, 1996; Tichen & Binnie, 1993).

> At the outsider end [is] the sociological approach of testing out theory in a real situation and Lewin's (1946) traditional approach of the researcher as professional expert entering the situation to facilitate and evaluate change. At the continuum's other end, termed endogenous research by DePoy & Gitlin (1994), lie those approaches where practitioner and researcher collaborate loosely, or are even the same person. (Badger, 2000, p. 202)

Coghlan and Casey (2001) share that the insider is sometimes the nurse working in his or her own situation: "Rarely is there much consideration of action by the permanent insider" (p. 675), in this case, the nurse who sees a situation in his or her workspace that needs a change.

To assist in the understanding of action research, four specific approaches will be described. These are cooperative inquiry, community-based action research, participatory action research, and action science or action inquiry.

Cooperative inquiry is a type of action research that values above all else the notion that individuals are self-determining, and as such, cannot be researched without their full participation. John Heron first advanced the ideas related to cooperative inquiry (Brown, 2001; Reason, 1998). According to Reason (1998),

> one can only do research on persons in the full and proper sense of the term only if one addresses them as self-determining, which means that what they do and what they experience as part of the research must be to some significant degree determined by them. (p. 264)

Therefore the implementation of cooperative inquiry requires that both researchers and informants cooperate to derive new knowledge.

As suggested earlier, the definitions/descriptions of the approaches presented here are not fundamentally different. The emphasis in all action research studies is the reciprocity between researchers and informants and empowerment of those who have not traditionally had a voice. Participatory action research (PAR), as described by William Foote Whyte (1984), is a type of action research that is best known because of its interdisciplinary focus. Also, it is known because of its political aspects (Reason, 1998). In more recent years, researchers have sought to remove the strong political overtones that characterize the method. According to Tetley and Hanson (2001), "it is the issues of creation, control and power that makes participatory research different from other types of social research" (p. 71). In PAR, the emphasis is on relinquishing control, learning through mutual inter-actions between researcher and participants, and giving voice to those who would otherwise not be heard.

Community-based action research represents the ideas advanced by Stringer (1999). Like PAR, community-based action research has faced some difficult times because of its association with radical political activism.

> It has reemerged in response to both pragmatic and philosophical pressures and is now more broadly understood as "disciplined inquiry (research) which seeks focused efforts to improve the quality of people's organizational, community and family lives" (Calhoun, 1993, p. 62). Community-based action research is also allied to recent emergence of practitioner research (e.g., Anderson et al., 1994) new paradigm research (Reason, 1988), and teacher-as-researcher (Kincheloe, 1991) (Stringer, 1999, p. 9).

As a research method, its most frequent application has been in problem solv-ing by practitioners: educators, social workers, nurses, organizational leaders, and human service workers. According to Stringer (1999), researchers "engage 'sub-jects' as equal and full partners" (p. 9). The method can be used to improve work activities, resolve problems or crises, and develop special projects. The overall goal is to deal with the problems that practitioners face in their everyday lives.

Action science or action inquiry is described by Reason (1998) as "forms of inquiry into practice" (p. 273) with the greatest emphasis being on developing action that will lead to systemic change within organizations, ultimately leading to "greater effectiveness and greater justice" (p. 273). The emphasis is on identifying theories of action that guide behavior (Reason, 1998). According to Argyris, Put-nam, & Smith as cited in Reason (1998), theories-in-use are rendered explicit by reflection on action. Therefore, action science concerns "itself with situations of uniqueness, uncertainty, and instability which do not lend themselves to the mode of technical rationality. It would aim at the development of themes from which...practitioners may construct theories and methods of their own" (Schon, 1983, p. 319). Ultimately, the reflection in action that is part of the action science process leads to a fuller understanding of how theory guides practice.

Holter and Schwartz-Barcott (1993) offer three classifications of action research. These are technical collaboration, mutual collaboration, and enhance-ment. In the technical collaboration approach, the researcher has a predetermined agenda that often involves intervention or theory testing; in the mutual collabora-tion approach, the researcher and participants identify the focus of the research together and together decide how to study and ultimately manage the problem; finally in the enhancement approach, the researcher and participants work together but move beyond the collaborative approach to engage in critical dia-logue to raise group consciousness (Sturt, 1999, p. 1059). According to Holter & Swartz-Barcott (1993) and Kendall & Sturt (1996), most reported nursing action research studies use the technical collaboration approach.

Given a basic understanding of the multiple definitions and descriptions of action research, it is important to examine the historical roots of this important research methodology. It is only through understanding of the method that nurse–researchers will have an appropriate framework to determine its applicability to problems faced in practice.

ACTION RESEARCH ROOTS

Action research is a method that might well be described as a research method that has gone through several phases. The early work is attributed to Kurt Lewin. Lewin, a social psychologist, is noted frequently as the first person to coin the term *action research*. Most nurses know Lewin as the person who described change theory. Lewin's theoretical ideas about change were very basic. Lewin said that in order for a change to occur, individuals would need to unfreeze—give up their ideas about something or give up the dominant structure. They would then need to change. The change would require the acceptance of new ideas or a new structure. Finally, once the new ideas were formally in place, the individuals involved in the change would refreeze or hold the new ideas or structure as permanent. Lewin's change model remains an influential model for social change up to the present (Greenwood & Levin, 1998).

Lewin, based on his ideas about change, saw action research as a process by which a researcher could achieve a goal by constructing a social experiment (Greenwood & Levin, 1998). "This research approach...fell very much within the bounds of conventional applied social science with its patterns of authoritarian control, but it was aimed at producing a specific, desired social outcome" (p. 17). As action research has developed, there is less emphasis on the stagnant manner of change, that being a process with a definitive ending point. Current action researchers believe the process is open with ongoing dialogue and that the refreezing described by Lewin is not a permanent condition.

Another group who worked on the ideas of action research in its early development was the Tavistock group. This group advanced Lewin's ideas in the post-World War II period. Following the war, when the English were rebuilding their industrial base, they found that traditional methods were not effective (Greenwood & Levin, 1998). To help with the understanding of why pre-war strategies no longer worked, the British government called on the Tavistock Institute of Human Relations to study the problem. "Tavistock brought Lewin's work on the concept of natural experiments and [action research] (Gustavsen, 1992) back to the United States, and committed itself to doing direct experiments in work life" (Greenwood & Levin, 1998, p. 20). The works of Tavistock led to additional exploration of the work environment and change process in Norway. The Norwegian Industrial Democracy Project used the ideas of Lewin and further developed by Tavistock to advance understanding of the work environment. For a complete description of this period, the reader is directed to Greenwood and Levin (1998).

The expansions of Lewin's work in Norway led to yet other modification in Sweden. The term used to describe the application of action research in the work environment was labeled *socio-technical thinking* (Greenwood & Levin, 1998). This type of organizational thinking and action spread to the United States. Trist (1981) identified the new paradigm of socio-technical design for organizations as follows: Person was complementary to machine, people were resources to be developed, people should have broad skills and grouped by tasks, people were internally motivated, organizations should be flat and represent participative models of functioning, activity should be collaborative and collegial, the people in the organization should be supported in their commitment to the organization, and individuals should be rewarded for innovation. Ultimately, it was discovered that if individuals were part of identifying and creating their work environments, then based on the interaction between all concerned parties, positive action and direction for the organization would be achieved.

Brown (2001) states Argyris and Schon represent the present day transformation based on their conceptualization of action research as action science. Both Argyris and Schon are most interested in theory in action as described earlier in this section.

As it occurs today, action research has a number of permutations. The most important facet of the design is its focus on emancipation of others and the collaborative nature of the research process. In the next section, the fundamental characteristics of the method will be explored.

FUNDAMENTAL CHARACTERISTICS OF THE METHOD

Similar to the definitions of action research, there is no one method of doing action research. However, there are some fundamental characteristics about the method and the way that it is executed. Common to all descriptions is the fact that the research is context bound. Second, the process seeks to have full engagement by researchers and participants. The process is truly collaborative. Third, those engaged pay regular attention to the process and how it impacts the lives of others. Fourth, an action or change is the focal point of the process. And, finally, the decision to implement the action or change is in the hands of the stakeholders.

Like many types of qualitative research, the purpose is not to create a generalizable study but rather one that is locally important. When initiating an action research study, the researcher would ideally become engaged in the process when a local group finds a problem that they want to solve and seeks the insights of an individual with research expertise. Because the problem is local and the planned change is practical, the findings will most likely be local. This is not to suggest that a local problem may not develop ideas or theories that can be applied in other situations, but rather to state that the purpose of an action research study is to create a real change for the stakeholders involved in the situation.

The collaboration that is identified as fundamental is at the root of this emancipatory research process. Those engaged must be *equal* members of the research team. The use of a truly democratic process to create new knowledge is potentially liberating for those involved (Greenwood & Levin, 1998).

> The logic of [the] inquiry is linked to the inquiry process itself, in the struggle to make an indeterminate situation into a more positively controlled one through an inquiry process where action and reflection are directly linked. The outside researcher inevitably becomes a participant in collaboration with the insiders (p. 78).

For example, if a group of individuals from an low income housing development find that health services are not available to them because of limited local care and even more limited public transportation, the way to effectively deal with the problem is to bring all the stakeholders to the table to resolve the problem using the action research process. Rather than the power group deciding the best way to handle the situation, if all stakeholders work to develop a practical solution to the problem, then the needs of all should be met. The researcher facilitates the process but does not control it.

Those involved must be aware of the impact participation in the process will have on their lives. Those concerned must agree to be constantly aware of the differences in beliefs, values, needs, and objectives of those involved in order to support an effective process. Using the example above, if the health care providers come to the table with preconceived ideas based on their beliefs, cultural values, and class and are not attentive to those who live in the neighborhood, then the process will not yield an outcome that is in the best interest of all concerned. Similarly, if those from the neighborhood are unwilling to collaborate with the researcher, health care providers, or city officials because of preconceived notions about power, class, and existing systems, then again what is best for all concerned will not emerge. Once there is commitment on the part of all concerned to stay attuned to the needs of each person, then the process can proceed, ultimately leading to a change.

Implementation of an action or change is the fourth fundamental characteristic of the action research process. The purpose of the process is not to describe an existing situation but rather to construct new knowledge, a new way to deal with a practical problem (Winter & Munn-Giddings, 2001). "Participants are empowered to define their world in the service of what they see as worthwhile interests, and as a consequence they change their world in significant ways, through action" (Reason, 1998, p. 279). The action is developed based on what is discovered through the process of dismantling the problem. For example, in work completed by Ducharme, Le'Vesque, Gendron, and Legault (2001), a program to support the mental health of family caregivers was developed based on focus groups held with these individuals to discover what they needed to create a healthier space for themselves.

The last characteristic of action research is that the power to act is always in the hands of the stakeholders. If the process works as it should, the action determined through collaboration results in an outcome that is acceptable and can be implemented by those involved. The action is part of the continuing process of emancipation and democracy. No one outsider or no one insider can determine the action that needs to be taken. The conclusion and subsequent action must reflect the collective thinking of the group.

SELECTION OF ACTION RESEARCH AS METHOD

Nurses who choose to use action research as an approach to solve a particular problem should have a clear understanding of what the purpose of their research is. As described earlier, action research is specifically designed as a research method whose outcome is the implementation of an action or change. The types of action that can be considered include bringing about a change in behavior, developing a plan of action to deal with resistance to change, implementing new nursing practices, or empowering providers or those for whom they care (Hart & Bond, 1996; Jenks, 1999). In addition to dedication to action or change, the nurse interested in using action research must be committed to the development of local theory. The outcomes of an action research study will not be generalizable and will usually not have meaning outside of the context in which the study occurs.

Second, the nurse–researcher must be committed to collaboration. The collaboration in action research is different than that which generally occurs among researchers in a nursing research study. In action research, the collaboration is not between colleagues with equivalent knowledge and power but rather with individuals who may have little or no understanding of research. The participants usually represent members of groups different from the researcher's own experience. For instance, the participants have a different hierarchical status within the health care arena such as the nurse who is trying to help patients change the way they are treated by professionals in the health care system. The patients may have a different socioeconomic background. For example, a nurse–researcher may be interested in helping single mothers from a low-income housing development obtain access to transportation for health-related appointments. There may be any number of differences between the participants and researchers. What is most important in the collaboration is that nurse–researchers *must* view those with whom they engage in the research process as *equal* partners. Without this commitment another method of inquiry will be most helpful.

Another important consideration in the selection of action research is the value placed on empowerment and voice. Nurse–researchers interested in engaging in action research must be comfortable with regular self-reflection relative to the issues of power and control. One of the fundamental characteristics of action research is the empowerment of others. That empowerment can only occur honestly when the researcher constantly attends to the issues of power and control in the research process and the setting in which the research takes place. For instance, if the nurse–researcher is interested in studying student nurses and their difficulty in being part of the clinical education setting, then the researcher must be ready to listen carefully to what is said, help the participants find their voice, and assist them in the development of a process that will empower them to take action.

The final consideration in choosing action research is the realization that in action research, the power to act resides exclusively with those who engaged in the process. No amount of external pressure can force the participants to carry out the change or action that results from the conduct of the study.

Once the nurse–researcher is comfortable with the fundamental characteristics, understands the outcome of the method, and is willing to share the power and control, which is usually the purview of the principal investigator, then and only then should action research be selected. Action research has the potential to dramatically change the life experiences of many individuals. However, the study must be conducted with attention to the fundamental issues of empowerment and action.

ELEMENTS AND INTERPRETATIONS OF THE METHOD

Action researchers have many interpretations of method. This can be seen from the information provided earlier regarding the many terms and descriptions given to the process. There are, however, some basic elements to which most researchers engaged in action research subscribe. These will be shared in the hope that they give the novice who is interested in the methodology enough information to determine whether the approach will be useful in dealing with a specific problem. Once the decision is made to conduct an action research study, the neophyte is encouraged to read primary sources on the method and engage a research mentor.

Data Generation

Data generation begins as soon as the problem becomes apparent and a decision is made to conduct an action research study. The initial discussions about the problem will become an important part of data analysis, as will all of the other information collected in the course of the study.

Defining the Problem

Ideally, the problem to be examined in an action research study should come from those who are experiencing the problem. For example, a group of single mothers who recognize that they have a significant problem with making annual physical examination appointments with their children are in a position to request help. In this case, the mothers might approach a trusted individual to help them sort the problem out. The representative then would be in a position to contact a nurse–researcher to help the single mothers develop an action research study to deal with the problem. Generally, this is not how action research problems in nursing frequently are identified. More often, nurses see a problem in practice or a problem in the lives of those with whom they work and propose an action research approach to study and act on the problem. Regardless of who identifies the problem, it is likely that the stakeholders in an action research study will be more committed to an action or a change if they believe that the situation is important to them and that they can bring about a change in the situation.

It is important to recognize that there are two perspectives in any action research study. This is the insider or emic view and the outsider or etic view. This dichotomy exists because the insiders are living the problem and have a unique understanding of it. The outsider, the researcher, is the person who comes to the situation with the intention to assist those involved but usually is unable to internalize the situation because he or she does not live it. It is also important to remember that the insiders are the ones who will implement the change and thus have to live with the outcome. As can be seen, the insider's stake is much higher than the outsider's. The earlier discussion made it clear that collaboration is essential. Thus, there may be two views on the problem but both views are equally valuable because of the partnership that must be developed to fully understand the problem and create the change.

To fully define the problem and begin to understand it, the insiders will need to bring their personal knowledge of the problem to the researcher. The researcher will bring theoretical and practical information relative to the problem forward. Together, the participants and the researcher will work to clearly identify what the problem is. Ideally, the problem can be identified clearly. From a practical standpoint, clearly defining the problem will be an evolving process.

Planning

One of the important initial stages of an action research study is to identify all the stakeholders. It is essential to bring as many of the stakeholders forward for initial conversations about the existing problem as possible. All who may be affected in any way by the problem or the desired change need to be part of the early conversations.

Once the stakeholders are identified, it is important to determine how the investigation will proceed. Greenwood and Levin (1998) offer a model of action research that they call the Cogenerative Action Research Model. In the description of the model, Greenwood and Levin recommend that communication arenas be developed. Communication arenas are spaces where participants and researcher can come together for mutual learning. Developing these spaces will be one of the most important aspects of engaging all the stakeholders. "Arenas must be designed to match the needs of the issue" (p. 117). Therefore, there may be need for large group, small group, and one-on-one meetings. There may be a need for specific arenas for explicit purposes such as information sharing or team building. There also will be the need to develop spaces for reflection. Ground rules for participation will be essential. It is also important to work together to clearly describe how the feedback loop for communication will work. As an example, the researcher or a member of the group may record minutes; however, in what forum will there be the opportunity to discuss the interpretation of what was recorded?

In addition to deciding in what space communication will occur, it is also important to decide how information will be collected. Will interviews, observations, focus groups, and printed material comprise the major data collection methods or will survey and questionnaires be the major strategies? This decision must be a decision made by all members of the research team. It will be the responsibility of the researchers to bring as much information as possible forward so that the members of the team who are not skilled in the strategies for data collection or the research process are provided with the opportunity to learn about the various data collection strategies and the method so they can make informed decisions about how to proceed.

Greenwood and Levin (1998) describe the value of reflection throughout the action research process for all those involved. One of the ways to encourage reflection is to select journaling or keeping a diary as one of the data collection strategies. Using a self-reflective mechanism can help sort out the issues for all concerned.

Different from other qualitative methods, the participants in an action research study are not separate from the researcher. Those who are the stakeholders are the ones who can most effectively inform the study. However, there will be times when data need to be collected to reflect the experience of members of affected groups who are not intimately involved with the study. For example, using the single mother scenario presented earlier, all mothers with the problem may not be part of the research team, but from time to time, it will be essential to collect information from as many mothers experiencing the problem as possible. In this case, the sample for focused data collection will be purposive. Depending on which data collection strategies are used, a decision will need to be made regarding who will conduct the interviews, do the observations, or collect survey or questionnaire data. It is wise to select the researcher from those who have no direct connection to those from whom data are being collected. Using an outsider to collect these data provides a potentially more open-minded and detached view of the situation.

Jenks (1999) recommends that at least three strategies of data collection be utilized to assure that there is cross-validation of information. All strategies will not need to be identified before the study begins. Since the question may not be clearly defined, data collection strategies not originally identified may need to be added because of evolving data. For instance, using the situation described earlier of the single mothers with transportation issues, a survey may have been selected as one of the data collection strategies. However, as the study progresses, it is discovered that there is information that the survey is not capturing. Focus group interviews then may be recommended.

The preparations that have been described represent the planning phase of the action research study. Stringer (1999) calls this developmental phase "setting the stage" (p. 43). Regardless of what name is given to the initial planning phase, all participants need to agree on how best to proceed.

Once the decisions are made regarding how best to collect data, data collection should commence. As stated earlier, the process of planning, data collection, and data analysis does not proceed in a linear manner. The process is dynamic and as such needs to respond to the changing needs of all involved.

Data Treatment and Analysis

As data are collected, they will be analyzed using the appropriate methodology for the strategy selected. For instance, if interviews were used, analysis can proceed using the constant comparative method. Jenks (1999) states that this method is useful in analysis of action research data. For a complete description of the constant comparative method, the reader is directed to Chapter 7.

The analysis phase of the study should include all stakeholders. Interpretations and explanations cannot be offered unless the context is fully understood. The participants in the study will be the individuals who can most accurately reflect the context. Also, by doing analysis as a joint activity, the entire research team can bring its perspectives to the discussion, providing the opportunity for dialogue and debate about the findings and their respective meaning.

The researcher will have primary responsibility for leading the data analysis phase based on knowledge of the process and experience. However, it will be the team that will draw the final conclusions.

Action

Unlike some of the other types of qualitative research, action research does not end with documentation of the findings. When data analysis is completed, the team decides on an action or a change that they want to occur. The change is a result of and based on the findings. The outsiders take no active role in the change. They may remain part of the team by contributing to guiding the process or assisting with reflection but they have no formal role in the change (Jenks, 1999).

In some instances, the action research process may start with the action or change and the study is conducted to assess the change as it is implemented. When the study is implemented in this way, it is conducted as an evaluation study with all members of the research team contributing. Modifications in implementation of the change can take place, as the research team deems appropriate.

An important part of the change or action phase of the research process is reflection. Reflection is used in this stage of the process as a way of gaining insights about the change and its impact on those who are part of it. Reflection can be conducted as a one-on-one activity, in a group or in a personal diary. "Data recorded during reflection are important contributions to the theory that emerges from the action research study" (Jenks, 1999, p. 260). Winter and Munn-Giddings (2001) speak to the cycle of action and reflection that is based on the work of Lewin. This spiral cycle includes planning, action, and fact-finding. The cycle repeats itself to more effectively understand some aspect of the research process.

According to Jenks (1999), reflective critique can be used to facilitate reflection.

> Reflective critique is based on an understanding that all statements made during data generation—including participants' and researchers' written and verbal language—are subject to reflexivity. Reflexivity describes the belief that the language individuals use to describe an experience reflects that particular experience and also all other experiences in each individual's life. Knowing that observations and interpretations are reflexive creates two assumptions for action researchers: (1) a rejection of the idea of a single or ultimate explanation for an event and (2) the belief that offering various explanations for an experience explicitly increases understanding of the experiences (p. 260).

Another process that can be used to assist in reflection is dialectical critique. In contrast to reflective critique, dialectical critique "probes data to make explicit their internal contradictions rather than complementary explanations" (Jenks, 1999, p. 261). The ultimate goal of each process is to ask important questions about data as they are revealed.

Evaluation

Evaluation of the action research process takes place throughout the study and at its end. A timeline for evaluation should be established during the planning phase. The timeline gives specific direction in order to keep evaluation in front of all members of the team. During evaluation, the process is assessed. Questions such as: Are we using the correct instruments?; Are we getting the data we need?; Who else do we need to interview?; and Is the process working? can be asked. These questions and others that the research team develops will keep the project focused.

Researchers have the responsibility to guide the evaluation process. This should not be done without consultation or the consent of the entire research team (Jenks, 1999).

Writing the Report

The report that results from the study will be a document prepared by the team. Information to be included and excluded should be agreed upon by all members of the team. The report is not necessarily the end of the action or change but it does represent the end of the formal study. Hopefully, if the action is effective, the change will be evaluated for its long-term impact on the individuals involved and be part of the formal report.

One important feature of the report will be to make recommendations. These recommendations are meant to be helpful and give direction for long-term implementation of the change. The recommendations should be determined collaboratively and be based on a solid understanding of the problem, careful data collection, and analysis and review of appropriate literature. Review of the literature is an activity that takes place throughout the study. It should be part of informing the planned change or action in concert with the data that are collected. It is also an activity that can place the study in the context of what is already known at the end of the study. Because action research focuses on local problems, the literature review most likely will not yield directly applicable information. However, the researcher may find conceptual connections that can help make sense of the action or provide support for the local theory.

Rigor

All research should be evaluated for its rigor. Action research is no exception. Stringer (1999) suggests that action researchers establish the rigor of their research by utilizing the trustworthiness criteria recommended by Lincoln and Guba (1985). These include credibility, transferability, dependability, and confirmability.

According to Stringer (1999),

> credibility is established by *prolonged engagement* with participants; *triangulation* of information from multiple data sources; *member checking* procedures that allow participants to check and verify the accuracy of the information recorded; and *peer debriefing* processes that enable research facilitators to articulate and reflect on research procedures with a colleague or informed associate (p. 176).

Transferability is established by creating thick descriptions that when read by another researcher can be applied in other contexts. It is the researcher's responsibility to describe as fully as possible the means for applying the information in other contexts (Stringer, 1999).

Dependability and confirmability is established through an audit trail. The researcher is responsible for providing enough information so that another researcher reading the study would come up with similar conclusions.

Waterman (1998) recommends that action researchers focus on the validity of their research. She offers three types of validity: dialectical, critical, and reflexive.

Dialectical validity "refers to the constant analysis and report of movement between theory, research and practice in examining the tensions, contradictions and complexities of the situation" (Badger, 2000, p. 204).

Critical validity involves analyzing the process of change. "The measure of validity is not the change effected but rather the analysis of intentions and actions, their ethical implications and consequences" (Badger, 2000, p. 204). "Action researchers tend to demonstrate a sense of timing or a sensitivity to the situation which has been cultivated through an intimate understanding of the context and the people involved" (Waterman, 1998, p. 103).

Reflexive validity is the attempt by the researcher to constantly be examining the biases, suppositions, and presuppositions of the research. It is only through constant attention to the researcher's view that a true understanding can result. The researcher must be certain that in the end he or she has told the story of the insider.

The very real concern in any qualitative research study is that the story that emerges is the story of the people. Action research is no exception. Action research is useful because of it fundamental characteristics. It would be inadvisable to apply criteria for rigor that subtract from the value of the fundamental characteristics. The rigor of an action research study should be measured by how well the researcher has attended to the fundamental characteristics of the method.

Ethical Considerations

An action research study has inherent ethical dilemmas that may not be seen in most other types of research. For example, one of the characteristics of an action research study is the focus on cooperation and collaborative decision making among stakeholders with the goal of carrying out a change or action project. For this reason, parties involved in the study may become involved in the study not being aware of the potential problems inherent in group process. For instance, individuals who share contrasting opinions from those in the dominant membership may find that although a consent form clearly stated the option to withdraw from the study at any time, pressure from within the group may be such that this is impossible to do so. The action researcher should try to identify as many of these dilemmas as possible. It may not be possible, however, to identify them all. The best that the researcher may be able to guarantee is a regular review of what the participants have agreed to. Munhall (2001) refers to this as process consent. Process consent is a procedure that allows the researcher and participants to renegotiate aspects of the informed consent based on the changing nature of the inquiry.

Kelly and Simpson (2001) offer another ethical dilemma that may occur—the feelings of vulnerability felt by those who are invested in making a change. There are always those who are invested in maintaining the status quo who will work relentlessly to maintain their position. To limit the potential for oppression, Kelly and Simpson recommend that action researchers seek as much consultation as necessary with relevant authorities and provide for close inclusion of all participants throughout the process.

Ethical issues can arise despite the most meticulous planning. Action researchers need to be cognizant of all the potential problems that may arise and inform their co-researchers of as many of them as can be identified before and during the study.

SUMMARY

Action research is a dynamic approach to inquiry. The researcher who opts to adopt the approach as a way to study a problem and assist in making a change in the lives of those who live in a particular situation must be willing to accept the important characteristics of this method. An attitude of collaboration, a commitment to cooperation, and an obligation to democracy and empowerment will be essential for the researcher who chooses the method. If the nurse–researcher understands the possibilities that exist when adopting the method and is willing to participate in research that is locally meaningful, then action research can be an invigorating process that can create *real* change. According to Jenks (1999), "when used appropriately, action research can result in lasting change that creates a more meaningful nursing practice" (p. 263).

REFERENCES

Anderson, G., Herr, K., & Nihlen, A. (1994). *Studying your own school: An educator's guide to qualitative practitioner research*. Thousand Oaks, CA: Corwin.

Badger, T. G. (2000). Action research, change and methodological rigor. *Journal of Nursing Management, 8,* 201–207.

Bennett, O. M. (2000). Action research: Reflective practice in occupational therapy education. Education: *Special Interest Section Quarterly, 19*(4), 1–2.

Brown, C. L. (2001). Action research: The method. In C. L. Munhall (Ed.), *Nursing research: A qualitative perspective* (3rd ed., pp. 503–522). Sudbury, MA: Jones and Bartlett.

Calhoun, E. (1993). Action research: Three approaches. *Educational Leadership, 51*(2), 62–65.

Coghlan, D., & Casey, M. (2001). Action research from the inside: Issues and challenges in doing action research in your own hospital. *Journal of Advanced Nursing, 35*(5), 674–682.

DePoy, E., & Gitlin, L. N. (1994). *Introduction to research: Multiple strategies for health and human services*. St. Louis: Mosby.

Ducharme, F., Le'Vesque, L., Gendron, M., & Legault, A. (2001). Development process and qualitative evaluation of a program to promote the mental health of family caregivers. *Clinical Nursing Research, 10*(2), 182–201.

Gustavsen, B. (1992). *Dialogue and development*. Assen-Maastricht: Van Gorcum.

Greenwood, D. J., & Levin, M. (1998). *Introduction to action research: Social research for social change*. London: Sage.

Hart, E., & Bond, M. (1996). Making sense of action research through the use of a typology. *Journal of Advanced Nursing, 23,* 152–159.

Holter, I. M., & Swartz-Barcott, D. (1993). Action research: What is it? How has it been used and how can it be used in nursing? *Journal of Advanced Nursing, 18,* 298–304.

Jenks, J. (1999). Action research method. In H. J. Streubert & D. R. Carpenter (Eds.), *Qualitative research in nursing: Advancing the humanistic imperative* (2nd ed., pp. 251–264). Philadelphia: Lippincott Williams & Wilkins.

Kelly, K., & Simpson, S. (2001). Action research in action: Reflections on a project to introduce clinical practice facilitators to an acute hospital setting. *Journal of Advanced Nursing, 33*(5), 652–659.

Kendall, S. A., & Sturt, J. A. (1996). Negotiation access into primary health care: Insights from critical theory. *Social Sciences in Health, 2*(2), 107–120.

Kincheloe, J. (1991). *Teachers are researchers: Qualitative inquiry as a path to empowerment*. London: Falmer.

Lewin, K. (1946). Action research and minority problems. *Journal of Social Issues, 2,* 34–46.

Lincoln, Y. S., & Guba, E. G. (1985). *Naturalistic inquiry*. Beverly Hills, CA: Sage.

Munhall, P. L. (2001). *Nursing research: A qualitative perspective* (3rd ed.). Sudbury, MA: Jones and Barlett.

Reason, P. (1994). *Participation in human inquiry*. London: Sage.

Reason, P. (1988). *Human inquiry in action: Developments in new paradigm research*. New York: Wiley.

Reason, P. (1998). Three approaches to participative inquiry. In N. K. Denzin & Y. S. Lincoln (Eds.), *Strategies of qualitative inquiry* (pp. 261–291). Thousand Oaks, CA: Sage.

Rolfe, G. (1996). Going to extremes: Action research, grounded practice and the theory-practice gap in nursing. *Journal of Advanced Nursing, 24,* 1315–1320.

Schon, D. (1983). *The reflective practitioner: How professionals think in action.* New York: Basic Books.

Stringer, E. T. (1999). *Action research* (2nd ed.). Thousand Oaks, CA: Sage.

Sturt, J. (1999). Placing empowerment research with an action research typology. *Journal of Advanced Nursing, 30*(5), 1057–1063.

Tetley, J., & Hanson, L. (2001). Participatory research. *Nurse Researcher, 8*(1), 69–88.

Tichen, A., & Binnie, A. (1993). Research partnerships: Collaborative action research in nursing. *Journal of Advanced Nursing, 18,* 858–865.

Trist, E. (1981). *The evolution of socio-technical systems* (Occasional Paper No. 2). Toronto: Ontario Quality of Work Life Council.

Waterman, H. (1998). Embracing ambiguities and valuing ourselves: Issues of validity in action research. *Journal of Advanced Nursing, 28*(1), 101–105.

Winter, R., & Munn-Giddings, C. (2001). *A handbook for action research in health and social care.* London: Routledge.

Whyte, W. F. (1984). *Learning from the field: A guide from experience.* Beverly Hills, CA: Sage.

Action Research in Practice, Education, and Administration

"Action research is an approach to research that aims at both taking action and creating knowledge or theory about that action" (Coghlan & Casey, 2001, p. 675). Frequently, nurses find themselves faced with problems in practice, education, or administration that require a change in behavior to affect a positive outcome for those with whom they work. Action research is a method of inquiry that provides a framework for action, knowledge generation, empowerment, and reflection. This chapter presents nursing research studies that have used action research to solve an identified problem. Table 14.1, a summary of recent action research studies, is provided to educate the reader about the types of practice areas that have been studied using the methodology. In addition, a critical review of three studies will be shared to give the reader a perspective on what is important in reporting action research. Box 14.1 provides a list of questions that are used for the review of the articles presented. The intent is to provide direction for critical review of action research studies specifically to determine the merits of the study and the overall utility and practical application of the findings. A reprint of Ducharme, Lévesque, Gendron, and Legault's (2001) article is offered at the end of the chapter to facilitate the reader's understanding of the critique process.

APPLICATION TO PRACTICE

Health care as an industry is in constant fluctuation. Nurses are called on routinely to readjust the way that care is delivered. Sometimes change is necessary without adequate time to thoroughly study all the issues that surround the needed action. Action research represents an opportunity for nurses to implement needed clinical changes while at the same time conducting much needed research to understand the implications of their actions. Nurses who are committed to empowerment of others; understanding the problem through the eyes of the stakeholders; sharing power, information and resources; and co-creating an action or change should consider using action research.

Clinical nursing practice is considered by some to be the place where nurse–researchers should focus their resources. The problems in the clinical practice area deal specifically with the focus of nursing care: individuals, families, groups or com-

text continues on page 274

TABLE 14.1 SELECTIVE SAMPLING OF ACTION RESEARCH STUDIES

Author	Domain	Purpose
Ainley, Barlow, Houldin, et al. (2000)	Administration	To develop and implement a process of clinical supervision
Anderson, Nyamathi, McAvoy, Conde, & Casey (2001)	Practice	The discovery of adolescent perception of risks and their consequences as well as identified dangers in neighborhoods in a population of men and women in juvenile detention
Berman, McKenna, Arnold, Taylor, & MacQuarrie (2000)	Practice	To develop a national action plan to address violence directed toward young girls
Chan & Wai-tong (2000)	Education	To implement and evaluate contract learning as a strategy for students in clinical settings
Dickson & Green (2001)	Practice	To study the health needs of Aboriginal grandmothers and respond to them through development of health promotion programming

Co-researchers	Data Generation	Findings
Representatives from each locality, health visitors who attended the Health Visitors' Association course, and a university lecturer	Group meetings	Clinical supervision was initiated under the steering group's facilitation. Members successfully implemented a group-designed process for supervision that was reported as still being successfully in place 18 months after the initiation of the study.
42 adolescents in juvenile detention and researchers	Focus groups and individual interviews	These adolescents focused on the more pressing dangers they encountered in their daily lives.
Girls from rural and urban settings, community leaders, researchers and activists	Focus groups	Young girls are sexually harassed in a variety of ways. Empowerment programs need to be developed and women need to become part of the political struggle against male dominance.
Students and clinical faculty	Questionnaire survey and semistructured interviews	Contract learning has benefits and difficulties. With careful consideration of the difficulties and attention to skillful implementation, contract learning can increase students' motivation and autonomy.
Aboriginal grandmothers, project advisory committee, project staff, research associates, external researcher, reflection committee	Individual and group interviews, observations, journal	"Action was taken on numerous individual and social issues, making the direct link between research and community action and change, giving the grandmothers a voice and connecting them with others created alliances, and building skills and organization for ongoing activities" (p. 480).

(continued)

TABLE 14.1 ° SELECTIVE SAMPLING OF ACTION RESEARCH STUDIES (CONTINUED)

Author	Domain	Purpose
Ducharme, Lévesque, Gendron, & Legault (2001)	Practice	Development and evaluation of an intervention program to promote mental health of women caregivers of institutionalized family members
Higgs, Bayne, & Murphy (2001)	Practice	To provide an information base on health care access for policy formation in a Spokane, Washington neighborhood
Hilton, Crawford, & Tarko (2000)	Practice	To describe the experience of men in three specific roles when their wives are going through chemotherapy for breast cancer

Co-researchers	Data Generation	Findings
Daughters and spouses of institutionalized adults and researchers	Focus groups, observations, audiotaping, semistructured interviews, diaries, informal group discussions	An educational and support program was developed based on the input from participants. Topics of the program included getting to know one another, how to feel good with your relative, how to avoid emotional turmoil, how to deal with losses on a daily basis and prepare for the eventual loss of the relative, how to reorganize your life after the placement of the relative, and how to identify and call on your support network.
Individuals living in the low-income neighborhoods	Interview, focus groups	Health care systems need to be developed that empower community residents, incorporate their ideas into planning, are funded at necessary levels, and help establish meaningful community benchmarks.
Spouses of women experiencing breast cancer treatment, nurses, social workers, an oncologist, the women with breast cancer	Semistructured interviews	Two main themes—focusing on wife's illness and care and focusing on the family to keep it going—were identified. There were 9 subthemes: being there, relying on health care professionals, being informed and contributing to decision making, trying to keep patterns normal and family life going, helping out and depending on others, being positive, putting self on hold, adapting work life, and managing finances.

(continued)

TABLE 14.1	SELECTIVE SAMPLING OF ACTION RESEARCH STUDIES (CONTINUED)	
Author	**Domain**	**Purpose**
Jones (2000)	Administration	To explore the problems in development and implementation of a care pathway for inpatients with schizophrenia
Kelly & Simpson (2001)	Administration	To introduce, develop, and evaluate the clinical practice facilitator role in acute care
Smith, Masterson, Basfore, et al. (2000)	Education	To disseminate and implement a philosophy of health in four schools of nursing and midwifery

munities who need health promotion, health maintenance, disease prevention, or treatment for health deviations. In the article entitled "Development Process and Qualitative Evaluation of a Program to Promote the Mental Health of Caregivers," Ducharme et al. (2001) share how they used action research to develop a program to improve the mental health of family caregivers based on collaboration with those who were affected. This article will be critically reviewed using the questions in Box 14.1 to demonstrate the quality of the work.

Ducharme et al. (2001) begin the description of their study by clearly describing the practice situation. The authors begin their report by providing a substantive overview of the life of individuals who care for elderly institutionalized relatives. They also share some important statistical information that demonstrates the impact of caregiving on the caregivers. It is clear to the reader at the completion of the literature review that the problem exists and that an action research approach to the problem is indicated. In the case of this study, the action occurs later in the study after a substantial fact-finding period.

The researchers explain that they used a three-step action research process to explore the problem. The steps include assessment of sources of stress, co-construction of the program, and experimentation and qualitative evaluation. During

Co-researchers	Data Generation	Findings
All members of the multidisciplinary team on a 16-bed, psychiatric mixed-sex adult psychiatric ward in a deprived borough in London	Interviews, participant observation, diaries, work groups	The major problem in developing and implementing the care pathway was staff turnover. Also identified as potential problems were lack of motivation of the staff to implement the care pathway, staff being unable to understand the implementation of the pathway and the practicalities of implementing the care pathway on a busy unit.
Nursing staff, clinical practice facilitators	Group meetings, questionnaires, diaries	Clinical practice facilitators were positively evaluated by nursing staff in acute care.
Six nurse educators, two researchers	Workshops, group and one-on-one discussions	"Interpretation and implementation of a philosophy of health in nursing had been variable" (p. 563).

Step One, the researchers used focus groups to collect data. This is an appropriate strategy given that the purpose of Step One is to "explore the main sources of stress of family caregivers" (Ducharme et al., 2001, p. 185). According to Goldman and Schmalz (2001), a focus group is used when the researcher wants to use an interactive strategy to gain insight into the perceptions, beliefs, and opinions of an intended audience on a specific program, issue, or service. In this case, Ducharme et al. (2001) are interested in the caregivers' perceptions of what causes their stress.

During Step Two, work meetings were used to develop a program to improve the well-being of the caregivers. This program was a collaborative effort by the participants and the researcher based on data collected during Step One. Field observations were conducted during this step as well. The researchers do not provide an explanation for doing the observations.

In Step Three, Experimentation and Qualitative Evaluation, data were collected through semistructured diaries completed by the group leader, audio taping of group sessions, semistructured interviews with 20 predetermined questions, and informal group discussion. The audiotapes of the sessions were reviewed at the conclusion of the session. A structured grid was used to assess "the adequacy of the initial design of the session with regard to its actual content" (Ducharme et al.,

2001, p. 190). The semistructured diaries were used to provide data on the intervention process. Data collected from the semistructured interviews were used to obtain general perceptions of the program by the participants. The informal group interviews served the same purpose as the semistructured one-on-one interviews. All the data collection strategies identified were appropriate.

Individuals were recruited to participate based on their experience with caregiving. These included a daughter or spouse of an elderly patient institutionalized for not

---

Box 14.1

CRITIQUING GUIDELINES FOR ACTION RESEARCH

Planning

1. Does the researcher justify the use of action research?
2. Does the study begin with an analysis of the practice situation or does it begin with implementation of the action?
3. Analysis of the practice situation
   a. Is the practice setting described in sufficient detail?
   b. What methods of data generation are used to describe the practice situation?
      • Are qualitative techniques used to study human qualities?
      • Are quantitative techniques used to study nonhuman factors?
   c. Are procedures for selecting participants described?
   d. What is the extent of collaboration between researchers and participants during the analysis of practice phase?
   e. Is protection of human subjects documented?
   f. Are strategies for data analysis described?
   g. Are participants involved in the interpretation?
   h. Does the description reflect understanding of the practice situation?
4. Action planning
   a. Is the planned change described in detail?
   b. Are methods of implementing the planned change described?
   c. Are methods for evaluating the planned change described?
   d. Are participants included in action planning?

Acting

1. Is the planned change implemented in the practice setting where the problem occurred?
2. Is the period for implementation specified?

(continued)

Box 14.1

Critiquing Guidelines for Action Research (Continued)

Reflecting

1. Are methods for facilitating reflection specified?
2. Are the results of reflection described?

Evaluating

1. Are strategies for evaluating the change described?
2. Are the processes for implementing the change and the outcomes of the change evaluated?
3. Are data evaluation methods appropriate to factors evaluated?

   a. Are qualitative techniques used to evaluate human factors?

   b. Are quantitative techniques used to evaluate technologic factors?
4. Are participants included in the evaluation?
5. Are appropriate methods used to analyze evaluation data?
6. Does the research address validity and reliability of quantitative findings and trustworthiness of qualitative findings?

Conclusions, Implications, and Recommendations

1. Do the conclusions reflect the findings?
2. Is a local theory formulated from the findings?
3. Are implications described in sufficient detail?
4. Has the researcher discussed ethical and moral implications of the study?
5. Are recommendations for research and practice included?
6. Does the researcher describe the benefits participants gained from the study?

---

less than 6 months and not more than 36 months who suffered from dementia. The individuals were recruited from three long-term care facilities in Montreal. There is no mention of protection of human subjects. One could infer that since the study was funded by Health Canada that its authors had to provide information relative to human subjects' protection before it was funded. Explicit statements reflecting institutional review would preclude the reader from having to make this assumption.

It is clear from the report that caregivers were co-participants in the construction and refinement of the program. The researchers also report that following Step One, validation of the content analysis was completed with participants.

The primary method of data analysis used in this study was content analysis. This strategy was used mostly during Steps One and Three. Content analysis is defined by LoBiondo-Wood and Haber (2002) as "a technique for the objective, systematic, and quantitative description of communications and documentary evidence" (p. 490). As presented, the information collected and analyzed in Steps One and Three is reflective of communication or subjective data and so content analysis is an appropriate method of data analysis.

Ducharme et al. (2001) clearly identify throughout their article the role that participants played in data collection and analysis. For example, after Step One, the authors report that two members of the research team carried out coding and categorization. This activity completed by the researchers is followed by "validation of the content analysis together with the participants (p. 187). This is an excellent example of a way to maintain the integrity of the empowering process and still utilize the expertise of group members in the most effective way. The researchers (formally trained) provided the initial coding and categorization; however, all members of the study participate in validating the analysis. Using this type of process of verification is also a meaningful way to document the trustworthiness of the process. It is clear from the reading of this report that collaboration led to a description of the situation, the mental health of caregivers, that reflects a thorough understanding of the dynamics at work.

Based on the development of an understanding of the informants' situations, the researchers and caregivers collaborated in the development of an education program that would be used to teach others about the experience of caregiving and its effect on mental health of caregivers. A joint decision was made by the team to experiment with the program using a group of caregivers other than those who were part of its development. The authors provide the reader with information related to how the program was evaluated. These included the following: (1) audio taping of each group session; (2) a semistructured diary completed by the group leader after each session; (3) informal group discussions; and (4) a semistructured individual interview with each caregiver after the sessions. These are appropriate methods to evaluate the program. The authors also could have included a pretest, posttest design if they wanted to include a quantitative evaluation strategy as well.

As stated earlier, the co-investigators decided to use individuals other than the caregivers who developed the program to implement it. The authors state that the educational program was provided to one group and then evaluated. Reflection is reported as being part of the journaling process used by the group leaders for the educational programs. However, based on the repeated references to group meetings for the purpose of developing, implementing, and evaluating the process, it is appropriate to imply that reflection was part of the process. However, the report would be stronger if it specifically addressed reflection as a unique concept.

Similar to Steps One and Two, content analysis was used to analyze the data collected in Step Three. Again, since the data collected are subjective statements, this is an appropriate strategy. Trustworthiness of data is demonstrated consistently through the use of strategies such as triangulation of data and validating findings as a part of the research process. Using criteria described by Badger (2000) to assure rigor, Ducharme et al. (2001) demonstrate dialectical validity by illustrating constant analysis and attention to the tensions and complexity in the situation and also critical validity through the authors' descriptions of analysis of the process of change.

The conclusions reported represent a local theory for providing a means to support caregivers before, during, and after the caregiving activity. The educational program is described in detail and certainly represents a program that can be implemented in similar practice settings. Ducharme et al. (2001) report that the use of action research "was coherent with the goal of empowering caregivers in the institutional setting and raising their awareness of their own health problems and rights" (p. 198). The researchers also share the difficulties included in conducting an action research study including the significant time and energy required and also the challenge of sharing power and changing one's world view about who should be in charge of conducting research.

The findings are offered within context and the implications are realistic and well stated. The authors offer that the study provides new information on nursing interventions for caregivers and also illustrates the relevance of the action research approach in valuing the contributions of family as part of the health care experience. In addition, Ducharme et al. (2001) discuss the moral and ethical concerns that arise from studying a group that has traditionally not had the power to control its environment. Finally, while sharing their conclusions, the researchers offer that the next step for this work will be to collect further evidence of the efficacy of the program that was developed as part of the study.

Ducharme et al. (2001) provide an excellent example of action research in their report of this study. They are honest in sharing the strengths of the method as well as the challenges. Most important, the study exemplifies the collaborative, empowerment process that is the hallmark of action research.

APPLICATION TO EDUCATION

Based on the literature reviewed, it is evident that the primary application of action research in nursing has been and continues to be in clinical practice. However, action research is an effective approach for looking at issues in education and administration. To help the individual new to action research evaluate its utility in nursing education, an action research study completed by Smith, Masterson, Basford, et al. (2000) entitled "Action research: A suitable method for promoting change in nurse education" will be reviewed using the critiquing criteria provided in Box 14.1.

The first question that is important to ask of any qualitative research study is: Why has a particular approach been selected to conduct the study? The researchers should convince you that they have selected the study approach for the appropriate reason. In the study by Smith et al. (2000), the authors do an excellent job of sharing the reason for selecting action research. They state that the approach was chosen for the following reasons: "1) its emphasis on participation and partnership and 2) its compatibility with a philosophy of health which promoted participatory forms based on equity and empowerment" (p. 564). These two statements reflect the fundamental characteristics of the approach and provide evidence for the reader that the researcher understands the characteristics of the approach. As part of the introduction, the researchers describe the education situation in England and help the reader appreciate why the action planned will be valuable.

Unique to the report is the fact that the published article does not share the results of the entire project but focuses on the first phase of the study, which was to enlist six nurse educators to assess the implementation and evaluate the integration of the concept of health into the preregistration nursing curriculum. Furthermore, the findings section of the report is focused on the process and outcomes of the study as well as how participants handled challenges and opportunities in implementing the curricular change. Therefore, all critiquing criteria suggested may not be able to be evaluated given the abbreviated presentation of the study.

The co-researchers in this study were six nurse educators from four centers and two researchers who had been part of an original research study that was commissioned by the English National Board of Nursing to facilitate the integration of health into preregistration and midwifery nursing curricula. These nurses came together on a regular basis to discuss the challenges and opportunities they faced in implementing health as a curricular concept. The specific procedures for selecting the six nurse educators are not shared.

Data were generated from workshop participation and in one-to-one discussions. There is little description of data analysis methods and no reference to human subjects' protection. The authors do share that based on reflective discussions, the categories of challenge and opportunity were identified and then themes were illuminated under each of these categories. Similar to the practice study reported earlier, the reader can assume that since the research was part of a study commissioned by the State Board of Nursing in England that human subjects' protection was assured; however, a statement reflecting institutional review would strengthen the report.

It is clear from the article that the co-participants were responsible for data generation and analysis. Reading their descriptions of the challenges and opportunities gives the reader a good idea of what the issues surrounding the integration of health into the curricula were. It is also clear that this information was generated as a result of reflection as evidenced by the authors' statement about the themes, "these headings are based on the key themes, which were identified during reflective sessions between the participants" (p. 565) as well as this statement about the nature of their reflections, "participants' experiences of undertaking action research demonstrated that findings constantly evolve and change as they are renegotiated and reinterpreted as the project progresses" (p. 568).

In this study report, the action has taken place already and the action research approach is being applied to identify the challenges and opportunities identified as part of the implementation. So, there is little information about how the action came about or its implementation. Since this report is intended to communicate the evaluation of the action, most of the data are descriptive of the evaluation process. In this case, action research is used as the way to evaluate the action brought about as a result of an earlier study.

The researchers and participants are clearly full collaborators in the evaluation process. This is evident in the report and also in the fact that all eight group members author the publication. There is no description of trustworthiness in the report provided.

The conclusions support action research as a strong method for conducting this follow-up study. The results are presented within context. They have generated some important information that will be useful in understanding the variable response to the implementation of health as a concept in the preregistration curriculum. No clear statements about the ethical and moral implication of the study are presented. The recommendations for use are focused on how to successfully use the action research process. The researchers presented the benefits to the participants throughout the study.

The research report offered by Smith et al. (2000) is not an easy article to follow for the reader who does not possess a working knowledge of action research. However, the work is important because it demonstrates the usefulness of action research as an approach to evaluation.

APPLICATION TO ADMINISTRATION

The roots of action research are in organizational change.

> Issues of organizational concern such as quality patient care, systems improvement, organizational learning and the management of change are suitable subjects for action research, as (a) they are real events, which must be managed in real time, (b) they provide opportunities for both effective action and learning and (c) can contribute to the development of theory of what really goes on in hospitals and to the development of nursing knowledge (Coghlan & Casey, 2001, p. 676).

Despite the opportunities that exist to conduct organizational studies in nursing, a current review of the literature reveals a limited number of action research studies that focus on organizational change. In this section, one of the articles identified during the literature search will be critiqued using the criteria found in Box 14–1. The publication by Kelly and Simpson (2001) is entitled "Action research in action: Reflections on a project to introduce clinical practice facilitators to an acute hospital setting."

The aims of the study conducted by Kelly and Simpson (2001) were "to introduce, develop and evaluate clinical practice facilitator (CPF) posts, whose remit [charge] was to work alongside newly qualified health care assistants (HCAs) to enhance their clinical skills" (p. 652). Since the aims include developing the role of the CPF and implementing it, action research seems an appropriate method to conduct the study. The researchers share a limited review and analysis of the practice situation. Similar to the article critiqued in the education section, this report is focused on both the research and reflections on the action research process. Therefore, the ability to critique all aspects of the study using the criteria offered may be limited.

Kelly and Simpson (2001) identify three phases to their approach to action research. These include assessment, action, and evaluation. Prior to initiating the assessment phase, the study was approved by a research ethics committee to ensure protection of human subjects. The views of all nursing staff in the areas where the project was to be implemented were solicited using the Ward Culture Questionnaire published by Adams, Bond, and Arber (1995). Findings from this questionnaire were examined by all CPFs to assist them in developing their roles. Also, "personal development reviews" (p. 654) were conducted with the CPFs to identify their strengths, weaknesses, and personal goals both long and short term. Finally, educational audits were reviewed to determine other factors that might potentially influence the planned intervention.

The participants in the study included the researchers, CPFs, and some "influential others" (Kelly & Simpson, 2001, p. 656) from within the institution. The specific procedures for including these individuals are not explicitly stated. Collaboration between the research partners is described. Kelly and Simpson reported that the "influential others" (p. 656) were less inclined to participate because of their fear of the costs associated with creating the new position.

During the action phase, the role of the CPFs was instituted. The actual time period for implementation is not offered. Reflective diaries were maintained by the CPFs as a way of providing documentation of key incidents. These offered the trigger for discussions during monthly project meetings. There is no description of how the diaries were analyzed. These data were meant to assist in negotiating or modifying the role as implemented.

Collaboration between the CPFs and researchers is evident. The researchers report that one of the ways collaboration was carried out was in the revision of the original role description for the CPFs. It is not clear how the role was developed or the process of its implementation.

Kelly and Simpson (2001) disclose that in addition to reflective diaries, reflective critique was undertaken. Reflective critique included "discussions of practical problems and identification of possible solutions" (p. 654). The results of the reflections were used as a way to conduct personal development review.

The evaluation plan is described. However, there is no reference to the role' that the CPFs played in development of the questionnaire that was used. The authors report the results of the questionnaire using percentages. Only one percentage figure is reported to demonstrate the positive response to the new role by nursing staff and managers in the affected areas. The authors do not specifically address the reliability or validity of their instrument. However, they do report the trustworthiness of their data by using triangulation of "qualitative accounts of the CPFs' experiences, supplemented with quantitative data from the assessment and evaluation questionnaires"(Kelly & Simpson, 2001, p. 654).

The conclusions of this study are reported within context and do reflect the findings. Local theory is evident. The implications of the study are clearly stated. The researchers offer recommendations for research and practice. A second phase of the reported project is already under way.

Kelly and Simpson (2001) "stress that it is essential for action researchers to consider the ethical dimensions of their work, and provide ways of ensuring that the ethical issues which do arise are discussed as openly as possible" (p. 658). Further they report that the participants gained from being involved by demonstrating considerable growth and development.

This report is a very good example of how the action research approach can be used effectively in administration. Nurse administrators who are interested in creating organizational change should feel confident that the approach offers a unique opportunity to co-create democratic and empowering change in real situations.

SUMMARY

In 1999, Jenks reported, "nurse-researchers in the United States rarely use action research because they do not regard it as a rigorous form of research" (p. 263). In this section, each of the studies offered demonstrates that action research can be useful in creating change and completed in a rigorous manner. Today, increasing numbers of nurses in the United States are utilizing action research because of its value in creating positive change in real situations. As this trend continues, nurse consumers should be careful to understand the characteristics of the method and the value of studying change in process.

In this chapter, critique has been the focus. Through rigorous review of published studies and careful implementation of the action research process, those unfamiliar with the method will gain an understanding and appreciation of the method as a valuable approach to nursing research.

REFERENCES

Adams, A., Bond, S., & Arber, S. (1995). Development and validation of scales to measure organizational features of acute hospital wards. *International Journal of Nursing Studies, 32,* 612–627.

Ainley, B., Barlow, P., Houldin, R., Miller, J., Potter, K., Reypert, A., & Wilson, S. (2000). Primary care: Action research in the implementation process. *Community Practitioner, 73*(2), 470–472.

Anderson, N. L. R., Nyamathi, A., McAvoy, J., Conde, F., & Casey, C. (2001). Perceptions about risk for HIV/AIDS among adolescents in juvenile detention. *Western Journal of Nursing Research, 23*(4), 336–359.

Badger, T. G. (2000). Action research, change and methodological rigor. *Journal of Nursing Management, 8,* 201–207.

Berman, H., McKenna, K., Arnold, C. T., Taylor, G., & MacQuarrie, B. (2000). Sexual harassment: Everyday violence in the lives of girls and women. *Advances in Nursing Science, 22*(4), 32–46.

Chan, S. W., & Wai-tong, C. (2000). Implementing contract learning in a clinical context: Report on a study. *Journal of Advanced Nursing, 31*(2), 298–305.

Coghlan, D., & Casey, M. (2001). Action research from the inside: Issues and challenges in doing action research in your own hospital. *Journal of Advanced Nursing, 35*(5), 674–682.

Dickson, G., & Green, K. L. (2001). Participatory action research: Lessons learned with aboriginal grandmothers. *Health Care of Women International, 22,* 471–482.

Ducharme, F., Lévesque, L., Gendron, M., & Legault, A. (2001). Development process and qualitative evaluation of a program to promote the mental health of family caregivers. *Clinical Nursing Research, 10*(2), 182–201.

Goldman, K. D., & Schmalz, K. J. (2001). Focus on focus groups. *Health Promotion Practice,* *2*(1), 14–19.

Higgs, Z. R., Bayne, T., & Murphy, D. (2001). Health care access: A consumer perspective. *Public Health Nursing, 18*(1), 3–12.

Hilton, B. A., Crawford, J. A., & Tarko, M. A. (2000). Men's perspectives on family coping with their wives' breast cancer and chemotherapy, *Western Journal of Nursing Research, 22*(4), 438–459.

Jenks, J. (1999). Action research method. In H. J. Streubert & D. R. Carpenter (Eds.), *Qualitative research in nursing: Advancing the humanistic imperative* (2nd ed., pp. 251–264). Philadelphia: Lippincott Williams & Wilkins.

Jones, A. (2000). Implementation of hospital care pathway for patients with schizophrenia. *Journal of Nursing Management, 8,* 215–225.

Kelly, D., & Simpson, S. (2001). Action research in action: Reflections on a project to introduce clinical practice facilitators to an acute hospital setting. *Journal of Advanced Nursing, 33*(5), 652–659.

LoBiondo-Wood, G., & Haber, J. (2002). *Nursing research: Methods, critical appraisal, and utilization.* St. Louis: Mosby.

Smith, P., Masterson, A., Basford, L., Boddy, G., Costello, S., Marvell, G., et al. (2000). Action research: A suitable method for promoting change in nurse education. *Nursing Education Today, 20*(7), 563–570.

RESEARCH ARTICLE

Development Process and Qualitative Evaluation of a Program to Promote the Mental Health of Family Caregivers

Francine Ducharme • Louise Lévesque • Marie Gendron
• Alain Legault

The purpose of this study was to develop and evaluate, through a participatory approach, an intervention program to promote the mental health of women caregivers in institutions. Focus groups were first organized to explore sources of stress for daughter and spousal caregivers. Workshops in which caregivers developed the content of a group program were then organized. The aims of the program were to increase empowerment and self-efficacy and to decrease stress and psychological distress of caregivers. Experimentation and qualitative evaluation of the program led to 10 weekly meetings covering the following topics: how to feel good with my relative, how to discuss with staff, how to appraise my experience differently, coping with my relative's losses, how to reorganize my life, and how to identify and ask for social support. This study provides a structured program to support family caregivers and a research method empowering families.

It is well recognized that caring for an elderly relative can have a negative impact on the mental health of family caregivers. Psychological distress, depression, perceived stress, sense of burden, and burnout have all been widely documented (for a review, see Guberman, 1999; Schulz, O'Brien, Bookwala, & Fleissner, 1995). Despite evidence that family caregivers continue to be involved in the care of elderly relatives even after they have been institutionalized (Aneshensel, Pearlin, Mullan, Zarit, & Whitlach, 1995;

Francine Ducharme, Ph.D., is a professor at the Faculty of Nursing, Université de Montréal, Québec, Canada, and a researcher at the Centre de Recherche, Institut Universitaire de Gériatrie de Montréal. She is director of the Nursing Research Chair in Nursing Care for the Elderly and Their Families.

Louise Lévesque, M.Sc., R.N., is a professor at the Faculty of Nursing, Université de Montréal. She is also a researcher at the Centre de Recherche, Institut Universitaire de Gériatrie de Montréal, a health research center on aging.

Marie Gendron, Ph.D., R.N., is director of "Baluchon Alzheimer," a community organization aimed at offering respite care for family caregivers of Alzheimer's patients.

Alain Legault, M.A., R.N. is a nursing doctoral student in the Université de Montréal–McGill University joint program.

Authors' Note: This project was funded by Health Canada through the Centre of Excellence for Women's Health Program.

Naleppa, 1996), most studies have limited their scope to the caregiving experience of families whose relative lives at home (Buck et al., 1997; Naleppa, 1996). One reason for this may be that admission to an institution is believed to reduce ipso facto the stress of caregiving (Zarit & Whitlach, 1992). The few empirical studies that have focused on family caregiving after institutionalization challenge this assumption and suggest that the caregiving experience continues to be associated with poor psychological well-being and that these caregivers remain an at-risk group that merits the attention of the health care system (Almberg, Grafstrom, & Winblad, 1997; Aneshensel et al., 1995; Buck at al., 1997).

Studies have shown that caring for an elderly relative suffering from dementia is more demanding and stressful than caring for a relative without this affliction (Lévesque, Ducharme, & Lachance 1999; Tennstedt, LeeCaffetera, & Sullivan, 1992). Dementia is characterized by a cognitive and functional deterioration that affects emotional expression and produces depressive moods and disruptive unpredictable behaviors that family members have difficulty coping with. The Canadian Study on Health and Aging (1994) showed the incidence of institutionalization of persons with dementia: Half of the elders with dementia in the 65 to 84 age-group and two thirds in the 85 plus age-group are institutionalized. According to this same survey, 71% of family caregivers of an institutionalized relative are women (i.e., spouses or daughters), and the depressive symptoms of these caregivers increase as their elderly demented relative deteriorates.

These results underscore the importance of further studying this specific group of women caregivers. Research into the sources of stress and the specific needs of these family caregivers of institutionalized elders with dementia has been scarce. The few authors that have addressed the issue have emphasized that caregivers must cope with new sources of stress associated with their relative's institutional setting (Aneshensel et al., 1995; King, Collins, Given, & Vredevoogd, 1991; Stephens, Kinney, & Ogrocki, 1991; Townsend, 1990; Zarit & Whitlach, 1992). These include adjustments in the relationship with the relative after placement, difficulty finding enough time and energy for visits, loss of social support, concerns about what to do or talk about during visits, and conflicts with staff due to unclear expectations regarding the family caregiver's involvement.

A literature review revealed that very few mental health promotion programs that could be offered by nurses have ever been designed and tested for this at-risk group of caregivers (Linsk, Miller, Pflaum, & Ortigara-Vicik, 1988; Maas et al., 1994; McCallion, Toseland, & Freeman, 1999; Wiancko, Crinklaw, & Mora, 1986; Wilken, Farran, Hellen, & Boggess, 1992). These few programs were analyzed using the conceptual perspective proposed by Twigg (1989) that entails three models of caregiving. In the first model, caregivers are considered key coworkers who can provide care to their relatives and relieve staff overload. In the second model, caregivers are seen as resources for the health care system, as they can provide staff with useful information for health care planning and quality of care. In the third model, caregivers are perceived as coclients of the health care system, whose own health needs are the focus of interventions aimed at promoting their well-being. The results of this analysis reveal that existing programs consider caregivers coworkers or resources, but not coclients.

These findings highlight the need to develop innovative and effective interventions for family caregivers (Canadian Association on Gerontology, 1999). Within this context, the purpose of this study was to develop and evaluate an intervention program to promote the mental health of family caregivers of institutionalized elders with dementia.

METHOD AND RESULTS

A constructivist inductive approach was used to develop and evaluate the program (Guba & Lincoln, 1989) with a view to gain knowledge of stressors and strategies to promote mental health from the perspective of caregivers. Based on a philosophy of empowerment (Tozer & Thornton, 1995), a participatory action-research model (Henderson, 1995) was selected. The research process entailed three steps in which participants were considered stakeholders, experts, and coinvestigators in the construction and refinement of a program to promote their own mental health (see Figure 1).

Step 1: Assessment of Sources of Stress

Given the little knowledge available on the specific needs of this particular group of caregivers, the first step in the research process sought to explore the main sources of stress of family caregivers. Focus groups (Morgan, 1998) were organized for the purpose of ensuring that the eventual program would be developed on the basis of the participants' own caregiving experience. This approach is generally used to obtain the opin-

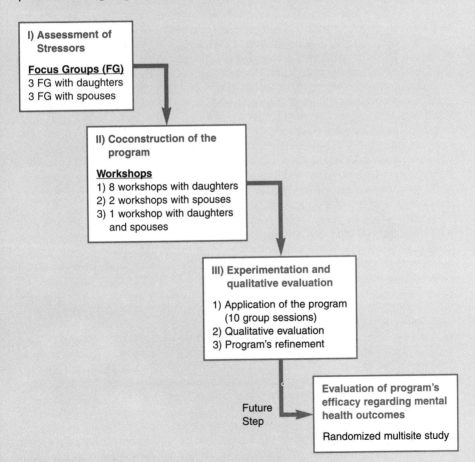

FIGURE 1 Steps in the research process.

ions and impressions of small groups of people (4 to 12) regarding a given problem, experience, or phenomenon (Krueger, 1998). It considers the benefit of group synergy (i.e., the interaction within the group) and facilitates the emergence of information that would not surface as easily without the group context (Carey, 1994). Focus groups have been recognized as a means to develop intervention programs (Krueger, 1998).

Sample and procedure. To participate in this first step, a family caregiver had to be the daughter or spouse of an elderly patient suffering from irreversible dementia and institutionalized for more than 6 but less than 36 months. Participants were recruited from various sampling sources to ensure a diversity of opinions and points of view (Krueger, 1998). The purposive sample was recruited in three long-term care institutions in the Montreal metropolitan area.

A total of nine daughters and eight spouses took part in this first step without attrition. The daughters had a mean age of 53 years (range of 39 to 69) and a mean duration of caregiving for their elderly parent of 9 years (range of 2 to 20). Five of the nine had children at home, and four of the nine were employed outside the house. Only two had previous experience with a support group. For the spouses, the mean age was 74 years (range of 57 to 87) and the mean duration of caregiving was 12 years (range of 2 to 47). All eight had children, but only one had a child living at home. Only one was employed outside the house and had previously been to a caregiver support group.

The group discussions were facilitated by a trained nurse expert in the field of caregiving for Alzheimer's patients and in group dynamics. Broad, open-ended questions were used to explore the participants' sources of stress and unmet health needs. Focus groups were conducted separately with daughters and spouses as their respective caregiving experiences may differ (Montgomery & Kosloski, 1994). A researcher was present at each session to collect data on the group dynamics (i.e., tacit acquiescence, body language, group's mood, contradictory statements). The sessions lasted 90 minutes, were held at night in three long-term care institutions, and were audiotaped while the researcher took field notes. Each focus group was followed by a debriefing session between the nurse facilitator and the researcher. Three focus groups were conducted, with each caregiver group. This number was determined by data saturation or redundancy of emerging themes across sessions and groups (Krueger, 1998).

Data analysis. As per the recommendations made by Huberman and Miles (1994), data collection and data analysis were combined into an interactive process. A preliminary content analysis of the verbatim transcript of the first group session was carried out by two members of the research team. A coding and categorization system was elaborated and a within-session analysis completed. This preliminary phase was followed by validation of the content analysis together with the participants (i.e., experts) using excerpts from the verbatim transcript to illustrate how their statements were coded and categorized. The results of the first focus group served as the starting point for the next focus group, and the data collected then were analyzed using the same process. The coding scheme was applied to all the focus groups and refined to avoid overlap, ambiguity, and lack of clarity. Analysis of reflective remarks based on field notes and memos (i.e., insights or ideas related to transcripts or codes) was also part of the analysis, as was identification of similar and different sources of stress across the two caregiver groups.

Results. The results of this first step led to the identification of stressors by the caregivers. Most stressors were common to the two caregiver groups. The five major stressors that emerged from the focus groups (i.e., daughters and spouses) and that were validated with the participants were the following: bereavement and sadness associated with the relative's deterioration, sense of powerlessness in the institutional setting due to loss of primary caregiver role (difficulty participating in decision making concerning relative's care, difficulty dealing with staff), sense of loneliness (difficulty finding appropriate social support), difficulty reorganizing own life after many years of primary caregiving, and feeling of fatigue and difficulty maintaining a personal life. The most salient stressors for daughters and wives, respectively, were role overload (i.e., daughter, wife, and worker) and sense of loneliness following husband's institutionalization.

Step 2: Coconstruction of the Program

Based on the focus group results (i.e., identification of sources of stress experienced by caregivers), the second step of the research process involved developing the program through workshops. Working meetings were organized in which caregivers themselves developed a program to promote their own well-being as coclients of the institutional health care setting. This approach was proposed to involve stakeholders as principal actors in the process of coconstruction of programs aimed at meeting their needs (Guba & Lincoln, 1989), in accordance with the principles of participatory action research (Henderson, 1995; McWilliam, 1997).

Sample and procedure. Volunteer spouses and daughters who took part in the focus groups were recruited for the weekly workshops. The same trained nurse acted as facilitator intent on encouraging the expression of ideas, proposals, opinions, needs, and expectations of the caregivers, as coinvestigators, concerning the future program. The same researcher collected field observations. Eight workshops with five daughters were followed by two workshops in which three spouses were asked to comment on the work done by the daughters and to add content with regard to their specific needs. There was no attrition. The number of workshops was determined by data saturation (i.e., when new ideas ceased to emerge concerning the content and structure of the program).

Data analysis. Data collected during each workshop were categorized and structured by the research team and validated by the participants at the beginning of the next workshop. As was the case with the focus groups, data collection and data analysis constituted an interactive process (see Figure 2).

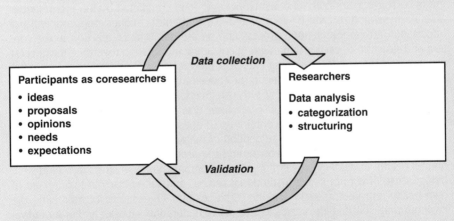

FIGURE 2 Interactive process of data collection and data analysis.

Finally, a refinement workshop was organized involving both daughters and spouses, in which a first version of the complete program was presented. Caregivers were asked to validate the adequacy of the program with respect to their needs.

Results. The results of this second step make it possible to clarify the goals of the program, as well as its content and structure. The following three goals were proposed by the participants: to increase their empowerment in the institutional setting, to increase their perceived self-efficacy relative to their abilities to take care of themselves and to find appropriate social support, and to decrease their perceived stress and psychological distress. The proposed program comprised ten 90-minute group sessions with five to eight caregivers and was structured according to six topics: coping with losses, appraisal of the caregiving experience, social support, life reorganization, taking care of self, and feeling in control. Empirical and conceptual data related to the above topics were considered in developing each group session. The stress and coping model of caregiving proposed by Pearlin, Mullan, Semple, and Skaff (1990), as well as conceptual and theoretical knowledge on social support (Stewart, 1993), empowerment (Jones & Meleis, 1993), and their relationship to mental health outcomes, were the underpinnings of the program. Role-playing, short theoretical presentations, individual and group exercises, readings, and discussions regarding concrete case examples were the strategies proposed by the caregivers to be used during the sessions. As the stressors identified and the content proposed by daughters and spouses were very similar, one program was developed taking into account the specificity of each group.

Step 3: Experimentation and Qualitative Evaluation

The final step of the research process was experimentation of the program coconstructed by caregivers and its qualitative evaluation.

Sample and procedure. The program was experimented with, as coinvestigators, a different sample of caregivers was made up of five daughters (mean age of 61 years) and one 73-year-old spouse. Only one daughter was single and only one was employed outside of the home. The program was offered at night in one institutional setting by the same trained nurse who once again acted as group leader.

Four data collection methods were used to evaluate the program: (a) audiotaping of each group session; (b) a semistructured diary completed by the group leader after each session, in which were recorded comments, critiques, suggestions, and information on the intervention process and on the participants' reaction to the content and structure of each group meeting (including information regarding reasons for absence and reasons for not doing exercises); (c) an informal group discussion at the last session aimed at soliciting feedback concerning the whole program; and (d) a semistructured individual interview with caregivers after completion of the program. To avoid social desirability, this last interview was conducted by an external interviewer using an interview guide containing 20 questions pertaining to the feasibility of the program; its acceptability; perception of the adequacy of its content and structure; satisfaction of participants concerning the program's achieved goals regarding mental health; and finally, perception of postprogram change in stress level and well-being, sense of control in the institutional setting, and self-efficacy in taking care of own health and finding social support. Critiques and suggestions for modifying the program were solicited (i.e., topics to add or avoid, duration, number and order of topics, exercises and readings, optimal number of participants, setting, and resources).

Data Analysis. The facilitator and the research team listened to the audiotapes after each session and, using a structured grid, assessed the adequacy of the initial design of the session with respect to its actual content. A content analysis of the facilitator's diary was performed simultaneously to provide data on the intervention process and on specific case examples that could be discussed the following week to illustrate or reinforce the content. The tenth audiotaped session provided group data on the general perception of the program (i.e., difficulties, relevance to this new group of caregivers). Finally, a content analysis of the verbatim transcripts from each individual interview was undertaken to provide in-depth qualitative evaluative data on each topic of the program. Data from all these sources were used to modify and refine the program.

Results. Analysis of the audiotapes of the 10 sessions shows that the program was administered as originally planned in terms of content, order of topics, and methods used. The duration of the sessions, however, exceeded initial plans (i.e., 2 hours instead of 1½). The length of time devoted to each topic was also more flexible. For instance, "Coping with my relative's losses," in which strategies to deal with the multiple losses associated with dementia and the eventual death of the loved one, took up more time than expected as caregivers were particularly vulnerable with regard to this sensitive topic. The caregivers participated actively in the complete program, asking for homework, particularly reading material on selected topics such as different ways to take care of oneself and prevent burnout, and rights and privileges as users of the health care system. There was no attrition. Moreover, although two elderly institutionalized relatives passed away during the course of the program, their caregivers continued their involvement in the group sessions.

The program received a positive assessment by the group at the last session. The comments gathered concerned the following: possibility of doing social comparisons during the sessions, value of exchanging coping strategies to deal with the losses of one's relative and reorganization of one's life, learning of new tools to cope with chronic stressors, a positive feeling of seeing things differently, and acquired knowledge of rights.

Analysis of individual interviews shows that the program met the various needs and expectations of the caregivers and achieved its goals. Although the content of the program addressed different ways to cope with loss and death, caregivers still had difficulty talking about these issues at the end of the program. All caregivers, however, considered this topic essential to the program.

Content analysis of the individual interviews makes it possible to identify five redundant themes in the participants' discourse. These themes are illustrated by the following excerpts from the verbatim transcripts:

Importance of being conscious of my needs and of taking care of myself:

To go through the exercise of trying to find time for yourself, force yourself to take five, it's not always obvious, but becoming aware of it is already a big step because once you're aware of it, you'll try to find a way of taking care of yourself.

The section "Taking care of myself" helped me most…laughing does me a lot of good, I don't always have time for that, taking care of myself…but at the same time, we managed to look at different aspects, how to try to find the time.

Taking care of yourself, that's always saying a mouthful when you're a caregiver, it's not always obvious, for me it's a big question mark. Taking care of others, sure, but there isn't always a whole lot left over for yourself. Just coming here is tak-

ing time off for you. You tell yourself: "Alright, I'm going to go to a meeting tonight and I'm going to take time off for myself, to sort a bunch of things out in my head, instead of taking care of..."

Becoming aware of my strengths and capacities:

There's one thing that I've become aware of, it's that I realized I had certain strengths that I didn't think I had. Maybe it's because I put them into practice and I saw that, yeah, I'm just as capable as the next person.

One of the positive aspects of the program...becoming aware of my strengths and abilities.

Recognition of my social support system:

I think we don't often stop to ask ourselves who might be able to help us out along the way or we simply don't dare ask for help.

We went through an exercise and it helped us a bit to open our eyes...just thinking about it can give us something...yeah, it's true, this or that person could hear me out....

We're better equipped, so we then know what to do, which door to knock on...who to talk to...

Need to know my rights and assert myself in the institution:

You can't be shy either, even in the nursing home, you can't be afraid to speak up or to say something when things don't suit you. The program helped me out in this department...it gave me a certain confidence, it made me realize that I am able to do this and that I am not alone...you can't be afraid cause living with your fears can really weigh you down day to day. It's quite a load to carry when you know there's a problem there and you can't fix it cause you don't know what to do about it...eventually it becomes quite a burden.

We talked about empowerment, and I put into practice on a couple of occasions...one moment, I was afraid and then the next I said, no, this is my mother and it's important that she be comfortable here...so I went to speak to the nurse...I put what we learned into practice and it helped.

Difficulty talking about the care, losses, and eventual death of my relative:

It's hard to talk about the care that our loved ones receive...we have certain concerns in this regard. You tell yourself: They're in the hands of strangers...we worry cause we ask ourselves: What can happen? And we don't know. We always feel a certain reticence, and we worry because we're handing over those we love, but we hand them over here cause we don't have a choice, but the question remains, What goes on when I'm not there?

They're our parents, we love them very much and we'd like to have them around forever...we know they have to go someday, but we'd like to put off the moment as long as possible.

It's pretty heavy stuff, we ask ourselves, how's it going to happen? (the death of a relative). We can't help worrying, it's heartrending, it's quite emotional.

Data from all these sources were used to refine the program and make a number of minor changes. The content of each session was more tightly linked to the central topic "Taking care of myself." Two sessions were planned on the difficult topic "Coping with the losses of my relative," and they were placed later on in the program after participants had had time to adjust to the group dynamics and build trust in one another. Finally, as caregiver empowerment was deemed an important topic, emphasis was placed on how to discuss the relative's care with staff. The final topics covered in the 10 sessions were the following:

- Getting to know one another
- How to feel good with your relative
- How to communicate your point of view to staff
- How to avoid emotional turmoil
- How to deal with small losses on a daily basis and prepare for the eventual loss of your relative
- How to reorganize your life after placement of your relative
- How to identify and call on your support network

The specific objectives and the content summary of each session are presented in Table 1.

DISCUSSION AND APPLICABILITY OF THE RESEARCH FINDINGS TO THE CLINICAL SETTING

The purpose of this study was to develop and evaluate an intervention program to promote the mental health of family caregivers of institutionalized elderly patients with dementia. It sought to contribute to the reconceptualization of services offered to family caregivers. As mentioned earlier, most programs consider caregivers either as coworkers or as resources of the health care system, not as coclients (Twigg, 1989). The participatory research process used in this study was congruent with its ultimate aim, that is, the development of a program to address the needs of family caregivers as coclients of the institutional setting.

The results of this study emphasize the importance of taking into account the health needs of family caregivers after the institutionalization of an elderly relative. The focus groups revealed that caregiver stress is not relieved after placement and that new sources of stress associated with the institutional setting emerge. Various difficulties specific to the new health care environment were described by the caregivers: participating in decision making concerning the relative's care, finding appropriate social support, reorganizing one's life after placement, and maintaining a personal life. These results support the fact that family caregivers continue their caregiving "career" even after placement of their relative and share major health needs.

Nurses are key players in supporting family members of long-term care patients. For a long time, they have been recognized for providing family-centered care in the form of instrumental assistance, information, and emotional support (Wright & Leahey, 1984). However, there are few systematic intervention programs available that have been tested for their efficacy on health of family caregivers. This project was an attempt to address this gap.

In this study, caregivers were allowed to voice their needs and desires. They asked for a greater say in the health care setting, greater self-efficacy in taking care of themselves and in finding social support, and relief from their stress and psychological distress. Nurses have the theoretical and clinical expertise to address these needs. The content of the program, coconstructed with the expert caregivers, concerns the four ingredients of the nursing metaparadigm, namely, health, person, environment, and

TABLE 1	TAKING CARE OF MYSELF: SPECIFIC OBJECTIVES AND CONTENT SUMMARY OF THE PROGRAM	
Topic of Meetings	**Specific Objectives**	**Content**
Session 1: Getting to know one another	• Introduce participants to objectives, content, and course of program • Allow participants to share their caregiver experience in the nursing home setting with respect to their health	• Participants' expectations • Presentation of the program • Exchanges among caregivers
Session 2: How to feel good with your relative	• Improve caregivers' perceived competence in their interactions with relatives	• Impact of illness on the relative's behaviors: perception of sources of stress; ways of improving communication
Sessions 3 and 4: How to communicate your point of view to staff	• Improve caregivers' ability to express their opinions regarding the care provided to their relatives and to take part in the decisions concerning them	• Relations with staff • Problem solving • Empowerment • Rights of family members • Complaint-handling procedure
Sessions 5 and 6: How to avoid emotional turmoil	• Enable caregivers to appraise their caregiving experience differently and to cope with difficult emotions	• Thought-modification strategy (e.g., reframing a difficult situation)
Sessions 7 and 8: How to deal with small losses on a daily basis and prepare for the eventual loss of your relative	• Facilitate awareness of the many losses caused by the illness of the relative and improve caregivers' ability to cope with these losses • Enable caregivers to cope with the eventual loss of their relative	• Losses caused by illness • Grieving process • Strategies for dealing with losses and grieving; thought modification • Preparing for the eventual loss of the relative
Session 9: How to reorganize your life after placement of your relative	• Increase caregivers' self-confidence in their ability to reorganize their life and to take care of themselves	• Reorganizing one's life • Strategies for taking care of oneself
Session 10: How to identify and call on your support network	• Increase caregivers' ability to call on their support network to meet their own needs	• How to ask for support

care (Fawcett, 1984). Communication, empowerment, coping with stress and grieving, self-efficacy, mental health, and social support are widely documented nursing concerns and concepts with a sound theoretical basis. In terms of its structure, the proposed program is convenient, does not call for substantial resources, and could be implemented in long-term care settings by nurse clinicians as part of their role within the family system.

During the course of this study, we were able to note that the relationship between the caregivers and the nurse clinician is just as important as the content of the program per se. The role of the nurse clinician was to form an alliance with the caregivers as they unfold their experience. She needs to consider these caregivers as active, meaning-giving persons to raise awareness of their existing abilities to change and control their own situation-in other words, to increase their empowerment. Two requirements appear to be particularly important to ensure the quality of this relationship between the nurse and the caregivers: openness and flexibility. The nurse clinician is exposed to a whole range of emotions and difficult situations during the program (e.g., issues related to the loss of a loved one and death) that can call into question her own value system. To maintain her openness, the clinician must be aware that her own values may influence her interpretation of the caregivers' statements and thus prevent her from exploring them further. Flexibility means to respect the readiness of the caregivers to change their coping behaviors, as well as sensitivity to the caregivers' rhythm and hesitations. In fact, the nurse clinician has to make the linkages between the various concepts proposed in the content of the program and participants' specific caregiving experiences and daily realities; a well-integrated knowledge of the program is not, by itself, sufficient.

Audiotaping was used as a self-assessment tool for the nurse clinician. The tapes gave important information on the content and the process of the intervention. It was also essential in preparing each session and in choosing relevant data for further discussion with the caregivers, considering their specific caregiving experience. This approach is convenient and could be used more widely when implementing such a program in clinical settings.

The process-oriented design used in this study deserves consideration in future nursing research. Its potential for social change and empowering clients and families in different settings and domain areas is noteworthy. Participatory research addresses how research should be conducted rather than which techniques should be used in gathering data. It is both an intervention per se and a means of studying an intervention. It is an alternative approach to conducting research that integrates science with education and political action (Henderson, 1995). In the participatory process, researchers share the power and control of decision making to construct, to implement, and to evaluate programs (Green et al., 1995). This approach ensures the ongoing involvement of participants in all phases of research.

As an integral part of the systems under investigation, subjects, considered experts, play an important role in gathering research data from the "real world" (McWilliam, 1997). Therefore, involving the stakeholders can potentially make a positive difference in achieving change. Such a participatory approach recognizes that for research to be usable, it must reflect the values and interests of those affected by it (Lomas, 1990). Involving participants in the research process also brings constituency values and interests to refining research questions, thereby ensuring that emerging knowledge reflects participants' priorities and beliefs.

As a practice discipline, nursing needs to focus on methods that can provide useful data for practice or data that can be rapidly transferable to the practice setting. As evidence mounts that the participation of service users strengthens interpersonal relationships and the sense of personal and political competence, namely, empowerment (Zimmerman, 1995), there has been a growing emphasis on participatory approaches in nursing interventions (American Academy of Nursing, 1993). In participatory nursing research, individuals become empowered to explore the connections between the social system and their own impaired health situations and to take action when these connections are uncovered (Henderson, 1995). In our study, the use of this approach was coherent with the goal of empowering caregivers in the institutional setting and raising their awareness of their own health problems and rights.

Nevertheless, despite its numerous advantages and its relevancy to nursing, it is important to recognize certain difficulties of this approach for clinical nursing research. Participatory research projects require time and energy from both partners involved, that is, the professional and indigenous researchers. The nurse researcher acts not only as a researcher but also as an educator, a mediator, a consultant, and sometimes an activist. This requires access to organizational resources, sharing of power, and a change in world view. Many nurses, like other health care professionals, assume that their training confers to them a status of expert and authority that becomes a barrier to considering their clients as collaborators. To be able to do participatory nursing research, nurses must give "power to the powerless and voices to the silent" (Comstock & Fox, 1993, p. 112). From a more systemic perspective, such a move favors social change in long-term care institutions.

It is also important to underscore the limits of this study. The sample size used was small. It was particularly difficult to recruit elderly spouses as their participation in the research process required time, energy, and a means of transportation. Also, although this study documented the program's feasibility and its acceptability to caregivers, further evidence of its efficacy is needed. The next step in the research process will be to test its effects on the mental health of caregivers. Selected outcome measures such as perceived stress and overload, psychological distress, self-efficacy, use of coping strategies, empowerment, and salivary cortisol level as a common physiological measure of stress used in caregiving research (Kiecolt-Glaser, Dura, Spreicher, Trask, & Glaser, 1991) will be considered. A randomized multisite study will provide empirical data in this regard (see Figure 1).

Finally, despite its limits, this study was interesting for two main reasons. First, it provided valuable empirical data on the sources of stress experienced by female caregivers of institutionalized elderly patients suffering from dementia, as well as a structured program inductively constructed to promote their own well-being. These results contribute new knowledge to the field of nursing intervention with family caregivers. Second, this study provided an illustration of a relevant approach coherent with a major nursing value: the importance of considering the family as an expert-client in its health experience (Parse, 1998).

Research article taken from: Ducharme, F., Lévesque, L., Gendron, M., & Legault, A. (2001). Development process and qualitative evaluation of a program to promote the mental health of family caregivers. *Clinical Nursing Research, 10*(2), 182–201. (Reprinted with permission.)

References

Almberg, B., Grafstrom, M., & Winblad, B. (1997). Caring for a demented elderly person: Burden and burnout among caregiver relatives. *Journal of Advanced Nursing, 25,* 109–116.
American Academy of Nursing. (1993). *Health care access, problems and policy recommendations.* Kansas City: Author.

Aneshensel, C., Pearlin, L., Mullan, J., Zarit, S., & Whitlach, C. (1995). *Profiles in caregiving.* San Diego: Academic Press.

Buck, D., Gregson, B., Bamford, C., McNamee, P., Farrow, G., Bond, J., & Wright, K. (1997). Psychological distress among informal supporters of frail older people at home and in institutions. *International Journal of Geriatric Psychiatry, 12,* 737–744.

Canadian Association on Gerontology. (1999). Canadian Association on Gerontology Policy Statement on home care in Canada. *Canadian Journal on Aging, 18,* i-iii.

Canadian Study on Health and Aging. (1994). Study methods and prevalence of dementia. *Canadian Medical Association Journal, 150,* 899–913.

Carey, M. (1994). The group effect in focus groups: Planning, implementing, and interpreting focus group research. In J. Morse (Ed.), *Critical issues in qualitative research methods* (pp. 224–241). Thousand Oaks, CA: Sage.

Comstock, D., & Fox, R. (1993). Participatory research as critical theory: The North Bonneville, USA experience. In P. Park, M. Brydon-Miller, & T. Jackson (Eds.), *Voices of change: Participatory research in the United States and Canada* (pp. 112–125). Westport, CT: Bergin & Garvey.

Fawcett, J. (1984). The metaparadigm of nursing: Present status and future refinements. *Image: The Journal of Nursing Scholarship, 16,* 84–89.

Green, L., George, M., Daniel, M., Frankish, C., Herbert, C., Bowie, W., & O'Neill, M. (1995). *Study of participatory research in health promotion: Review and recommendations for the development of participatory research in health promotion in Canada.* Ottawa: The Royal Society of Canada.

Guba, E., & Lincoln, Y. (1989). *Fourth generation evaluation.* Newbury Park, CA: Sage.

Guberman, N. (1999). *Caregivers and caregiving: New trends and their implication for policy* (Research Report prepared for Health Canada). Montréal, Canada: Université du Quebec à Montréal.

Henderson, D. (1995). Consciousness raising in participatory research: Method and methodology for emancipatory nursing inquiry. *Advances in Nursing Science, 17,* 58–69.

Huberman, A., & Miles, M. (1994). Data management and analysis methods. In N. Denzin & Y. Lincoln (Eds.), *Handbook of qualitative research* (pp. 428–444). Thousand Oaks, CA: Sage.

Jones, P., & Meleis, A. (1994). Health is empowerment. *Advances in Nursing Science, 15,* 1–14.

Kiecolt-Glaser, J., Dura, J., Spreicher, C., Trask, J., & Glaser, R. (1991). Spousal caregivers of dementia victims: Longitudinal changes in immunity and health. *Psychosomatic Medicine, 53,* 345–362.

King, S., Collins, C., Given, B., & Vredevoogd, J. (1991). Institutionalization of an elderly family member: Reactions of spouse and non-spouse caregivers. *Archives of Psychiatric Nursing, 5,* 323–330.

Krueger, R. (1998). *Analyzing and reporting focus group results.* Thousand Oaks, CA: Sage.

Lévesque, L., Ducharme, F., & Lachance, L. (1999). Is there a difference between family caregiving of institutionalized elders with or without dementia? *Western Journal of Nursing Research, 21,* 472–497.

Linsk, N., Miller, B., Pflaum, R., & Ortigara-Vicik, A. (1988). Families, Alzheimer's disease, and nursing homes. *Journal of Applied Gerontology, 7,* 331–349.

Lomas, J. (1990). Finding audiences, changing beliefs: The structure of research use in Canadian health policy. *Journal of Health Politics, Policy and Law, 15,* 525–542.

Maas, M., Buckwalter, K., Swanson, E., Specht, J., Tripp-Reimer, T., & Hardy, M. (1994). The caring partnership: Staff and families of persons institutionalized with Alzheimer's disease. *American Journal of Alzheimer's Care and Related Disorders and Research, 9*(6), 21–30.

McCallion, P., Toseland, R., & Freeman, K. (1999). An evaluation of a family visit education program. *American Geriatrics Society, 47,* 203–214.

McWilliam, C. (1997). Using a participatory research process to make a difference in policy on aging. *Canadian Journal on Aging, Supplement Bridging Policy and Research,* 70–89.

Montgomery, R., & Kosloski, K. (1994). A longitudinal analysis of nursing home placement for dependent elders cared for by spouses vs. adult children. *Journal of Gerontology, 49,* S62-S74.

Morgan, D. (1998). *Planning focus groups.* Thousand Oaks, CA: Sage.

Naleppa, M. (1996). Families and the institutionalized elderly: A review. *Journal of Gerontological Social Work, 27,* 87–111.

Parse, R. (1998). *The human becoming school of thought: A perspective for nurses and other health professionals.* Thousand Oaks, CA: Sage.

Pearlin, L., Mullan, J., Semple, S., & Skaff, M. (1990). Caregiving and the stress process: An overview of concepts and measures. *The Gerontologist, 30,* 583–594.

Schulz, R., O'Brien, A., Bookwala, J., & Fleissner, K. (1995). Psychiatric and physical morbidity effects of dementia caregiving: Prevalence, correlates, and causes. *The Gerontologist, 35,* 771–791.

Stephens, M., Kinney, J., & Ogrocki, P. (1991). Sources of stress for family caregivers of institutionalized dementia patients. *Journal of Applied Gerontology, 10,* 328–342.

Stewart, M. (1993*). Integrating social support in nursing.* Newbury Park, CA: Sage.

Tennstedt, S., LeeCaffetera, G., & Sullivan, L. (1992). Depression among caregivers of impaired elders. *Journal of Aging and Health, 4,* 58–76.

Townsend, A. (1990). Nursing home care and the family caregivers' stress. In M. A. Stephens (Ed.), *Stress and coping in later-life families* (pp. 267–280). New York: Hemisphere.

Tozer, R., & Thornton, P. (1995). *Having a say in change.* York, U.K.: University of York, Social Policy Research Unit.

Twigg, J. (1989). Models of carers: How do social care agencies conceptualize their relationship with informal carers? *Journal of Social Policy, 18,* 53–66.

Wiancko, D., Crinklaw, L., & Mora, C. (1986). Nurses can learn from wives of impaired spouses. *Journal of Gerontological Nursing, 12*(11), 28–33.

Wilken, C., Farran, C., Hellen, C., & Boggess, J. (1992). Partners in care: A program for family caregivers and nursing home staff. *American Journal of Alzheimer's Care and Related Disorders and Research, 7*(4), 8–15.

Wright, L., & Leahey, M. (1984). *Nurses and families: A guide to family assessment and intervention.* Philadelphia: F. A. Davis.

Zarit, S., & Whitlach, C. (1992). Institutional placement: Phases of transition. *The Gerontologist, 32,* 665–672.

Zimmerman, M. (1995). Psychological empowerment: Issues and illustrations. *American Journal of Community Psychology, 23*(5), 581–598.

15

Triangulation as a Qualitative Research Strategy

*T*riangulation is an approach to research that uses a combination of more than one research strategy in a single investigation. Researchers describe four types of triangulation for qualitative research: (1) data, (2) investigator, (3) theory, and (4) methods (Denzin, 1970). Mitchell (1986) has suggested a fifth type, multiple triangulation, whereby a combination of triangulation strategies is used. This is a complex approach, using a combination of two or more triangulation techniques in one study. For example, using multiple triangulation, the study design may include more than one data source as well as more than one researcher. (Denzin, 1970; Polit, Beck, & Hungler, 2001).

Navigators use the term *triangulation* to describe a technique of plotting a position using three separate reference points. Navigators must know the exact location of a ship or plane at any given time. However, navigation is not an exact science, particularly when the vessel is moving. Imagine the difficulty of describing the exact location of a ship when it is in the deep ocean far from shore. The ship navigator takes a compass reading between the boat and one reference point, often a star. This reading makes it possible for the navigator to draw a line on a map. The navigator knows the position of the ship is somewhere on the line drawn. That position on this line is far from accurate. To increase accuracy, the navigator then takes a compass reading between the boat and a second reference point, often a second star. This reading makes it possible for the navigator to draw a second line on a map that intersects with the first. The intersection of the two lines, still not an exact point, provides a more accurate location of the boat. This second location is inaccurate because both the first compass reading and the second compass reading have a margin of error. To decrease the margin of error, the navigator takes another compass reading from a third reference point. The line from this reading intersects the previous two lines at the location of the boat, providing a more exact location.

Campbell and Fiske (1959) were the first to apply the navigational term *triangulation* to research. The metaphor is a good one because a phenomenon under study in a qualitative research project is much like a ship at sea. The exact description of the phenomenon is unclear. To gain clarity about the phenomenon, researchers study the phenomenon from a particular vantage point, from which they learn additional information about the phenomenon. However, the information at this point is not precise. Like navigators, researchers then move to a different vantage point to study the phenomenon. Information from the second vantage point provides additional data about the phenomenon, hence making the description clearer. A third vantage point makes the description of the phenomenon far clearer than either of the first two vantage points. As in compass readings, techniques of qualitative research have their margins of error. The goal in choosing different strategies in the same study is to balance them so each counterbalances the margin of error in the other (Fielding & Fielding, 1989).

CHOOSING TRIANGULATION AS A RESEARCH STRATEGY

Qualitative investigators may choose triangulation as a research strategy to ensure completeness of findings or to confirm findings (Campbell & Fiske, 1959; Miles & Huberman, 1989; Patton, 1983). Completeness provides breadth and depth to an investigation, offering researchers a more accurate picture of the phenomenon (Denzin & Lincoln, 1994). Triangulation reveals the varied dimensions of a phenomenon and helps create a more accurate description (Fielding & Fielding, 1989). The metaphor of a group of visually impaired people describing an elephant based on the area they touch provides a good description of completeness. The person touching the trunk describes the elephant based on what that person feels. The person touching the foot provides a different description because of what he or she feels. The person touching the tail provides a third description. The most accurate description of the elephant comes from a combination of all three individuals' descriptions. None of the three alone is complete or accurate. Combining data from the vantage point of all three people results in a more complete and holistic description of the elephant.

Researchers might also choose triangulation to confirm findings and conclusions. Any single qualitative research strategy has its limitations. By combining different strategies, researchers confirm findings by overcoming the limitations of a single strategy (Breitmayer, Ayres, & Knafl, 1993). Confirmation occurs when investigators compare and contrast the information from different vantage points. Uncovering the same information from more than one vantage point helps researchers describe how the findings occurred under different circumstances and assists them to confirm the validity of the findings. In this case, researchers do not use validity to find an ultimate truth but, rather, to provide increased understanding and a more accurate picture.

TYPES OF TRIANGULATION

Investigators have the option of using several different types of triangulation to confirm or ensure completeness of findings. The choice of type depends on the research question asked and the complexity of the phenomenon under study. When planning a study, researchers carefully consider the research methodology necessary to adequately answer a research question. Qualitative researchers may choose to use triangulation as a strategy in any investigation in which their goal is to provide understanding or to obtain completeness and confirmation. In designing their study, researchers may use data triangulation, methodological triangulation, investigator triangulation, and theory triangulation, or a combination. Each type of triangulation possesses both strengths and weaknesses. Table 15.1 illustrates the strengths and weaknesses for each approach. A discussion of each triangulation type follows.

Data Triangulation

Using data triangulation, researchers include more than one source of data in a single investigation. Denzin (1970) described three types of data triangulation: (1)

TABLE 15.1   STRENGTHS AND WEAKNESSES OF FOUR TYPES OF TRIANGULATION

Type of Triangulation	Strengths	Weakness
Data Triangulation	Extensive data Data convergence and divergence Increased confidence in the research data Creative, innovative ways of phenomena	False interpretation due to overwhelming amount of data Difficulty dealing with vast amounts of data Fitting qualitative data into a quantitative mold
Investigator Triangulation	Expertise of more than one researcher in more than one methodology Decreased potential for bias Increased credibility of findings	Investigator bias Disruptive during interview Potential disharmony based on investigator biases
Method Triangulation	Exposing different types of information that contribute to overall understanding of the research problem Unique findings	Multimethod research is expensive Difficulty meshing narrative and numerical data
Theoretical Triangulation	Broader analysis of findings	Adds to confusion if concepts are not defined Conflicts due to theoretical frameworks Lack of understanding as to why triangulation strategies were used

Adapted from: Thurmond, V. A. (2001). The point of triangulation. *Journal of Nursing Scholarship, 33*(3), 253–258.

time, (2) space, and (3) person. Researchers choose the type of data triangulation that is relevant to the phenomenon under study. Using *time triangulation*, researchers collect data about a phenomenon at different points in time. Time of day, day of week, or month of year are examples of times researchers would collect data for triangulation. Studies based on longitudinal designs are not considered examples of data triangulation for time because they are intended to document changes over time (Kimchi, Polivka, & Stevenson, 1991).

Space triangulation consists of collecting data at more than one site. For example, a researcher might collect data at multiple units within one hospital or in multiple hospitals. At the outset, the researcher must identify how time or space relates to the study and make an argument supporting the use of different time or space collection points in the study. For example, a researcher studying decision making on a nursing unit might collect data on six different nursing units to triangulate for space. The researcher might also collect data on each shift and on weekdays and weekends to triangulate for time. The rationale for using the various collection spaces and times is to compare and contrast decision making at each time and in each location. By collecting data at different points in time and in different spaces, the researcher gains a clearer and more complete description of decision making and is able to differentiate characteristics that span time periods and spaces from characteristics specific to certain times and spaces.

Using *person triangulation*, researchers collect data from more than one *level of person*, that is, a set of individuals, groups, or collectives (Denzin, 1970). *Groups* can be dyads, families, or circumscribed groups. *Collectives* are communities, organizations, or societies. Investigators choose the various levels of person relevant to the study. In the previous example of studying decision making on a nursing unit, the level of person might be individual nurses, the staff working on a given shift, or the staff assigned to a given unit. Researchers use data from one level of person to validate data from the second or third level of person. Researchers might also discover data that are incongruent among levels. In such a case, researchers would collect additional data to reconcile the incongruence.

Reising (2002) conducted a grounded theory study to explore the early socialization of new critical care nurses. She used data triangulation in her research by interviewing both critical care nurses and their preceptors regarding the experience of socialization to the critical care area. The interviews with the preceptors were conducted following the conclusions of data collection with the critical care nurses. This was done "to help clarify the orientation process from the preceptors' points of view" (p. 21). Person triangulation added to the trustworthiness of the Reising's findings by confirming and clarify data.

When carried out responsibly, data triangulation contributes to the rigor of a qualitative study. When planning a study, investigators should consider their data carefully. They should decide if time, space, or level of person is relevant to the data. They should plan to collect data from all appropriate sources, at all appropriate points in time, and from all appropriate levels of person. The result will be a broader and more holistic description of the phenomenon under study.

Methods Triangulation

Qualitative researchers use methods triangulation when they incorporate two or more research methods into one investigation. Methods triangulation can occur at the level of design or data collection (Kimchi et al., 1991). Methods triangulation at the design level has also been called *between-method triangulation*, and methods triangulation at the data collection level has been called *within-method triangulation* (Denzin, 1970). Design methods triangulation most often uses quantitative methods combined with qualitative methods in the study design. Sometimes triangulation design method might use two different qualitative research methods. For example, Wilson and Hutchinson (1991) described how researchers might use two qualitative research methodologies, Heideggerian hermeneutics and grounded theory, in qualitative nursing studies. They explained that using two unique methods in one study can explicate realities of the complex phenomena of concern to nursing that might remain illusive if researchers used either method alone. "Hermeneutics reveals the uniqueness of shared meanings and common practices that can inform the way we [nurses] think about our practice; grounded theory provides a conceptual framework useful for planning interventions and further quantitative research" (p. 263).

When researchers combine methods at the design level, they should consider the purpose of the research and make a cogent argument for using each method. Also, they should decide whether the question calls for simultaneous or sequential implementation of the two methods (Morse, 1991). If they choose *simultaneous implementation*, they will use the qualitative and quantitative method simultaneously. In *sequential implementation*, they will complete one method first, then, based on the findings of the first technique, plan and implement the second technique. Using simultaneous implementation, researchers must remember that they must limit interaction between the two data sets during data generation and analysis because the rules and assumptions of qualitative methods differ (Morse, 1991, 1994). For example, it is usually impossible to implement qualitative and quantitative methods on the same sample. Qualitative methods require a small, purposive sample for completeness, whereas quantitative methods require large, randomly selected samples. In simultaneous triangulation, the qualitative sample can be a subset of the larger quantitative sample, or researchers might choose to use different participants for each sample. An exception occurs if the quantitative measure is standardized. In this case, researchers would have the participants in the qualitative sample complete the quantitative measure and then would compare the findings with the standardized norms (Morse, 1994). If the measure is not standardized, then researchers must use a sequential triangulation technique as well as a much larger sample for the quantitative measure.

Morgan and Stewart (1997) used simultaneous methods triangulation at the design level in their study on the effects of the client care unit design on the care of elderly residents with dementia. The researchers designed a large study that compared the effects of a low-density special care unit with those of a high-density special care unit. They gathered quantitative data from staff and family caregivers in a quasi-experimental study. A smaller subset of the original sample participated in the qualitative portion of the study, which the researchers designed to provide complementary data on questions raised by the quantitative data. The qualitative data, which provided detailed descriptions of clients' behavior that the researchers did not obtain using the quantitative measures, was particularly valuable in providing information about the effects of the social environment on that behavior. The researchers found the combination of methods provided a more complete picture of the effects of the unit design than either method would have provided alone. Although the researchers did not provide the information necessary to determine if one researcher was a quantitative expert and the other was a qualitative expert, they did analyze the quantitative and qualitative data separately and provided for rigor in both methods.

Skillen, Olson, and Gilbert (2001) used method triangulation to study personal risk in public health nursing with regard to organizational factors and work hazards. They conducted a thematic analysis of "unanalyzed semistructured interview segments from data that emerged during an earlier exploratory descriptive study" (p. 664). Combining methods once again provided a more complete understanding and description of the problem. Butcher, Holkup, and Buckwalter (2001) also used method triangulation in their study dealing with caring for family members with Alzheimer's disease.

In contrast, researchers using a sequential triangulation technique begin by collecting either quantitative or qualitative data. If substantial theory has already been generated about the phenomenon, if the researchers can identify testable hypotheses, or if the nature of the phenomenon is amenable to objective study, the investigation would begin with a quantitative technique. If there is no theory, the theory is not well developed, or the phenomenon is not amenable to objective study, researchers would begin with a qualitative technique (Morse, 1991). Researchers who begin a study with a qualitative approach do so to further explore unexpected findings following the completion of a quantitative analysis. A study might begin with a qualitative technique to generate testable hypotheses that a researcher will then study quantitatively.

Morrison (1997) used sequential methods triangulation at the design level in an investigation intended to identify nursing management diagnoses. The study began with qualitative focus group interviews of 35 nurse-managers to determine the problems of managing nursing units and to ground the diagnoses in the nurse-managers' practice. The nurse-managers also described typical judgments they might make while managing a nursing unit. An initial listing of potential management diagnoses emerged from the managers' descriptions of problems and judgments. The researchers then used a quantitative Delphi technique to determine a final listing of nursing management diagnoses. The investigators completed the quantitative portion of the study with 400 randomly selected nurse-managers.

When combining research methods, it is essential that investigators meet standards of rigor for each method. Using qualitative methods, researchers should ensure sampling is purposive and should generate data until saturation occurs.

Using quantitative methods, researchers should ensure sample sizes are adequate and randomly chosen. Theory should emerge from the qualitative findings and should not be forced by researchers into the theory they are using for the quantitative portion of the study (Morse, 1991). Likewise, investigators should appropriately use validity and reliability measures to assure rigor of quantitatively derived data. Analysis techniques should be separate and appropriate to each data set. The blending of qualitative and quantitative approaches does not occur during either data generation or analysis. Rather, researchers blend these approaches at the level of interpretation, merging findings from each technique to derive a cohesive outcome. The process of merging findings "is an informed thought process, involving judgment, wisdom, creativity, and insight and includes the privilege of creating or modifying theory" (Morse, 1991, p. 122). If contradictory findings emerge or researchers find negative cases, the investigators most likely will need to study the phenomenon further. If knowledge gained is incomplete and saturation has not occurred, additional data collection and analysis should reconcile the differences and result in a more complete understanding.

In another study, Dreher and Hayes (1993) used methods triangulation at the design level to study the effects of marijuana use during pregnancy and lactation on children from birth to school age. The researchers planned to study two groups of Jamaican women: marijuana users and non-marijuana users. However, the tool they had expected to use had been developed in the United States and, thus, was culturally inappropriate to Jamaican society. Instead, the researchers used ethnographic interview and observation of Jamaican women to revise the tool for culture appropriateness. The ethnographic data helped the researchers refine the language and relevancy of the instruments and modify the manner in which the tool was administered. By administering the tool in a culturally appropriate manner, the researchers were able to elicit valid and reliable responses.

Using methods triangulation at the level of data collection, researchers use two different techniques of data collection, but each technique is within the same research tradition. In a qualitative study, researchers might combine interview with observation or diaries with videotaping. The purpose of combining the data collection methods is to provide a more holistic and better understanding of the phenomenon under study. When combining methods at this level, researchers must first carefully consider the advantages and disadvantages of each method. Then, they should combine methods so that each overcomes the weaknesses in the other. For example, observation is an excellent technique for qualitative data generation. However, using observation, researchers cannot determine the reasons behind actions observed. Interview is an excellent method for determining reasons behind behavior. However, researchers can never be sure that individuals' actions mirror what they say they would do in an interview. By combining the techniques, investigators can see behavior in action and hear the participants describe the reasons behind behavior.

Miles and Huberman (1989) described methods triangulation at the data collection level as a state of mind. They suggested that a rigorous qualitative researcher automatically checks and double checks findings and uses multiple data generation techniques to ensure accuracy and completeness of findings. For this reason, many qualitative researchers do not specifically identify their use of triangulation when combining data collection techniques. However, designing qualitative research with multiple data collection methods requires careful planning. Researchers must carefully incorporate each data collection technique into the research design and state the rationale for the use of each technique. They also should delineate the strengths and limitations of each technique. Researchers may not always create the design a priori. A study may begin with two data generation techniques, each designed to overcome the weaknesses of the other. After collecting data, the researchers may realize an additional limitation in the data. At this point, the researchers may add a third data collection technique to the design. For example, an investigator studying a phenomenon using interview and observation might realize that participants have a sketchy memory of past experiences. To get a more accurate view of experiences that have occurred over time, the researcher might decide to add diaries to the research design.

Carr and Clarke (1997) reported using methods triangulation at the data collection level in their study on the phenomenon of vigilance in families who stay with hospitalized relatives. The researchers used informal, semistructured interviews and participant observation of the caregivers to confirm and complete the data. The interviews provided insight into the caregivers' perceptions of what it meant to have the day-to-day experience of staying with a hospitalized relative. The investigators also observed the family members as they interacted with their relative to gain insight into patterns of interaction. Participant observation allowed the investigators to observe the environmental aspects of the client unit, relationships, processes, and events. The observational data confirmed the interview data; that is, observations confirmed families' verbalized commitment to their hospitalized relative. In their report, the researchers indicated that the combination of interview and observation data resulted in a more complete and holistic picture of vigilance than either method would have provided alone.

It is not an easy task to use methods triangulation; it is often more time-consuming and expensive to complete a study using methods triangulation (Begley, 1996). The study design is more complicated, complex, and difficult to implement, and imprecise use may actually increase error and enhance the weaknesses of each method, rather than compensate for weaknesses (Fielding & Fielding, 1989; Morse, 1991). Often a single researcher is not expert in using more than one technique; consequently, investigator triangulation is required.

Investigator Triangulation

Investigator triangulation occurs when two or more researchers with divergent backgrounds and expertise work together on the same study. To achieve investigator triangulation, multiple investigators each must have prominent roles in the study and their areas of expertise must be complementary (Kimchi et al., 1991). Having a second research expert examine a data set is not considered investigator triangulation. Rather, all researchers need to be involved throughout the entire study so they may compare and neutralize each other's biases.

The choice of investigators depends on the nature of the phenomenon under study. Research method, data generation technique, data analysis, or theory may drive the choice. For example, the use of multiple theories in a study directs the choice of investigators when a researcher expert in parenting and a researcher expert in homelessness collaborate to study what parenting means to homeless women. In this example, each investigator brings theoretical expertise to the study. Or using methods triangulation, research method drives the choice of investigators-investigators expert in each method used in the study participate in the study. When each investigator participates fully in the investigation, his or her expertise contributes to every aspect of the study. Each investigator ensures that he or she has properly implemented the research method, data generation technique, or theory to formulate the ultimate study outcome. Then, all the investigators discuss their individual findings and reach a conclusion, which includes all findings.

Use of methods triangulation usually requires investigator triangulation because few investigators are expert in more than one research method (Oberst, 1993). Researchers experienced in each method need to collaborate to design and implement the study, particularly when combining qualitative and quantitative methods because the philosophical orientation and the requirements for rigor are so different between the two methods. An understanding of the phenomenon under study will increase as each researcher combines his or her differing perspectives and approaches. Through this collaboration, the researchers will synthesize new understandings and theories. It is vitally important that researchers representing each discipline approach the investigation with open minds. Ideally, each will come with his or her discipline-specific biases but, simultaneously, will be open to hearing other investigators' approaches. Open dialogue with articulation and acceptance of biases will result in unique understandings.

Theoretical Triangulation

Theory triangulation incorporates the use of more than one lens or theory in the analysis of the same data set (Duffy, 1987). In a quantitative study, researchers identify two theories a priori and articulate rival hypotheses. Through the investigation, the researchers test and compare the rival theories. The result might be accepting one theory over the other or merging the theories to form a new, more comprehensive theory. In qualitative research, more than one theoretical explanation emerges from the data. Researchers investigate the utility and power of these emerging theories by cycling between data generation and data analysis until they reach a conclusion. By considering rival explanations throughout analysis of qualitative data, researchers are more likely to gain a complete or holistic understanding.

Lev (1995) used theory triangulation to investigate efficacy in clients who were receiving chemotherapy. The investigator triangulated the Orem's self-care theory and Bandura's self-efficacy theory because she believed neither theory completely explained efficacy in this client population. From the combined theories, the researcher designed an efficacy-enhancing intervention that she applied to clients who were receiving chemotherapy. The researcher implemented a combination of qualitative and quantitative methods to investigate the effectiveness of the intervention, using a form of methods triangulation at the level of data collection. Because the researcher used both theory triangulation and methods triangulation, the study is also an example of *multiple triangulation*, the use of more than one method of triangulation in a single study (Mitchell, 1986).

In another example of theoretical triangulation, Boutain (2001) combined critical social theories, African American studies and critical discourse concepts in her qualitative study on hypertension in rural south Louisiana. Her rationale was related to the fact that multiple perspectives intersect in the development of knowledge about African American health.

Clearly, each type of triangulation has both strengths and weakness. As Boutain (2001) noted, "Appropriately used, triangulation might enhance the completeness and confirmation of data in research findings of qualitative research. The use of both quantitative and qualitative strategies in the same study is a viable option to obtain complementary findings and to strengthen research results. However, researchers must articulate why the strategy is being used and how it enhances the study" (p. 257).

SUMMARY

Triangulation can be a useful tool for qualitative as well as quantitative researchers. Used with care, it contributes to the completeness and confirmation of findings necessary in qualitative research investigations. As researchers plan and carry out investigations, they should strive to provide the most complete understanding possible, using triangulation only when appropriate in their search for understanding. Nursing phenomena are complex and multifaceted. Clearly there are times when a multidimensional perspective will provide rich, unbiased data that are reliable and valid. This chapter has explored the various types of triangulation strategies that may be applied to a research study, their disadvantages, and their benefits. Ultimately, the fundamental design of the study must be strong. Qualitative researchers should approach investigations with openness to philosophic approaches. If different philosophical and research traditions will help to answer a research question more completely, then researchers should use triangulation.

REFERENCES

Begley, C. M. (1996). Using triangulation in nursing research. *Journal of Advanced Nursing, 24*, 122–128.

Breitmayer, B. J., Ayres, L., & Knafl, K. A. (1993). Triangulation in qualitative research: Evaluation of completeness and confirmation purposes. *Image, 25*, 237–243.

Boutain, D. M. (2001). Discourse of worry, stress and high blood pressure in rural south Louisiana. *Journal of Nursing Scholarship, 33*(3), 225–230.

Butcher, H. K., Holkup, P.A., & Buckwalter, K. C. (2001). The experience of caring for a family member with Alzheimer's disease. *Western Journal of Nursing Research, 23*(1), 33–55.

Campbell, D. T., & Fiske, D. W. (1959). Convergent and discriminant validation by the multitrait-multimethod matrix. *Psychological Bulletin, 56,* 81–105.

Carr, J. M., & Clarke, P. (1997). Development of the concept of family vigilance. *Western Journal of Nursing Research, 19,* 726–739.

Denzin, N. K. (1970). Strategies of multiple triangulation. In N. K. Denzin (Ed.), *The research act* (pp. 297–313). New York: McGraw-Hill.

Denzin, N. K., & Lincoln, Y. S. (1994). Entering the field of qualitative research. In N. K. Denzin & Y. S. Lincoln (Eds.), *Handbook of qualitative research* (pp. 1–17). Thousand Oaks, CA: Sage.

Dreher, M. C., & Hayes, J. S. (1993). Triangulation in cross-cultural research of child development in Jamaica. *Western Journal of Nursing Research, 15,* 216–229.

Duffy, M. E. (1987). Methodological triangulation: A vehicle for merging quantitative and qualitative research methods. *Image, 19,* 130–133.

Fielding, N. G., & Fielding, J. L. (1989). *Linking data.* Newbury Park, CA: Sage.

Kimchi, J., Polivka, B., & Stevenson, J. B. (1991). Triangulation: Operational definitions. *Nursing Research, 40,* 364–366.

Lev, E. L. (1995). Triangulation reveals theoretical linkages and outcomes in nursing intervention study. *Clinical Nurse Specialist, 9,* 300–305.

Miles, M. B., & Huberman, A. M. (1989). *Qualitative data analysis.* Newbury Park, CA: Sage.

Mitchell, E. S. (1986). Multiple triangulation: A methodology for nursing science. *Advances in Nursing Science, 8*(3), 18–26.

Morgan, D. G., & Stewart, N. J. (1997). The importance of social environment in dementia care. *Western Journal of Nursing Research, 19,* 740–761.

Morrison, R. S. (1997). Identification of nursing management diagnoses. *Journal of Advanced Nursing, 25,* 324–330.

Morse, J. M. (1991). Approaches to qualitative-quantitative methodological triangulation. *Nursing Research, 40,* 120–123.

Morse, J. M. (1994). Designing funded qualitative research. In N. K. Denzin & Y. S. Lincoln (Eds.), *Handbook of qualitative research* (pp. 220–235). Thousand Oaks, CA: Sage.

Oberst, M. T. (1993). Possibilities and pitfalls in triangulation. *Research in Nursing & Health, 16,* 393–394.

Patton, M. Q. (1983). *Qualitative evaluation methods.* Beverly Hills, CA: Sage.

Polit, D. F., Beck, C. T., & Hungler, B. P. (2001). *Nursing research: Methods, appraisal and utilization* (5th ed.). Philadelphia: Lippincott Williams & Wilkins.

Reising, D. L. (2002). Early socialization of new critical care nurses. *American Journal of Critical Care, 11*(1), 19–26.

Skillen, D. L., Olson, J. K., & Gilbert, J. A. (2001). Framing personal risk in public health nursing. *Western Journal of Nursing Research, 23*(7), 664–678.

Thurmond, V. A. (2001). The point of triangulation. *Journal of Nursing Scholarship, 33*(3), 253–258.

Wilson, H. S., & Hutchinson, S. A. (1991). Triangulation of qualitative methods: Heideggerian hermeneutics and grounded theory. *Qualitative Health Research, 1,* 263–276.

Ethical Considerations in Qualitative Research

Ethical issues related to professional nursing practice arise daily in the constant struggle to do good for the patient and avoid harm. All that we do in the name of patient care is wrought with tension between these two principles. As science and technology provide avenues to intervene in ways we never thought possible, unanticipated and more complex ethical dilemmas will continue to arise in our practice settings. The ethical dilemmas that emerge are grounded in the fact that direct relationships with human beings are the heart of nursing's important work. Understanding ethical principles in theory combined with life experience in practice prepares the nurse to make sound ethical and moral decisions on a daily basis. This knowledge and experience can be transferred to an understanding of ethical issues with regard to the research process.

Ethical issues and standards must be critically considered in any research study. Nurse researchers have a professional responsibility to ensure the design of both quantitative and qualitative studies that maintain ethical principles and protect human rights. The profession of nursing has a code of ethics that provides guidelines related to practice issues (American Nurses Association, 2001). Silva (1995) provides an explicit account of the roles and responsibilities of nurses in the conduct, dissemination, and implementation of nursing research. The principles addressed by Silva (1995) can be transferred to a discussion of ethical issues in qualitative research.

There has been an ongoing discussion in the nursing literature pertaining to the ethical variances that have arisen in qualitative investigations. A number of authors have noted that guidelines established for quantitative research investigations require an expanded scope of discussion when applied to qualitative research endeavors (Demi & Warren, 1995; Haggman-Laitila, 1999; Orb, Eisenhauer, & Wynaden, 2001; Robley, 1995). These authors have examined in depth specific ethical issues related to the conduct of qualitative research. Given that understanding, this chapter will address ethical issues that require critical consideration in any qualitative research endeavor. Table 16.1 provides qualitative researchers with an "ethics checklist" to use as a guide in the constructive critique of the ethical aspects of a research study.

Discussions are devoted to ethical issues related to informed consent, participant-researcher relationships, gaining access, confidentiality, anonymity, sample size, and data analysis. The ethical issues considered in this chapter are relevant to

TABLE 16.1	THE "ETHICS CHECKLIST": A GUIDE FOR CRITIQUING THE ETHICAL ASPECTS OF A QUALITATIVE RESEARCH STUDY

Topic	Guiding Questions
Phenomenon of interest	1. Is the research study relevant, important, and most appropriately investigated through a qualitative design? Explain.
	2. Are there any aspects of the research or phenomenon of interest that appear to be misleading either in terms of the true purpose or misleading to participants? Explain.
	3. Is the research primarily being conducted for personal gain on the part of the researcher or is there evidence that the research will somehow contribute to the greater good? What are the benefits to the participants or society as a whole?
Review of the literature	1. Has all the available literature been reviewed?
	2. Are all citations accurate in terms of referencing and quoting?
	3. Is the basis for inclusion of the articles referred to explicit?
Research design	1. How did the researcher protect the physical and psychological well-being of the participants?
	2. Is consent freely given?
	3. How were vulnerable populations recruited and protected?
	4. Did an Institutional Review Board approve the research?

(continued)

each of the methods presented in the text and should be considered within the context of the method selected for a particular investigation. Ultimately, qualitative researchers must remain sensitive to the possibility of ethical issues arising that may not have been anticipated.

It is critical that qualitative researchers maintain an ongoing dialogue regarding ethical dilemmas encountered during qualitative investigations so that all researchers can benefit from the experience of others. Despite the most vigilant attempts to ensure ethical conduct during a qualitative investigation, new and important considerations are always emerging. For example, Boman and Jevne (2000) report on an experience of being charged with an ethical violation in the conduct of a qualitative investigation. The article centers on a frank discussion of a qualitative research endeavor in which the identity of a study participant was disclosed (Boman & Jevne, 2000). There is much to be learned from this open and honest sharing of the researcher experience.

TABLE 16.1	THE "ETHICS CHECKLIST": A GUIDE FOR CRITIQUING THE ETHICAL ASPECTS OF A QUALITATIVE RESEARCH STUDY (CONTINUED)

Topic	Guiding Questions
Sampling	1. How was the confidentiality of participants protected?
	2. Is there any evidence of coercion or deception?
Data generation	1. If more than one researcher collected data, were they adequately prepared?
	2. Is there evidence of falsified or fabricated data?
	3. Is there intentional use of data collection methods to obtain biased data?
	4. Was data collection covert? If so, does the researcher explain why?
	5. Have the participants been misled with regard to the nature of the research?
Data analysis	1. Was data analysis conducted by more that one person?
	2. Is there evidence of data manipulation to achieve intended findings?
	3. Is there evidence of missing data that may have been lost or destroyed?
Conclusions and recommendations	1. Is there evidence of intentional false or misleading conclusions and recommendations?
	2. Is confidentiality broken given the presentation of the findings?

Adapted from Firby, P. (1995). Critiquing the ethical aspects of a study. *Nurse Researcher, 3*(1), 35–41.

Similarly, Lawton (2001) discusses ethical concerns related to informed consent and role conflict that emerged during a participant observation study of dying patients. Lawton (2001) and Boman and Jevne (2000) provide relevant examples from personal experience that will serve to enhance the ethical integrity of future studies. Their open and frank discussions leave all researchers in a better position to address ethical issues that present during the conduct of a qualitative investigation.

ETHICAL ISSUES IN QUALITATIVE RESEARCH

Distinct and conceivably unanticipated ethical issues emanate from the unpredictable nature of qualitative research. As Robley (1995) so aptly noted, "ethical considerations relevant to quantitative research impact qualitative investigations in unique and more fragile ways" (p. 45). The ethical dilemmas inherent in issues surrounding informed consent, anonymity and confidentiality, data generation, treatment, publication, and participant-researcher relationships are reviewed in light of the unique issues that emerge in the design and conduct of qualitative investigations. The content presented is comprehensive; however, the researcher must remain open to the possibility of new and to date unexamined ethical concerns related to qualitative research. Ethical standards for qualitative investigations must evolve from a sense that the research is dynamic and a process that may result in unanticipated ethical concerns. Further, these standards must be grounded in the ethical principles of autonomy, beneficence, and justice.

Researchers must observe certain basic principles when conducting an investigation. First, participants must not be harmed, thereby supporting the principle of *beneficence*. In any qualitative investigation, if researchers sense that the interview is causing issues to surface that may result in serious consequences, they must protect the welfare of the participants, perhaps by ending the interview or providing follow-up counseling and referrals. Researchers must obtain informed consent, and informant participation must be voluntary, thereby supporting the principle of *autonomy*. Furthermore, researchers must assure participants that confidentiality and anonymity will be upheld and that participants will be treated with dignity and respect. The principles of *beneficence* and *justice* are upheld in this regard (Beauchamp & Childress, 1994). The three ethical principles of autonomy, beneficence, and justice provide the organizing framework for a meaningful dialogue regarding ethical issues that pertain to qualitative investigations.

INFORMED CONSENT

Informed consent is a topic of regular discussion in health care settings. There is an expectation that, in the clinical setting, when clients sign a consent form, they are fully aware of both the health benefits and the actual or potential risks to their health (hence, the term *informed consent*). Informed consent in research holds similar meaning, with added inherent dimensions.

Any dialogue referencing informed consent must be grounded in the ethical principle of autonomy that encompasses the notion of being a self-governing person with decision-making capacity. Polit, Beck, and Hungler (2001) defined informed consent as follows: "Informed consent means that participants have adequate information regarding the research; are capable of comprehending the information; and have the power of free choice, enabling them to consent voluntarily to participate in the research or decline participation" (p. 78). The researcher is obligated to provide the participant with relevant and adequate information when obtaining informed consent. The emergent design of a qualitative investigation, however, presents qualitative researchers with ethical considerations that have the potential to violate the basic premise of informed consent.

Of particular concern is the notion that participants will have adequate information regarding the research study. Although a participant may consent to a study on the life experience of open heart surgery, new issues may emerge within the context of the interview for which the participant and, perhaps, even the researcher were unprepared. Research with vulnerable populations or topics that deal with sensitive subjects may change the direction of the research or reveal information that is not related to the original purpose of the study.

"As a minimum, it [informed consent] requires that prospective human subjects are given true and sufficient information to help them decide whether they wish to be research participants" (Behi & Nolan, 1995, p. 713). The open, emerging nature of qualitative research methods in most cases makes informed consent impossible because neither researchers nor participants can predict exactly how data will present themselves either through interview or participant observation (Holloway & Wheeler, 1995; Ramos, 1989; Robley, 1995). As Robley (1995) pointed out, "Questions of ethics arise within the context of the shifting focus of the study, the unpredictable nature of the research and the trust relationship between the researcher and the participant" (p. 45).

"The inherent unpredictability of the research process undermines the spirit of informed consent and endangers the assurance of confidentiality, two basic ethical safety nets in more quantitative research" (Ramos, 1989, p. 58). For example, in a study on the meaning of quality of life for individuals with type 1 (insulin-dependent) diabetes mellitus, data collection might begin with one open-ended question: "Tell me in as much detail as possible: What does it mean to have quality of life with type 1 insulin-dependent diabetes mellitus?" The researcher's probing questions to elicit a more detailed understanding can literally open a Pandora's box. Issues surrounding compliance or noncompliance may arise that endanger the client's health, or perhaps the client is depressed and concerned about issues related to loss, death, and dying. What may emerge is impossible to predict, but both researchers and participants must be informed and prepared to address issues that arise as data emerges.

The emergent design of qualitative research demands a different approach to informed consent. *Consensual decision making*, also called *process informed consent*, is more appropriate for the conduct of a qualitative investigation. This approach requires that researchers, at varying points in the research process, reevaluate participants' consent to participate in the study. According to Munhall (1988), process consent encourages mutual participation: "Because qualitative research is conducted in an ever-changing field, informed consent should be an ongoing process. Over time, consent needs to be renegotiated as unexpected events or consequences occur" (p. 156). Information about how the researcher enters the field, participants' time commitment, and what will become of the findings are all important components to process consent (Munhall, 1988). Participants must know from the beginning of and be reminded throughout the investigation that they have the right to withdraw from the research study at any time. A process consent offers the opportunity to change the original consent as the study emerges and change becomes necessary. "Common sense plays a large part in renegotiating informed consent. If our focus should change, we need to ask participants for permission to change the first agreement. Continually informing and asking permission establishes the needed trust to go on further in an ethical manner" (Munhall, 1988, p. 157).

It is essential that researchers and participants discuss and clarify their understanding of the investigation (Alty & Rodham, 1998; Raudonis, 1992). As Alty and Rodham (1998) have emphasized, "At the best of times, it is difficult to know if the person you are talking to really has the same understanding of the topic as you do, indeed, if the researcher has an accurate understanding of what the subject is expressing" (p. 277).

Covert participant observation, which results when participants are unaware they are being observed, presents another ethical concern for qualitative researchers. Covert participant observation is sometimes a necessary component to data generation in some qualitative investigations. The rationale from the researcher's perspective would be to ensure that collected data are true and accurate. This type of data generation is grounded in the idea that, when the participants are aware they are being observed, their behavior will change. For example, Clarke (1996) discussed the use of covert participant observation in a secure forensic unit and the ethical issues that emerged from this method of data generation. Clarke emphasized the need to obtain an "uncontaminated picture of the unit" (p. 37).

A researcher's integrity can become damaged if the researcher uses deception to generate data. Some researchers claim that deception in the form of covert observations—or not completely describing the aims of the study or its procedures—is sometime necessary to get reliable and valid data (Douglas, 1979; Gans, 1962). Punch (1994) agreed that field-related deception might be necessary, provided the interests of the subjects are protected. Others have argued that the need for covert research is exaggerated (Bulmer, 1982). The use of covert participant observation must be given serious consideration in the conduct of a qualitative investigation. Researchers must consider available alternative solutions for data generation provided those solutions will maintain the integrity of the study.

Confidentiality and Anonymity

The principle of beneficence, doing good and preventing harm, applies to providing confidentiality and anonymity for research study participants. According to Polit et al. (2001), "A promise of confidentiality to participants is a guarantee that any information the participant provides will not be publicly reported or made accessible to parties other than those involved in the research" (p. 138) and "anonymity occurs when even the researcher cannot link a participant with the data for that person" (p. 82).

The very nature of data collection in a qualitative investigation makes anonymity impossible. The personal, one-to-one interaction during the interview process allows researchers to know the participants in ways that are impossible and unnecessary in quantitative designs. Qualitative research methods such as participant observation and one-to-one interviews make it "impossible to maintain anonymity at all stages; in other words, when using these methods, becoming cognizant of the source of data is unavoidable" (Behi & Nolan, 1995, p. 713).

Small sample size and thick descriptions provided in the presentation of the findings can present problems in maintaining confidentiality (Behi & Nolan, 1995; Holloway & Wheeler, 1995; Lincoln & Guba, 1987; Ramos, 1989; Robley, 1995). Davis (1991) discussed thick descriptions as follows: "We learn from our experiences and we need to present the fruits of that learning in a full-bodied way that invites our audience to share that experience with us, and also to judge the legitimacy of our results" (p. 13). Robley (1995) emphasized that thick descriptions are extremely important to the meaning of the research and offered a solution supported by the works of Cowles (1988), Davis (1991), and Lincoln and Guba (1987): "If the narrative requires it, retain it and return to the respondent for permission, verification, and justification" (Robley, 1995, p. 48).

Often, if the research has been conducted close to home and the sample is familiar to others, the details given in the thick slices of data used to support and verify themes may reveal research participants' identities. The researcher must make every effort to ensure that confidentiality is a promise kept. "Guaranteeing confidentiality implies that the research subject's data will be used in such a way that no-one else but the researcher knows the source" (Behi & Nolan, 1995, p. 713). As Robley (1995) has pointed out, "Guarding against disclosure that may create unacceptable risks for the respondents is accomplished in part by respecting the need for withdrawal of revealing material during the interview process, and in part through the process of member checking and negotiated outcomes" (p. 46). In some instances, circulation of the research may need to be restricted to protect participants' identity (Orb, Eisenhauer, & Wynaden, 2001).

Orb, Eisenhauer, and Wynaden (2001) note that confidentiality and anonymity can be breached by legal requirements such as when researchers' data are subpoenaed for legal purposes (p. 95). Audit trails, commonly used to establish the confirmability of research findings, require that other researchers read the raw data. Participants need to know that this may occur within the context of data analysis.

The process of publication may also result in a breach in confidentiality or anonymity. Permission to use direct quotes must be acquired and the researcher must be sure that examples of raw data do not reveal the participant's identity. It is imperative that within the process of gaining consent that the participants know how the results will be used and whether they will be published (Orb, Eisenhauer, & Wynaden, 2001).

Ethical Considerations Related to the Researcher-Participant Relationship

The principle of justice concerns fair treatment and the right to privacy and anonymity. The data generation strategies associated with a qualitative investigation include such approaches as one-to-one interviews, focus groups, and participant observation. The private and intimate nature of this relationship imposes unique constraints and raises distinct ethical issues for investigators using qualitative methods. The researcher is the tool for data collection and, as such, comes to know participants in a personal way. The boundaries of the relationship may become blurred as the research progresses, and role confusion may lead to ethical concerns for the investigation. As Ramos (1989) explained, "The respondent and the investigator interact verbally, and their relationship can range from one of civil cooperation to camaraderie in problem-solving to the abiding trust and dependency of the therapeutic alliance" (p. 59).

"Nurses are legally, culturally, and historically bound to nurture and protect the health and welfare of their patients" (Ramos, 1989, p. 57). Therefore, when participants confuse the researcher's role with that of a counselor, therapist, or nurse as caregiver and unrelated issues of concern emerge, the protection of the participants' welfare must always take precedence over the research. Researchers must not move from the role of instrument in the investigation to that of counselor or therapist. "Research in nursing constitutes a delicate balance between the principles of rigorous investigation and a nurturing concern for patient welfare" (Ramos, 1989, p. 57). Investigators can attempt to guide the interview and maintain focus on the topic under investigation. Following the closure of the interview, researchers should recap for the participants issues of concern that emerged during the interview and should also provide follow-up.

Researchers must also consider the selection of participants for a qualitative research study from an ethical standpoint. "An ethical basis for selection would also involve attention to the inclusion of those whose voices need to be heard: women, minorities, children, the illiterate, and those with less personal or professional status. Social responsibility calls for attention to diversity" (Robley, 1995, p. 46).

SENSITIVE ISSUES ARISING IN THE CONDUCT OF QUALITATIVE RESEARCH

The interview may be one of the few opportunities participants have to discuss the issue at hand, and the topic may well be a sensitive one. Alty and Rodham (1998) have given perspective to sensitive issues:

> The ouch! factor is a term that describes certain experiences encountered in the process of conducting qualitative research. These experiences include those ranging from a short sharp shock to the researcher to those situations and experiences that can develop into a chronic ache if not addressed early (p. 275).

Sensitive issues also may arise in research conducted with vulnerable populations such as dying people (Raudonis, 1992), children and adolescents (Faux, Walsh, & Deatrick, 1988), families (Demi & Warren, 1995), lesbians and gay men (Platzer & James, 1997), HIV research in poor nations (Mabunda, 2001), and individuals with intellectual disabilities (Llewellyn, 1995). Certain topics such as the "sudden violent death of a loved one, controversial involvement in political activity, a crumbling relationship, legal incarceration, and a life-threatening illness" (Cowles, 1988, p. 163) are extremely sensitive and place participants in a vulnerable situation as the researcher asks the probing questions to elicit the necessary data. Given the intensity of the interaction between researcher and participant, the researcher also may be in a vulnerable position. As Robley (1995) has observed,

> Subjectivity and collaboration makes the researcher vulnerable. Emotionally immersed in the lived experience of others, continually sensitive to the potentially injurious nature of language, and experiencing the rights of passage as an interviewer/observer—all require an inner strength that can be enhanced by self care. The researcher can use the ethics committee as a guide and support throughout the process. [He or she] can use debriefing to explore personal responses and weigh risk/benefits. Personal education in ethics and consultation with experts when it is believed that the nurse researcher is being hurt is advocated (p. 48).

Similarly, James and Platzer (1999) discuss the risk of harm to both researcher and participant in a qualitative study with lesbians and gay men and their experiences with health care. Their account of the complex emotional and ethical issues that can arise in research with vulnerable groups emphasizes the need for researchers to pay attention to things that cause them discomfort and unease in the process of their research.

Do not stray from the focus of the investigation. Recognize that participants may need to talk but make clear that the researcher will address the issue after the interview. "All research (particularly that which focuses on sensitive issues) may stir up emotions of such intensity that failure to provide an opportunity for the respondent to talk may be perceived as irresponsible" (Alty & Rodham, 1998, p. 279). Allowing time for feedback and discussion of participants' feelings brings with it the possibility that the researcher will hear too much, but it must be done. After each interview, ask participants if they need follow-up. Provide a contact for additional help (Alty & Rodham, 1998; Holloway & Wheeler, 1995).

GATHERING, INTERPRETING, AND REPORTING QUALITATIVE DATA

Gathering, interpreting, and reporting qualitative research findings requires that researchers spend time planning how data will be collected and then reading and rereading verbatim transcriptions of interviews and field notes. Procedures such as bracketing (defined in Chapter 2) are required if researchers are to have any confidence in the final data analysis. Researchers must keep any presuppositions or personal biases separate or set aside throughout the entire investigation. Having a second researcher review the data and verify categories can also serve as a validity check. According to Ramos (1989),

The investigator, even with the validation of inferences afforded by the relationship with the respondent, imposes his or her logic and values onto the communicated reality of the respondent. He or she imposes his or her subjective reality upon the interpretation of meaning-data from the respondent. The researcher cannot extract correct meanings unilaterally. Without the validation afforded by member checking, a leap in logic could occur, and a serious misinterpretation of sensitive information can occur (p. 60).

Returning final descriptions to participants so that they may validate that the interpretation of the interview or observation is authentic and true further adds to final data analysis. This procedure can assist researchers in verifying that there were no serious misinterpretations or omissions of critical information.

Haggman-Laitila (1999) expands on the discussion of authenticity of data and overcoming the researcher's personal views. Haggman-Laitilla (1999) bases a discussion of data collection and analysis on the assumption that the researcher cannot detach from his or her own view in phenomenological research. The researcher is able to understand the experiences of an individual only through the researcher's own view. The research process is a balanced cooperative relationship between the subjects and the researcher (p. 13). Given this assumption, Haggman-Laitila offers practical guidelines for the purpose of data gathering and interpretation in a qualitative investigation.

During the process of data gathering, Haggman-Laitaila suggests that researchers plan key interview questions in advance, keep interviews open and discussion-like, verify interpretations by asking more questions and allowing additions and corrections, avoid rhetorical or leading questions, and keep a diary or videotape to facilitate recognition of the researchers' own views during the data analysis process. During data analysis the researcher must look for additional questions raised in the data, write down questions that emerge during the reading of the data, compare researcher and participant views, reexamine all experiences, and be sure that the presentation of findings is based on the views expressed by the participants.

SUMMARY

The process of conducting a qualitative investigation is complex, personal, and intense. Qualitative data collection strategies prevent anonymity and may result in the development of close, intimate relationships between participants and the researcher. In addition, presentation of the findings with thick descriptions and slices of raw data may complicate issues of confidentiality. Researchers must consider and address the vulnerability of certain populations. These issues are important in the ongoing development and use of qualitative research methods.

Although established ethical guidelines may give some direction, the ethical and moral picture of qualitative research is much more complicated. Even though an ethical review board may have approved a research study, problems may still arise. "We should not simply assume that because research has been accepted by a committee it is morally justifiable in its methods" (Firby, 1995, p. 36). Ethical guidelines for qualitative research will continue to emerge, and researchers must consider those guidelines from a different perspective than those associated with quantitative designs.

REFERENCES

Alty, A., & Rodham, K. (1998). The ouch! factor: Problems in conducting sensitive research. *Qualitative Health Research, 8*(2), 275–282.

American Nurses Association. (2001). *Code for nurses with interpretive statements*. Kansas City, MO: Author.

Beauchamp, T. L., & Childress, J. F. (1994). *Principles of biomedical ethics* (3rd ed.). Oxford, England: Oxford University Press.

Behi, R., & Nolan, M. (1995). Ethical issues in research. *British Journal of Nursing, 4*(12), 712–716.

Boman, J., & Jevne, R. (2000). Ethical evaluation in qualitative research. *Qualitative Health Research, 10*(4), 547–554.

Bulmer, M. (Ed.). (1982). *Social research ethics*. New York: Macmillan.

Clarke, L. (1996). Covert participant observation in a secure forensic unit. *Nursing Times, 92*(48), 37–40.

Cowles, K. V. (1988). Issues in qualitative research on sensitive topics. *Western Journal of Nursing Research, 10*(2), 163–179.

Davis, D. S. (1991). Rich cases: The ethics of thick description. *Hastings Center Report, 21*(4), 12–16.

Demi, A. S., & Warren, N. A. (1995). Issues in conducting research with vulnerable families. *Western Journal of Nursing Research, 17*(2), 188–202.

Douglas, J. D. (1979). Living morality versus bureaucratic fiat. In C. B. Klockers & F. W. O. Connor (Eds.), *Deviance and decency: The ethics of research with human subjects* (pp. 13–33). Beverly Hills, CA: Sage.

Faux, S. A., Walsh, M., & Deatrick, J. A. (1988). Intensive interviewing with adolescents. *Western Journal of Nursing Research, 10*(2), 180–194.

Firby, P. (1995). Critiquing the ethical aspects of a study. *Nurse Researcher, 3*(1), 35–41.

Gans, H. J. (1962). *The urban villagers: Group and class in the life of Italian-Americans*. New York: Free Press.

Haggman-Laitila, A. (1999). The authenticity and ethics of phenomenological research: How to overcome the researcher's own views. *Nursing Ethics, 6*(1), 12–22.

Holloway, I., & Wheeler, S. (1995). Ethical issues in qualitative nursing research. *Nursing Ethics, 2*(3), 223–232.

James, T., & Platzer, H. (1999). Ethical considerations in qualitative research with vulnerable groups: Exploring lesbians' and gay men's experiences of health care-a personal perspective. *Nursing Ethics, 6*(1), 73–81.

Lawton, J. (2001). Gaining and maintaining consent: Ethical concerns raised in a study of dying patients. *Qualitative Health Research, 11*(5), 693–705.

Lincoln, Y. S., & Guba, E. (1987). Ethics: The failure of positivist science. *Review of Higher Education, 12*, 221–240.

Llewellyn, G. (1995). Qualitative research with people with intellectual disability. *Occupational Therapy International, 2*, 108–127.

Mabunda, G. (2001). Ethical issues in HIV research in poor countries. *Journal of Nursing Scholarship, 33*(2), 111–114.

Munhall, P. (1988). Ethical considerations in qualitative research. *Western Journal of Nursing Research, 10*(2), 150–162.

Orb, A., Eisenhauer, L., & Wynaden, D. (2001). Ethics in qualitative research. *Journal of Nursing Scholarship, 33*(1), 93–98.

Platzer, H., & James, T. (1997). Methodological issues conducting sensitive research on lesbian and gay men's experience of nursing care. *Journal of Advanced Nursing, 25,* 626–633.

Polit, D. F., Beck, C. T., & Hungler, B. P. (2001). *Nursing research: Methods, appraisal, and utilization* (5th ed.). Philadelphia: Lippincott Williams & Wilkins.

Punch, M. (1994). Politics and ethics in qualitative research. In N. K. Denzin & Y. S. Lincoln (Eds.), *Handbook of qualitative research* (pp. 86–97). Thousand Oaks, CA: Sage.

Ramos, M. C. (1989). Some ethical implications of qualitative research. *Research in Nursing and Health, 12,* 57–63.

Raudonis, B. A. (1992). Ethical considerations in qualitative research with hospice patients. *Qualitative Health Research, 2*(2), 238–249.

Robley, L. R. (1995). The ethics of qualitative nursing research. *Journal of Professional Nursing, 11*(1), 45–48.

Silva, M. (1995). *Ethical guidelines in the conduct, dissemination, and implementation of nursing research.* Washington, DC: American Nurses Publishing.

A Practical Guide for Sharing Qualitative Research Results

Developing a qualitative research study is a significant activity. Identifying a problem suitable for qualitative investigation, following through with data collection and analysis, and disseminating the findings can be a lengthy process. Researchers using qualitative designs will need a degree of tenacity to complete a qualitative project. However, the enthusiasm generated from completion of the first study will certainly support continuing work within the qualitative paradigm. Sharing the results of a qualitative investigation with other nurse–researchers becomes a reality at the completion of the study. This is an exciting opportunity to provide new insights, receive thoughtful critiques, and learn from others with similar interests.

Once qualitative researchers develop a degree of comfort with research activities involved in the conduct of a qualitative project, they may become interested in developing a grant proposal using qualitative approaches. Grant writing requires qualitative researchers to develop additional skills, an effort well worth the time, especially when researchers' ideas are validated through the receipt of grant funds.

This chapter informs qualitative researchers about the differences in presentation style when a researcher submits a qualitative manuscript for publication, offers suggestions on how to submit a qualitative proposal for grant funding, and shares creative strategies for presenting qualitative research findings. In addition, a funded qualitative research proposal and critique are included at the end of the chapter.

PUBLICATION PREPARATION

All researchers are responsible for disseminating research findings. Sharing results with colleagues is an exciting opportunity. Whether they share ideas in a journal article or in a public forum such as a conference, qualitative researchers need to be aware of the audience's expectations as well as the best way to offer the findings of their studies.

Identifying an Audience

Upon completion of a study, when it is time to report results, researchers should clearly identify for whom they are writing. If the audience is comprised of primarily qualitative researchers, the manuscript will read differently than if the audience is made up of nurse-clinicians, educators, or administrators interested in the research. Be clear from the start who the audience is. By reviewing current journals, the researcher can begin to identify which journals support the publication of qualitative research and which ones don't. Some nursing journals include more qualitative research studies on average than others. Regular review of major research journals will alert investigators to these journals. Journals that publish qualitative studies on a regular basis include *Advances in Nursing Science, The Journal of Nursing Scholarship, Nursing Science Quarterly, Qualitative Health Research, Research in Nursing and Health*, and *Western Journal of Nursing Research*. This list is not exhaustive, nor is it offered to suggest that other journals do not publish qualitative studies. The purpose is to share the names of journals that have demonstrated a sustained and ongoing commitment to the publication of qualitative research.

In addition to identifying a journal that will be receptive to qualitative research approaches, it is essential to identify a journal with a focus on the content area of the study. For instance, the purpose of *Qualitative Health Research* is to disseminate qualitative research; however, the journal focuses on practice issues in health care and does not usually publish nursing education research articles. Therefore, an education study that utilizes qualitative methods would best be reported in an education journal such as *The Journal of Nursing Education* or *Nurse Educator*.

Once researchers have identified the potential journal, it is essential that they obtain a copy of the journal guidelines for authors. This document assists researchers to develop a manuscript that meets the editorial expectations of the selected journal. Most guidelines for authors do not offer specific recommendations for the presentation of qualitative findings. Reading qualitative studies published in journals is the best way to develop an understanding of how to meet editorial guidelines when submitting results of a qualitative study for publication. Regardless of the journal in which the findings will be published, qualitative researchers should follow certain guidelines.

Each group of readers has a specific purpose in reading a particular journal. Therefore, researchers must speak to the important facets of the research as they relate to the audience. These facets should reflect the purpose of the journal. For example, if researchers are writing for a scientific journal such as *Nursing Research*, detailing methods and data analysis will be as important as sharing the findings. In contrast, if they plan to publish in *Home Health Care Nurse*, the findings and implications for practice will be more important to the readership than the actual methods for conducting the study.

Most novice scholars are educated to submit query letters. A query letter tells the editor about what the author wishes to write. Many journal editors now report that query letters are unnecessary and may prolong the editorial process because of the time from submission of the query letter to response by journal staff. Often a phone call or e-mail will suffice to confirm whether the topic is of interest to the readership of a particular journal. Remember that, when developing a manuscript, you must be certain to present the research well. Poorly prepared manuscripts can set the stage for a rejection letter even if the study has significant merit.

Once researchers have submitted a manuscript, editorial staff will review the new submission and decide whether the content reflects the journal's purpose and is well written. If not, they will return the manuscript. Researchers are then responsible for identifying a more suitable periodical. Authors should expect to receive a postcard or letter within a few weeks of submission reporting on the status of the manuscript. The time from submission to publication may be more than 1 year. However, if after 3 or 4 months, authors have not received a progress report on the disposition of the manuscript (i.e., whether it has been accepted or rejected), they should follow up with a phone call, e-mail or letter.

Developing the Manuscript

The most difficult thing about writing is getting started. This statement is not intended to suggest that qualitative researchers have not been writing. However, documenting field notes and analyzing interviews are much different forms of writing than writing for publication. Documenting field notes or interviews is personal in nature and is not usually scrutinized by others. Researchers usually learn through the conduct of their projects that it is easy and even fun to write notes for themselves, but it is more difficult to transfer those personal ideas to paper for others to read.

The very nature of data collection and analysis requires that researchers write. Documenting their feelings, perceptions, observations, theoretical directions, or insights is part of the implementation of the qualitative research experience. Transforming diaries, memos, or transcripts into a publishable manuscript requires rigor and determination, as well as keen synthesis, writing, and organizational abilities.

Qualitative research generates a large amount of raw data. In raw form, the data are interesting but unusable for research reporting. Qualitative researchers must condense, analyze, and synthesize for readers the importance of the research while not losing the richness of the findings. This effort can be a real challenge because of the prolonged and intimate involvement of researchers with the participants.

One way to focus on research for publication in a journal is to break the study into parts. Researchers can develop more than one manuscript from a qualitative research study. If, for example, a researcher studies the culture of an open heart surgery unit over a 1-year period, he or she can develop a manuscript to examine the access and ethical considerations in this type of setting. The researcher may develop another manuscript that focuses on nurses, their activities, and artifacts that were discovered during the inquiry. Still another article might look at the interactions among clients, their families, and institutional structures. In addition, the researcher may develop a description of the process of conducting such an inquiry into yet another manuscript. Ideally, a book or several chapters of a book would provide researchers with the best opportunity for presenting an entire qualitative research study. As Morse and Field (1995) have pointed out, a book-length manuscript is best when researchers wish to share a description of the research process. However, time, commitment, and opportunity may limit publication in this format.

If researchers are uninterested in publishing the study in parts, then they can certainly develop the report so that it will be of greatest interest to readers. For instance, using the open heart surgery unit example, the researcher can present findings in the context of practice implications in critical care journals. A manuscript for publication in a practice journal would not require a great deal of emphasis on method or analysis but would require significant attention to findings and implications.

The most difficult obstacle to overcome in developing a qualitative manuscript for publication is the need to report the study in 12 to 15 pages, as required by most journals. With this limitation, it is critically important to be concise, focused, and logical rather than to try to report the entire study.

Once researchers have identified the journal and determined the focus, the next step is to logically develop the ideas they wish to convey. "An outline provides guidance in writing" (Field & Morse, 1985, p. 130). The purpose of the outline is to keep the writer directed. It is easy to drift away from the focus of the manuscript without an outline. Depending on the preference of the author, the outline may be more or less detailed.

When writing begins, remember to organize ideas in a logical manner but also in a way that provides readers with an appreciation of the richness of the data. For example, in Cote-Arsenault and Morrison-Beedy's (2001) phenomenological study, the authors wanted to share a narrative that reflected the theme "changing self: lifelong effects" (p. 243) to illustrate the effects of perinatal loss on subsequent pregnancies. The example offered is as follows:

> I was really afraid that I wouldn't have any life with any child...I was just petrified of that idea; that someday I would wake up and I would be 50, 60, or 70 and I would not have had that experience of raising a child. To me, that would have been the greatest loss; so, like everything was riding on that pregnancy...I wanted that experience...I really am so grateful that it happened to me. When I look around at other people and they seem to take it (parenting) so for granted and maybe would too, if I was like them (p. 243).

This excerpt provides readers with an insider's (emic) view of what it is like for a woman who has lost a child and the long-term effect of that experience. It gives readers a "feel" for or depth of the experience. This excerpt demonstrates one way in which qualitative reporting differs from quantitative reporting. Qualitative reporting demands documentation of ideas or conclusions in words rather than numbers. Using words to justify the researcher's position takes a significant amount of skill because, unlike the presentation of statistics, the significance of the findings is found in the writer's syntax, not in the statistical manipulation of numerical values.

On completion of the manuscript, authors should ask colleagues to critique the ideas presented. Too often, neophyte qualitative researchers make the mistake of believing that, because they have spent much time immersed in the data, writing about the data is merely a technicality. Qualitative research manuscripts are subjected to rigorous review. It is essential that the ideas be clear and demonstrate important findings to the nursing community. Review by knowledgeable colleagues will assist in assuring the logic, consistency, and importance of the findings.

Once the manuscript is submitted, researchers should be ready to revise as requested by the reviewers. Few manuscripts, qualitative or quantitative, sustain juried review without requests for revision. Morse (1996b) further suggests that, if researchers receive a request for revision in which reviewers' recommendations are contradictory, the researchers' responsibility is to attend to the most meaningful comments. Researchers should indicate why they did not use all of the reviewers' comments; however, when the comments do not reflect the truth of the study, researchers should not submit to revising based on those comments. Never be naive, though, to the point of not considering reviewers' comments. Researchers have a great deal to gain in positive and negative comments. They need to ask, Why did someone read this in a particular way? When asked to revise, researchers must work quickly. The sooner they return the revised manuscript, the sooner the acceptance, and the earlier the manuscript will be queued for publication (Morse, 1996b).

If the unfortunate circumstance occurs—receipt of a rejection letter—do not throw away the manuscript. Look carefully at the critique, use the comments to improve the manuscript, and try another journal. It is acceptable also to use the comments, revise the manuscript, and resubmit it to the same journal. Quality research should be published. Sometimes, it takes a fair amount of tenacity to see ideas through to publication. But once published, researchers will enjoy the thrill of having the work available in print for readers interested in the topic and particular research approach.

CONFERENCE PRESENTATION

Satisfaction results from the publication of a manuscript that shares the results of intensive investigation. Manuscript publication is just one of researchers' responsibilities in their dissemination of the findings. In addition to getting ideas in print, which may take between 10 and 18 months, researchers should present the findings to the scholarly community using other forums. One way to share results in an efficient and effective way is through a formal conference presentation as a paper or poster presentation. Whether presenting findings in a paper or poster, qualitative researchers need to address important guidelines for sharing results in public forums.

Most formal presentations result from a *call for abstracts*, which requires investigators to submit a synopsis of the research in a few paragraphs, with an average limit of between 150 and 500 words. Guidelines for abstract submissions generally are available from the group sponsoring the research conference or workshop. It is essential that responses to the call reflect the theme of the conference and meet the criteria for presentation. The guidelines for abstract submission usually include the study purpose, the method the researcher used to conduct the inquiry, the sample, the findings, and the significance of the findings to nursing. Inclusion of the information requested will greatly improve the chances for abstract acceptance. However, because the results of a qualitative study are rich and dense, the question becomes, how do I demonstrate the richness of my work and the significance in 150 to 500 words when I have trouble writing it in 15 pages?

When submitting an abstract, it is essential to convince reviewers that the work has been done well, will be interesting, and is significant to the profession. It is impossible to share the richness of the research in an abstract. What researchers should be striving for is to whet the reviewers' appetites so that they say they want to know more about this study.

A call for abstracts generally asks researchers to indicate the format in which they prefer to present: poster or paper. Neophyte researchers would be wise to indicate both. Podium presenters of a paper often have demonstrated their ability to successfully engage a group in their work through their ability to clearly articulate their ideas in the abstract. For individuals who have their abstracts rejected for podium presentation, poster presentations offer the opportunity to share the findings in a comfortable, relaxed atmosphere. A poster presentation provides neophyte researchers with the chance to develop skill and confidence in presenting research findings. More importantly, in some conference formats, posters are the only opportunity to present findings since podium presentations may be reserved for keynote speakers.

Preparing for an Oral Presentation

If their study is accepted for an oral presentation, researchers must keep in mind important aspects of sharing the results. They should present qualitative research so that they engage the conference participants in the work. Presentation of a portion of the work will allow researchers to share the richness of the findings. Because the average length of podium presentation is between 20 and 30 minutes, be careful not to spend too much time discussing the method used to conduct the inquiry. Although the method is essential information, the audience will be most interested in the findings. Inform the audience about the method to give them the context and direction of the study, but do not share so much information that presentation of the findings is rushed. It is essential that presenters not hurry the presentation of quotations from informants or the analysis of findings, because those elements *are* the study results. Share the quotations and analysis thoughtfully, giving the audience time to absorb the words. Slides, overheads, or a computerized multimedia presentation provides a visual representation of the quotes, giving the audience additional time to assimilate the meaning of the words. Photographs and illustrations add to the presentation as well. Be sure to leave adequate time for questions. If the research has been presented well, the audience will want to know more because its interest has been aroused. During the question-and-answer period, a unique opportunity is available to share additional findings and anecdotal information.

Be aware that not all questions will be easy or fun to answer. At times, the audience can demonstrate interest in the trustworthiness or ethical considerations in the study. If you have executed a well-designed study, you can handle these questions. If you have not been insightful enough to predict questions and do not have ready answers, be honest. Use the critique questions shared in this text as a developmental learning experience. In this way you, too, will have learned from sharing your results.

Preparing for a Poster Presentation

Presenting qualitative research in poster format is a unique challenge, but certainly one researchers can meet successfully. Many good articles are available on the mechanics of preparing and presenting a poster. Display poster presentations so that, in a glance, interested individuals can determine whether they want to know more or whether they prefer to move to the next poster. Anyone who has ever attended a poster session knows that the sheer volume of posters available limits interested parties from spending time with each poster presenter. Therefore, the poster must immediately capture the audience's attention. The title, color of the poster, size of print, and content should catch the passerby's interest first. However, the most important part of the poster is the title. It is essential to present a title that immediately informs readers of the topic and research approach. For instance, the title "Living in Fear" would attract individuals interested in the topic. Because the title is brief, passersby can decide in a moment whether they want to know more. Similarly, a title such as "Living with AIDS: A Cultural Examination" quickly informs people about the subject matter and research approach. Also of importance is the author's name and affiliation. There are situations when the poster presenter may not be available to answer questions related to the research. If the consumer can jot down the presenter's name and affiliation or pick up a business card, then he or she can contact the poster author at a later time.

In addition, researchers should present the content in a visually appealing way. At a minimum, the poster should include the title of the research, the researcher's name, the purpose, the sample, the method used, the findings, a summary, and the implications. Not all of this information will fit on the poster depending on the space provided. Therefore, it is up to the researcher to illustrate as much as possible and then indicate to the viewer the availability of additional information either on a handout or in a notebook. Pictures and illustrations capture the passerby's attention and give presenters an opportunity to verbally share results. For qualitative researchers, there is benefit in providing interested individuals with a handout

---

of the abstract or handouts highlighting the important research findings or offering an exhaustive description, if appropriate. On the printed handouts, researchers should include their names and addresses so that nurses interested in the findings or the method may contact them for additional information. Russell, Gregory, and Gates (1996) suggest researchers place a notebook on the table with the poster. In the notebook, the researcher can insert additional information, including narrative, pictures, and illustrations that are too cumbersome to place on the poster. The notebook provides people interested in additional information about the study an opportunity to get it "on the spot."

As well as using a matted poster format, some qualitative researchers have used audiovisual materials such as a multimedia projection system to give an added dimension to their presentations. The inclusion of sound and changing visuals connects consumers to the work. Presenting a poster using a multimedia system, however, requires access to electricity and additional space. Researchers interested in presenting a poster in this format need to contact the conference planners to see whether there is accessible electricity and adequate space.

Creativity is the key to the successful presentation of ideas. The nature of qualitative research supports creativity in presentation. Because of the type of data collected, the strategies used, and the rich narrative that results, researchers have much more to draw from in developing their poster. Nurses presenting a poster illustrating a qualitative research approach should take advantage of the possibilities open to sharing their findings and exploit those possibilities to share the interesting and exciting data revealed in the conduct of the inquiry. However, remember to do so in a logical and appealing manner.

GRANT WRITING

Although some graduate students are successful in submitting proposals for funding of their dissertation work before they have a publication history, the more frequent scenario is for a researcher to submit a grant proposal after having had one or more research studies published. The development of a competitive research proposal requires researchers to construct the project so they convince a panel of reviewers that they have the necessary knowledge, experience, and commitment to complete the proposed project. Reviewers will be looking at a researcher's credentials, the scientific merit of the project, and the potential contribution of the project to the profession.

Identifying Funding Sources

One of the first steps in developing a competitive proposal is to identify potential funding sources, a number of which are available to nurses interested in conducting a qualitative inquiry. Different organizations offer materials on the types of projects they fund and their submission guidelines. For researchers seeking their first funding dollars, small grants are the most useful and are generally easier to access. Examples of small grant programs include college or university funds, which are accessible through small grant proposals available on a competitive basis within institutions. The monies generally come from allocations to faculty development budgets, foundations, or alumni gifts.

In addition to college or university funding, several nursing organizations offer small grants. These organizations, among others, include Sigma Theta Tau International, National League for Nursing, American Nurses Foundation, American Association of Critical Care Nurses, and Association of Rehabilitation Nurses. Many corporations also offer small grants, including product companies such as infant formula or durable medical equipment firms. Health care organizations, such as hospitals and community health organizations, frequently fund research as well.

Nurses interested in receiving funding need to identify the available resources. This effort will require a moderate amount of time to first determine the available funding sources and then to select the source that will most likely be interested in funding the project. Nurses might use resource libraries found in universities that have established nursing research centers to identity potential funding sources. These institutions, where available and accessible, generally have a plethora of diverse materials and experienced staff to assist in locating the appropriate resources and developing the proposal. However, it is no longer necessary for potential grant writers to spend hours in the library: The Internet is a wellspring of funding sources. If university-based nursing research centers are unavailable, researchers may log onto the websites of organizations such as the American Association of Colleges of Nursing (AACN), National League for Nursing (NLN), Sigma Theta Tau International (STTI), and American Nurses Association (ANA), which have resource materials on their websites as well as links to other sites to help focus the search. In addition, sites such as http://fdncenter.org or http://www.internet-prospector.org/found.html might offer a starting point. These are more general sites and are not specific to nursing. They do, however, reference large foundations that provide funds for health-related projects, such as Kellogg or Coca Cola.

Individuals interested in developing larger projects should have completed and had published results of small, funded projects before seeking monies from organizations that offer larger funding support. Such organizations include the National Institute of Nursing Research (NINR), National Institutes of Health (NIH), American Education Association (AEA), Kellogg Foundation, Robert Wood Johnson Foundation, and National Science Foundation (NSF). In addition, many nonprofit organizations such as the American Heart Association, National Arthritis Foundation, and American Cancer Society provide moderate-to-large funding for projects. Critical to receiving larger sums of money and submitting a well-developed project is experience. Organizations that make large awards do not do so unless single researchers or research teams demonstrate significant, documented experience.

Developing the Proposal

Because Chapter 4 focuses on proposal development and grant writing, this section will not address the specific mechanics of developing a research proposal for funding. Instead, the section gives qualitative researchers ideas about the challenges and potential pitfalls in developing qualitative grant proposals. As Morse (1991) commented, "In comparison to the WYSIWYG (what you see is what you get) presentation of the quantitative application, the qualitative proposal is vague, obscure, and may even be viewed as a blatant request for a blank check" (p. 148). The idea of developing a proposal for funding, knowing beforehand that the ambiguities cannot be written out of the grant, presents a unique but not insurmountable challenge. Researchers interested in receiving funding for a qualitative study must convince reviewers not only of the merits of the project, which may seem obscure and undirected, but also of the researcher's experience.

There is inconsistency in the literature as to whether pilot work is important for qualitative research funding. Clearly, quantitative research proposals require pilot work to demonstrate the potential design strengths and weaknesses. Connelly and Yoder (2000) state that pilot work enhances the qualitative researcher's chances for funding. Given the inconsistencies in the literature and strong possibility of review by quantitative researchers, qualitative researchers are well served to state why they did or did not conduct pilot work.

In qualitative proposals, the number of participants is determined by data saturation, which can include as few as five or more than 50 people. In a quantitative study, the number of participants is determined by the design, projected outcome, and number of variables under study. Based on these parameters, researchers can establish a precise number of participants for inclusion in a study. In qualitative studies, data collection and analysis require flexibility. In quantitative studies, data collection and analysis are largely objective. The preceding comparisons focus on the precise and often predictable nature of a quantitative research proposal versus the often imprecise and unpredictable nature of a qualitative proposal.

Morse (1998) recommends "the first principle of grantsmanship is to recognize that a good proposal is an argument—a fair and balanced one" (p. 68). Therefore, qualitative researchers must clearly and persuasively present evidence that will convince grant reviewers the proposal is worth funding. To facilitate a clear understanding of the research ideas, proposal authors have the responsibility of explaining everything.

The second principle of grant writing offered by Morse (1998) "is that one should think and plan before starting to write" (p. 70). Planning before writing will give proposal authors an opportunity to clearly delineate the research plan, beginning with development of the research question and ending with the distribution of research results. In addition to assisting with writing the actual proposal document, planning conclusively before beginning to write allows authors time to draft a complete budget. Because the budget is the part of the proposal that provides researchers with the resources to fully operationalize a project, it is essential that researchers develop the budget well and detail all expenses. Items to include in the budget are personnel, such as research assistants, transcription services, secretaries, and consultants; equipment, such as a tape recorder, computer, and data analysis program; supplies, such as paper, printer cartridges, audiotapes or videotapes, and photocopies; and travel, including mileage between research sites, conference travel, presentation fees, and consultant travel. Carefully laying out the project will assist greatly in developing a proposal that is clear, succinct, and can be funded.

Identifying Investigator Qualifications

The challenge in obtaining larger sums for qualitative research is for prospective grant recipients to convince reviewers they are a risk worth taking. Proposal authors need to illustrate to reviewers a track record in scholarly publication, presentation, consultation, and success in acquiring small awards. "Granting bodies must [be made to] recognize the process nature of the research and that they are funding the *investigator* rather than the *proposal* per se" (Morse, 1991, p. 149). Morse added that "for major grant applications, evaluation of the *investigator* is critical and should be most heavily weighted" (p. 149). This is not to say that the research project does not need to have scientific merit and be described as fully as possible; rather, it illuminates the nature of the process that is decidedly imprecise when compared with a quantitative proposal.

In recent years, NIH and other funding agencies have begun requiring that research proposals include a qualitative component (Morse, 1994). This situation is confusing: Does this requirement support the value of qualitative research and reflect the belief that qualitative research will be driven into the system, or is this a strongly misguided request that reflects a definite misunderstanding of research and the qualitative research process in general (Morse, 1994)? In either case, it is up to grant developers to clearly provide the reasons why they have selected one paradigm over another and indicate how the paradigm and, more specifically, the method will provide the answers to the questions asked.

Furthermore, Morse (1996a) has pointed out that funding agencies have given the distinct impression that qualitative research is not an end but rather a means to an end. Based on the literature, qualitative researchers are led to believe that qualitative inquiry is a prelude to "good" quantitative design. This, too, may be a misguided belief. Researchers must make clear to funding agencies the project goal and clearly describe how the method selected is appropriate.

More than one researcher with expertise in quantitative methodology may be able to bring a dimension to an entire project that a qualitative researcher alone would be unable to do. It is up to the principal investigator to determine whether the study will be enhanced by the addition of a strong team with varied philosophical beliefs and interests. Based on this author's experience with recently funded projects, grant reviewers are frequently viewing research teams more favorably, particularly if the teams are multidisciplinary.

Identifying Mechanisms for Ensuring Participant Protection

Not only must qualitative researchers clearly demonstrate their expertise and qualifications, it is essential that their qualitative research proposals conclusively identify the mechanisms for assuring the protection of participants. One of the strengths of qualitative approaches is the unique opportunity to get to know individuals, groups, or communities over a long period. This strength creates its own potential hazards for participants' protection because the nature of the data—personal descriptions—precludes qualitative researchers from maintaining confidentiality, particularly when they publish quotes or use them as references in publications (Munhall, 1991). Nevertheless, qualitative researchers can assure anonymity. It is essential that they demonstrate how they will protect informants' identities. In some cases such as in ethnography or action research, participant identification may actually contribute significantly to the position of groups or their ability to access resources. In such cases, qualitative researchers must document that participants have agreed that researchers may make the informants' identities public. Audio taping interviews and taking photographs are additional examples of potential violations of participants' rights. Researchers must document informants' permission for such activities.

Although developing mechanisms for ensuring confidentiality and anonymity contributes significantly to a grant proposal, it is also important to clarify for institutional review boards and funding agencies that mechanisms are in place to deal with potentially sensitive outcomes. For example, if a researcher is living with a community and discovers that one of the group rituals involves physically isolating and abusing children who do not excel in academics, the researcher must be able to clearly define steps he or she will take to protect the vulnerable group (i.e., the children). It is essential to try to identify all the potentially sensitive situations and develop mechanisms to intervene or to have intervention available.

Connelly and Yoder (2000) identify a number of common problems with qualitative research proposals that are worth noting. These authors share that researchers should clearly demonstrate an understanding of the assumptions of the research approach they are using. "It is critical to write from the perspective of the appropriate assumptions" (p. 70). Often the proposal author will slip from qualitative terminology to quantitative terminology, which is the second common problem identified. Qualitative researchers must be very careful to fully understand the philosophical foundations of qualitative research in general as well as the specifics of the particular method selected. Sharing methodological information is important. It is especially important when the reviewer is unfamiliar with the assumptions of the method, terminology, and techniques used to collect and analyze data. Connelly and Yoder state qualitative researchers have a responsibility to respond to the outline presented for funding, albeit quantitative in orientation. It is the qualitative researcher's responsibility to explain why it is not possible to provide specific requested information.

Other common problems identified include no logical argument for why a qualitative research approach is warranted, no discussion of training data collectors, little or no discussion of methodological rigor, inadequate description of the unique nature of researcher/informant relationship and its impact on human subjects' protection, inadequately developed significance of the research, inexperienced researcher without adequate consultation, and underestimating budget requirements (Connelly & Yoder, 2000). Any one or more of these common problems can lead to an unsuccessful grant proposal.

SAMPLE GRANT

Following this chapter, a funded research grant proposal completed by Cathi Cox, Ph.D., is presented to illustrate the processes discussed in this chapter. The grant was funded by Department of Defense, Triservice Nursing Research Program. Also following is a critique of the funded grant that shares reviewers' comments to further illustrate issues that are important in the development of a qualitative research proposal.

SUMMARY

Qualitative research is an exciting opportunity to create meaningful nursing knowledge from individuals' lives and experiences. To make the knowledge accessible, researchers must share the findings in a significant way. Presenting a qualitative project in an article, poster, speech, or grant proposal requires imagination and refined presentation skills. Qualitative researchers have a responsibility to their consumers and to developing qualitative scholars to present their ideas in a clear and acceptable manner. They should share their research in a way that illustrates the richness and value of conducting research using the approaches described in this text.

The development of qualitative research projects and the refinement of social sciences approaches to human inquiry that are appropriate to nursing science establish a major research focus for the profession. Nurses interested in these projects have a unique opportunity to be on the cutting edge of the developments. It is an exciting time for nurses and for research. There is a vast and expansive qualitative research landscape waiting for interested nurse–researchers. This is a landscape of imagination that is colored by the lives and experiences of the individuals with whom nurses interact: clients, students, and other nurses. It is essential to document these unique experiences and share them to fully explore and describe the human experience. The challenge awaits those nurses who are willing to participate.

REFERENCES

Connelly, M. L., & Yoder, L. H. (2000). Improving qualitative proposals: Common problem areas. *Clinical Nurse Specialist, 14*(2), 69–74.
Cote-Arsenault, D., & Morrison-Beedy, D. (2001). Women's voices reflecting changed expectations for pregnancy after perinatal loss. *Journal of Nursing Scholarship, 33*(3), 239–244.

Dialogue: The granting game. (1991). In J. M. Morse (Ed.), *Qualitative nursing research: A contemporary dialogue* (rev. ed., pp. 240–244). Newbury Park, CA: Sage.

Field, P. A., & Morse, J. M. (1985). *Nursing research: The application of qualitative approaches.* Rockville, MD: Aspen.

Morse, J. (1991). On the evaluation of qualitative proposals [Editorial]. *Qualitative Health Research, 1*(2), 147–151.

Morse, J. M. (1994). Designing funded qualitative research. In N. K. Denzin & Y. S. Lincoln (Eds.), *Handbook of qualitative research* (pp. 220–235). Thousand Oaks, CA: Sage.

Morse, J. M. (1996a). Is qualitative research complete? [Editorial]. *Qualitative Health Research, 6*(1), 3–5.

Morse, J. (1996b). "Revise and resubmit": Responding to reviewers' reports [Editorial]. *Qualitative Health Research, 6*(2), 149–151.

Morse, J. M., & Field, P. A. (1995). *Qualitative research methods for health professionals* (2nd ed.). Thousand Oaks, CA: Sage.

Morse, J. M. (1998). Designing funded qualitative research. In N. K. Denzin & Y. S. Lincoln (Eds.), *Strategies of qualitative inquiry* (pp. 56–85). Thousand Oaks, CA: Sage.

Munhall, P. L. (1991). Institutional review of qualitative research proposals: A task of no small consequence. In J. M. Morse (Ed.), *Qualitative nursing research: A contemporary dialogue* (rev. ed., pp. 258–272). Newbury Park, CA: Sage.

Russell, C. K., Gregory, D. M., & Gates, M. F. (1996). Aesthetics and substance in qualitative research posters. *Qualitative Health Research, 6*(4), 542–552.

FUNDED GRANT PROPOSAL

The Lived Experience of Nurses Stationed Aboard Aircraft Carriers

This project (or research) is (or was) sponsored by the TriService Nursing Research Program, Uniformed Services University of the Health Sciences; however, the information or content and conclusions do not necessarily represent the official position or policy of, nor should any official endorsement be inferred by, the TriService Nursing Research Program, Uniformed Services University of the Health Sciences, the Department of Defense, or the U.S. Government.

*Currently, there are 12 aircraft carriers deployed worldwide in support of the United States' interests and commitments. In each carrier's Medical Department, there is one Navy nurse assigned to directly care for over 5,500 personnel. The purpose of this phenomenological research study is to describe the lived experiences of Navy nurses practicing aboard aircraft carriers. Using phenomenology, nurses previously stationed aboard aircraft carriers will be interviewed to explore their experiences as a ship's nurse. The question guiding this inquiry will be: "**What is your experience as a nurse on an aircraft carrier?**" Interviews will be conducted until data saturation is reached. The interviews will be tape recorded, transcribed, and analyzed in four steps:*

1. Carefully reviewing the interviews to obtain a general sense of the experience
2. Reviewing the transcripts to uncover essences
3. Apprehending essential relationships
4. Developing a formalized, exhaustive description of the phenomenon

Once data analysis is completed, credibility will be achieved by sharing the exhaustive description with each participant and validating whether or not it represents his or her experience. If the participant does not agree with the description as written, additional data will be collected, analyzed, and incorporated into the exhaustive description. Consistent with qualitative research, an extensive literature review will follow data analysis, placing the findings in the context of what is already known. Then, the results will be disseminated to the military and nursing communities. The significance of this study is that the findings will provide valuable insight into clinical care in service unique environments and potentially describe issues related to deployment and readiness. Finally, since there is currently a paucity of literature on this topic, the results will give a public voice to this extraordinary experience of operational nursing.

INTRODUCTION

Specific Aims

The purpose of this phenomenological research study is to describe the lived experiences of Navy nurses practicing aboard aircraft carriers. Using phenomenology, nurses previously stationed aboard aircraft carriers will be personally interviewed to explore their experiences as a ship's nurse. No explicit a priori hypothesis is formulated for this type of qualitative research. In fact, most qualitative studies are conducted without a hypothesis defined at the onset because the aim of most projects is to provide an opportunity for the human experience to be revealed without preconceived restrictions (Creswell, 1998).

The Navy has 12 aircraft carriers in operation at present. In each carrier's Medical Department, there is one Navy nurse assigned to directly care for over 5,500 personnel. It is difficult to envision what it would be like to be the only nurse available to a patient population in the thousands. Questions that come to mind include: What is it like? What might one learn about this type of operational nursing practice? Do these nurses think that they are prepared for this role? If not, should the Navy provide a transition program for them prior to reporting to these billets? What are their experiences with treating, holding, evacuating, and transporting patients aboard aircraft carriers? Do Navy nurses make a difference in the health outcomes of the patients stationed on aircraft carriers? With the integration of women on board ships, what is the experience of aircraft carrier nurses with women's health issues?

The phenomenon of interest—perceptions of nurses' experiences while stationed aboard aircraft carriers—has never before been explored, analyzed, or described from a research perspective. Because there is absolutely no research-based information available on nursing aboard aircraft carriers, this study will make a contribution to the dearth of knowledge available regarding this unique form of "operational nursing" (defined as nursing outside of traditional Navy hospitals in support of Navy operations).

The significance of this study is that the findings will provide valuable insight into clinical care in service unique environments and potentially describe issues related to deployment and readiness. Finally, since there is currently a paucity of literature on this topic, the results will give a public voice to this extraordinary experience of military nursing.

Background and Significance

The intended research cannot build on what has already been done because there has been no research conducted in this aspect of Navy nursing. This project is necessary because the characteristics of nursing practice on board aircraft carriers could provide valuable insight into the experiences of shipboard nurses (specifically those related to military deployment and readiness and clinical care in service unique environments).

True to qualitative methodology, researchers conduct an extensive literature review after data analysis so as not to influence their thoughts regarding the phenomenon of study (Streubert & Carpenter, 1995, 1999). However, an exploratory literature review may be conducted in order to ascertain what currently exists in the literature about the phenomenon of interest (Locke, Spirduso, & Silverman, 1993;

Taylor & Bogdan, 1998). An exploratory literature review revealed that as of August 1999, CINAHL Information Systems for Nursing the Allied Health had 537 citations available regarding the topic of Military Nursing. Of these 537 articles, only 42 were related to Navy nursing. Of the 42 remaining Navy nursing articles, only 9 were deemed appropriate for review regarding shipboard nursing. Of the 9 articles reviewed, only one addressed nursing aboard aircraft carriers—Austin (1993–1994). Austin's short article reported his experience as a nurse on board the aircraft carrier U.S.S. Enterprise and was written with job satisfaction as a major theme.

In another article, which does not specifically address nurses stationed aboard aircraft carriers but may have implications for this study, Shiffer (1990) reports information that pertains to the role of the shipboard nurse as both an expert nursing practitioner and naval leader. He writes:

> *The ultimate Navy nurse role would be described as the Nurse Corps officer who is known to be an expert nursing practitioner and simultaneously [meets] all role expectations as a naval leader. Unclear or inaccurate expectations regarding the traditional Navy Nurse role may originate from expectations of peers or superiors. Role stress and strain results when role expectations are not or cannot be met, which may lead to loss of commitment and professional values both as an officer and as a nurse (p. 208).*

Shiffer's article suggests that role stress and strain may occur in those nurses on board aircraft carriers because once they report to these billets, they are no longer hospital-based nurses. They are now division officers who no longer report to a senior Nurse Corps officer but rather to their Senior Medical Officer and, ultimately, the Commanding Officer of their aircraft carrier. Therefore, they become part of the Navy line community.

The Navy Nurse Corps' Strategic Plan's Mission states that the "Nurse Corps actively supports the Navy and Marine Corps Team and Navy Medicine with a community of active and reserve component professionals focused on accomplishing the readiness and health benefit missions." Its vision statement reveals that "By the year 2001, all Nurse Corps officers will fully understand, support, and be prepared for their peacetime and wartime roles." The three goals of the Navy Nurse Corps' Strategic Plan pertain to the qualifications of leadership, professional nursing practice, and operational readiness. Because aircraft carrier nurses incorporate all three of these characteristics into their job, it is postulated that the proposed study supports the goals of the Navy Nurse Corps.

Preliminary Studies/Progress Report

Anecdotal information expressed to the principal investigator (PI) from nurses previously assigned to aircraft carriers precipitated this proposal. Some of the nurses expressed a desire to be more senior (at least an 0–4 or 0–5) for this type of tour. They also voiced a desire to have personnel management classes prior to assuming this duty because they found that their role changed from critical care nurses to division officers immediately after they transitioned to the aircraft carrier. Those stationed aboard nuclear-powered aircraft carriers wished they had more radiation safety preparation prior to reporting to this billet. Finally, at least one spoke of the need to increase the billets for nurses aboard aircraft carriers from more than one because the demand for directing quality nursing care to over 5,500 shipmates is an impossible goal for just one nurse. To determine whether these comments are representative of more than one aircraft carrier nurse, the PI would like to interview former aircraft carrier nurses to identify their lived experiences in this role.

As requested by the TSNRP reviewers for the previous grant submission, the PI contacted the Navy Specialty Advisor for Operational Nursing to ascertain what life is like for nurses on aircraft carriers. She writes that a typical day may entail supervising inpatient care, conducting training, attending planning meetings, setting up and executing medical training drills, and conducting quality improvement activities. The ship's nurse is considered a Principal Assistant (PA) so he or she does not always fall within the medical chain of command. The ship's nurse does not have any direct subordinates except for the corpsmen who are assigned to the inpatient ward when the aircraft carrier is underway. He or she also coordinates the Medical Training Team (MTT). When the ship is underway, the ship's nurse is on-call 24 hours a day, seven days a week. Unlike the six or seven medical officers who share call and have duty every six or seven days, the nurse is always on duty. If there is a critical patient on the inpatient ward, the nurse will hand over the patient to one of the medical officers for a short sleep break, but other than that, it is up to the ship's nurse to provide nursing care to that critical patient. As for other inpatient care, the corpsmen perform most of the duties. The corpsmen also conduct most of the training throughout the ship; however, the ship's nurse is still ultimately responsible for all training exercises.

The qualifications for a ship's nurse are as follows:
- Preferably a senior lieutenant (03) or lieutenant commander (04)
- Completed at least two tours of duty
- Have two years of critical care experience
- Be certified in Basic Life Support (BLS) and Advanced Cardiac Life Support (ACLS)
- Have some teaching experience (such as a BLS or ACLS instructor)
- Have some administrative experience, (i.e., as a division officer), as well as other collateral duties such as quality improvement activities
- Possess a strong performance record that demonstrates good leadership and interpersonal skills
- Meet physical fitness standards

Unfortunately, the Navy Specialty Advisor for Operational Nursing reports that some nurses make it to these assignments without the qualifications identified and tend not to represent the Navy Nurse Corps to the best of their abilities.

True to qualitative methodology, the information shared by the Specialty Advisor for Operational Nursing has the potential for introducing bias into the project. Therefore, it will be "bracketed" (as described in the methods section below) prior to data collection.

The PI has taken course work on qualitative methods as part of her doctoral education and has experienced phenomenological data collection and analysis in these classes. This course work includes taking the following two classes at George Mason University (the descriptions were obtained from the on-line course catalog via http://www.gmu.edu):

920/HSCI 920 (through the College of Nursing and Health Science)—"Qualitative Research in Nursing and Health Care" (3 credits). Philosophical foundations and approaches to qualitative research in nursing and health care administration, health care policy, and health care ethics analyzed within the scholarship of discovery, integration, application, and teaching.

EDSR 895 (through the Graduate School of Education and Research)—"Emerging Issues in Qualitative Research" (3 credits). Examines current issues in qualitative research, such as designing and writing a qualitative research proposal, interviewing, collecting video data, using qualitative computer programs, analyzing data, and writing qualitative reports. Provides students with opportunities to apply new skills and knowledge to projects related to their own interests and to design relevant individualized components.

The PI's co-investigator is recognized as an expert in qualitative research and her consultant is the author of the book outlining the methodology that will be used for analyzing the data generated from the proposed interviews.

Research Design and Methods

Study Design

Polit and Hungler (1995) believe that "many qualitative studies are based on the premise that gaining knowledge about humans is impossible without describing human experience as it is lived and as it is defined by the actors themselves" (p. 517). The authors write that there is an ongoing debate about which type of study is better for advancing nursing science: quantitative or qualitative? They conclude that researchers now believe that both approaches are needed and that the structure of the study should be based on the nature of the research. Creswell (1998) points out that quantitative researchers work with few variables and many cases whereas qualitative researchers work with few cases and many variables. For this proposal, a qualitative approach using a phenomenological method of inquiry will be employed because the PI feels it is impossible to investigate this phenomenon using quantitative methods since the purpose is to describe the lived experiences of Navy nurses practicing aboard aircraft carriers.

The science of phenomenology describes particular phenomena as lived experience (Streubert & Carpenter, 1995, 1999). Streubert (1991) writes that "through sharing of experiences and identifying the commonalties or essences, as phenomenologists call them, individuals come to know themselves and all in contact with them....Through understanding of the essences or commonalties of phenomena, people come to know the experience....Essences, therefore, represent the basic units of common understanding of any phenomena" (p. 119).

Qualitative research is an inductive process. Because pure induction is impossible, "qualitative researchers operate within theoretical frameworks" (Taylor & Bogdan, 1998, p. 8). Edmund Husserl's (1859–1938) phenomenology provides the theoretical framework guiding this research study. (As suggested by the TSNRP reviewers for the previous grant submission, Benner's framework has been replaced.) Husserl was a German philosopher who was a key figure in the development of phenomenology. He purported that phenomenology was not a natural science and could not be equated or measured by the methodologies associated with the natural sciences. He believed that phenomenology was in a completely different realm from other sciences and that it needed to be approached and understood with different methodologies in order to attain the essence of knowledge. He felt that each experience has its own moment and must be described, refined, and revealed as one is conscious of it. Therefore, his phenomenological method sought to clarify and distinguish meaning as it was presented to the conscious (Natanson, 1973).

There are a number of methodological approaches available for analyzing phenomena. The PI will adopt that of Streubert (Streubert & Carpenter, 1995, 1999) who synthesized the work of several phenomenological researchers (Speigelberg, Colaizzi, Patterson & Zderad, Oiler, and van Manen) in order to develop a clear and consistent method to investigate experiences. Streubert's method involves the following steps:

1. Explicating a personal description of the phenomenon of interest
2. Bracketing the researcher's presuppositions
3. Interviewing participants in settings comfortable to the participant
4. Carefully reading the transcripts of the interview to obtain a general sense of the experience
5. Reviewing the transcripts to uncover essences
6. Apprehending essential relationships
7. Developing formalized descriptions of phenomena
8. Returning to participants to validate descriptions
9. Reviewing the relevant literature
10. Distributing the findings to the nursing community (1999, p. 51)

The following description eloquently describes the qualitative research process that will be discussed in greater detail throughout this application:

One undertakes qualitative research in [a setting] where the researcher is an instrument of data collection who gathers words or pictures, analyzes them inductively, focuses on the meanings of the participants, and describes a process that is expressive and persuasive in language (Creswell, 1998, p. 14).

Sampling

The most common type of sampling utilized in phenomenology is purposive sampling because the purpose of the research is to accentuate specific information and not to generalize findings (Streubert, 1991). Once the appropriate group is identified, the researcher seeks access, provides informed consent, and then collects data until saturation. Saturation is described as the "sense of closure [one] experiences when data collection ceases to yield any new information" (Polit & Hungler, 1995).

According to Creswell (1998), phenomenological study requires in-depth interviews. It has been reported that these can last from one to two hours. The PI's review of qualitative research studies reveals that the typical size of a phenomenological sample is between seven and twelve. Therefore, it is planned that seven to twelve former aircraft carrier nurses will be needed to achieve saturation. Please refer to page 34 of this application for sample and recruitment procedures.

Data Collection

As requested by the TSNRP reviewers regarding the previous grant submission, the concept of bracketing will be further explored. Many terms have been utilized to transfer Husserl's concept of epoche—bracketing, reduction, suspension, disconnection, abstention, setting aside, and canceling have all been employed. For consistency's sake, the term "bracketing" will be used throughout this grant application. Natanson (1973) states that bracketing does not mean neglecting, rather it is simply accepting the obvious and is thus reflectively recognized "as a performance of consciousness and subjected to analysis" (p. 59). Natanson writes that few concepts in phenomenology have led to as much misunderstanding as the concept of bracketing and that even Husserl was not consistent in his writings on bracketing. Bracketing occurs prior to data collection, during data collection, and throughout the data analysis process.

So how does one accomplish the abstract concept of bracketing? Natanson (1973) illustrates the process beautifully:

> As I write these lines I am looking out over a view of the city. In sight are the rooftops of the neighboring houses, their chimney stacks jutting upward; some of the fences surrounding yards are visible, part of a school building can be seen, there are many trees about, and, in the far distance, a part of the bay can be glimpsed. I know who lives in some of the houses in the line of my vision, the kinds of trees around me, the style of the environing architecture...Each time I look out the window, I see once again the same sight, the same buildings and foliage. I know that they are reliable features of my prospect, part of my world. Now, [with bracketing], I choose to attend to the scene in a different way. I set aside the actuality of the houses and the details of their ownership and history. The house across the way has a mortgage, a roof in need of repair, and a freshly painted door. I concern myself only with its being there for me as something seen and noticed. The mortgage drops away; the roof presents itself as a patchwork...That Haskell lives next to Immerbind is no longer part of my viewing—that knowledge has been set aside. I see rectangular and oblong stretches of multicolored shapes...what is set aside in [bracketing] is becoming clear, but it is no less important to note what has not been altered: there is still the 'I' who looks over the view; there is still the past of that 'I', its history; there is still the scene set within the world which surrounds and includes it; and there is still the history of that world...Bringing all of these subtle elements into clarity is the first requisite of [bracketing], and refraining from positing and building upon those primordial grounds is the goal of that ultimate [bracketing] (pp. 65–66).

Seidman (1998) offers a very succinct description of bracketing:

> It is important that the researcher identify his or her interest in the subject and examine it to make sure that the interest is neither unhealthy nor infused with anger, bias, or prejudice. The interviewer must come to the transcript prepared to let the interview breathe and speak for itself (p. 100).

The PI will fully explicate her own pre-conceived ideas about the phenomenon of interest through documentation of these in a journal (Streubert & Carpenter, 1999). Further, it is proposed that journaling will occur prior to and following each interview. Through this procedure, the PI will maintain her ideas and conceptions about the phenomenon foremost in her consciousness prior to and during data collection and data analysis. Also, Locke, Spirduso, and Silverman (1993) recommend cross-checking the researcher's perceptions and decisions with a colleague whenever it appears that individual biases may influence the project. These processes support the concept of bracketing.

The primary data collection strategy will be the use of tape-recorded personal interview. In keeping with Streubert's (1999) recommendations, the interviews will take place in settings familiar (and comfortable) to the participants so that each respondent can share his or her perceptions freely. Taylor and Bogdan (1998) profess that most people feel comfortable and/or relaxed in their own homes and offices; thus, the PI will allow the participant to pick the place he or she feels most comfortable (and where privacy is assured) whether it be the home or office. Incidentally, telephone interviews were considered for this study. However, according to Polit and Hungler (1995), "when the interviewer is unknown, respondents may be uncooperative and unresponsive in a telephone situation, especially if the interview is long" (p. 188).

The participants will be contacted prior to the formal session to solicit their interest, address the nature of the study, provide an overview of informed consent, and give them time to reflect on the phenomenon of study. It is anticipated that a period of reflection will enable richer descriptions during the interview (Streubert, 1991). Prior to the start of the formal interview, the PI will document informed consent and obtain demographic data as follows:

- Age
- Gender
- Educational preparation
- Length of time in the Navy
- Current rank and rank while on the ship
- Current duty status—active duty, reservist, retired, or civilian
- Number of years on the ship
- Length of time since leaving the ship
- Number of tours of duty on a ship

The interview will begin with the question: **"What is your experience as a nurse on an aircraft carrier?"** The participants will be encouraged to fully describe their perceptions without being interrupted or led by the researcher. During the course of each interview, any descriptions which are deemed unclear will be clarified. Taylor and Bogdan (1998) caution the researcher to always clarify a participant's remarks (and never assume that the researcher knows what the participant means). They recommend using the following phrases when clarifying remarks:

- What do you mean by that?
- I don't follow you exactly.
- Explain that again (p. 63).

A successful interviewer knows when and how to probe (Taylor & Bogdan, 1998). According to Sorrell and Redmond (1995), two styles of probes may be used in an interview: the recapitulation probe and the silent probe. Recapitulation is used when the participant stops talking and the researcher directs the individual to return to previous comments in order to clarify or elaborate on his or her description. When participants are asked to retell parts of their stories by returning to the beginning, they often add new details. The researcher will also recognize periods of silence as being important because "powerful silence...may speak more than words" (Sorrell & Redmond, p. 1121). Thoughtful probes can also bring out important contextual details that are embedded in each participant's narrative. The following questions may help the respondent to reflect on the experience of interest:

- How were you feeling at that time?
- What else was going on then?
- Tell me more about that (Sorrell & Redmond, p. 1122).

Seidman (1998) offers some specific suggestions for the researcher regarding interviewing techniques:

- Listen more, talk less
- Follow-up on what the participant says but don't interrupt
- Ask questions when you do not understand
- Ask to hear more about a subject
- Avoid leading questions with tones that imply an expectation
- Ask open-ended questions
- Keep participants focused and ask for concrete details
- Avoid reinforcing your participants' responses
- Explore a participant's laughter (Seidman writes that laughter can be a cry of pain and silence may be a shout)
- Follow your hunches, trust your instincts
- Tolerate silence (pp. 63–78)

When the informant feels he or she has expended his or her description, the PI will offer the concluding question: "Is there anything that you have not offered, either positive or negative, about the experience that you would like to add?" If there are no additions, the interview will end. Based upon a review of qualitative research studies, it is anticipated that each interview will take approximately one to two hours to complete.

The interview approach planned for this study will be pilot tested twice prior to starting the interviews. These data will not be reported as part of the findings. According to Sorrell and Redmond (1995), "trying out a variety of openings and probes before undertaking the actual research interview will help the interviewer to avoid situations where a respondent reacts with long silences, confusion, or irrelevant chatter. Use of a pre-interview may also help to prepare both the interviewer and the respondent for the experience of the future interview" (p. 1118). Seidman (1998) writes that pilot interviews may alert researchers to elements of their own research techniques that either contribute or distract from the objectives of the study.

Finally, more than one type of data will be collected (as recommended by the TSNRP reviewers regarding the previous grant submission). This involves:

- Asking participants to bring any journals, diaries, letters, records, calendars, memorabilia, and/or photographs they wish to share regarding their experiences on the aircraft carriers (Taylor and Bogdan [1998] feel that personal documents can be used to guide interviews and that later in the interviews, they may even "spark memories and help people recall old feelings" [p. 105])
- Collecting demographic data information about the nurses in order to fully place the data into context
- Taking notes during the interviews (Seidman [1998] encourages noting all non-verbal signals such as coughs, laughs, sighs, pauses, outside noises, and interruptions [p. 98])

- Making arrangements for the participants to contact the PI after the interviews for "ah-ha" types of questions (the PI's e-mail address, phone and fax numbers will be made available to the participants in order to accomplish this goal)

Data Analysis

Data analysis includes four steps:

- Carefully reading the interviews to obtain a general sense of the experience
- Reviewing the transcripts to uncover essences
- Apprehending essential relationships
- Developing a formalized, exhaustive description of the phenomenon

The first step involves reading the transcripts while listening to the audiotapes so that the accuracy of the transcriptions can be verified. It also provides an important opportunity for the researcher to begin "dwelling in the data." Streubert (1991) describes dwelling in the data as the time and reflection committed to reading the interviews over and over and becoming immersed in their content. This process is also called immersion (Streubert & Carpenter, 1999).

The second step is reviewing the transcripts is to uncover the essences. This entails a sentence by sentence review to identify the essences. There is no attempt to order sentences into themes at this step.

During the third step, apprehending essential relationships, the researcher relates the themes to one another. It is at this point that the researcher shifts from Husserl's "natural attitude" to the "phenomenological attitude." Natanson (1973) describes this transition as follows:

> ...The turn from the natural to the phenomenological attitude is a shift in the direction of one's interests, not in the abandonment of one world for another. There is but one world, though there are different ways of attending to it. In the natural attitude...the individual lives spontaneously in his perception of what there is; in the phenomenological attitude, he makes of his perceptual life an object of inquiry. In Husserl's language, perceptual experience is thematized by the phenomenologist (p. 54).

This leads to the final step of developing a formalized, exhaustive description of the phenomenon. The exhaustive description is the result of the researcher's analysis of the data and the inter-relationship of the themes to one another resulting in a formalized view of the phenomenon. Organization of the data will be aided through the use of the computer program entitled ATLAS.ti.

In response to the TSNRP comments concerning the extent to which individual cases will be analyzed during data collection, in-depth analysis will commence after saturation has been achieved. Seidman (1998) reports that some researchers think that interviewing and analysis should be integrated so that each informs the other. However, he advocates avoiding any in-depth analysis of interview data until all have been completed to avoid imposing meaning from one participant's interview onto the next.

Validation/Trustworthiness

Trustworthiness is the term used by qualitative researchers to demonstrate rigor. According to Yonge and Stewin (1988), there are four criteria:

- Credibility
- Dependability
- Confirmability/Auditability
- Transferability/Fittingness

"Credibility includes activities that increase the probability that credible findings will be produced" (Lincoln & Guba, 1985; Streubert & Carpenter, 1999, p. 29). To confirm the credibility of the findings, the researcher shares the outcome with the participants. If the participants recognize the findings to be true to their experience, then credibility has been established (Yonge & Stewin, 1988). Lincoln and Guba call this activity "member checks." The TSNRP reviewers for the previous grant submission were concerned about a participant's disagreement with the exhaustive description. However, Taylor and Bogdan (1998) write that even if a participant rejects one's interpretation, the rejection may enhance the PI's understanding of the participant's perspective. Seidman (1998) reports that sharing the descriptions is crucial for credibility of the study; however, he "would not give the person automatic censure on matters of interpretation" (p. 54).

Dependability is a criterion of neutrality. There can be no dependability unless credibility has been established (Lincoln & Guba, 1985). "The question to ask is, 'How dependable are these results'" (Streubert & Carpenter, 1999, p. 29).

"Confirmability [audibility] is a process criterion" (Streubert & Carpenter, 1999, p. 29). The way the researcher confirms the findings is by leaving an audit trail (which was not addressed in the original grant application). The audit trail consists of raw data, memorandums, communications, thought processes, etc. The purpose of the audit trail is to document decisions made.

Transferability/fittingness refers to the likelihood that the findings will have meaning outside of the study situation. "The expectation for determining whether the findings fit or are transferable rests with potential users of the findings and not with the researchers" (Greene, 1990; Lincoln & Guba, 1985; Sandelowsi, 1986; Streubert & Carpenter, 1999, p. 29).

Context of the Phenomenon
Following the recommendations of Taylor and Bogdan (1998) and Streubert and Carpenter (1999), the major literature review for this study will occur after data analysis. This literature review also offers support for the described phenomenon as well as guides the researcher to ask other questions about the phenomenon under study and suggest recommendations for future research.

Dissemination of Findings
The findings will provide valuable insight into nursing care in service unique environments and potentially describe issues related to deployment and readiness. The PI plans to disseminate the findings via publication of a journal article, presentation at a national conference, and through her dissertation process.

Ethical Considerations
Qualitative research has some unique ethical considerations. Because the interviews are taped, anonymity is not possible. Therefore, the researcher must take all measures to ensure confidentiality. For this study, all participants will be asked to sign informed consent in order to participate in the study. Audiotapes will be erased

once accurate transcription has been verified. Data then will be stored in locked filing cabinets and, under no circumstances, will individual identities be revealed.

Because there is no way to know exactly what might transpire during each interview, the researcher will view consent as an ongoing transactional process. Streubert and Carpenter (1995) report several concerns that can occur with qualitative research such as awkward and embarrassing events, over-identification with the participants, and loss of composure. The PI will remember these concerns with each interview.

In an attempt to avoid a fear of coercion, the PI will not use her military rank when coordinating and conducting the interviews. She will wear civilian attire when meeting with the participants. Because the day-to-day activities of life on an aircraft carrier may involve classified information, the participants will be directed by the researcher not to reveal any information that may be deemed classified.

Finally, the PI was concerned that she might have to report sensitive information, (i.e., reports of fraternization, drug use, etc.) if revealed in an interview. However, after a telephone conversation, the PI learned that because she will be acting in a civilian capacity and not on official orders (or drilling for the Navy Reserves), the PI has no obligation to reveal and/or report such information.

Human Subjects

IRB Approval

In accordance with George Mason University's Office of Sponsored Programs (OSP), any research activity involving human subjects conducted by George Mason University personnel, including doctoral students, needs approval. OSP found this proposal exempt from review by the Human Subjects Review Board at George Mason University because it fell under the Department of Health and Human Services' (DHHS) Exempt Category 2 (See Appendix B).

As recommended by the TSNRP reviewers for the previous grant submission, the PI has obtained letters of endorsement from the Commander, Naval Air Forces, U.S. Pacific Fleet (COMNAVAIRPAC)—the command that governs aircraft carriers on the West Coast—and the Commander, Naval Air Forces, U.S. Atlantic Fleet (COMNAVAIRLANT)—the command that governs aircraft carriers on the East Coast (see Appendix C and Appendix D for copies of the letters). Both COMNAVAIRPAC and COMNAVAIRLANT revealed that individual letters from the commanding officers of the aircraft carriers are not necessary because the Force Medical Officers at COMNAVAIRPAC and COMNAVAIRLANT are the approval authority regarding research concepts. The PI will obtain assistance from the Force Medical Officers at COMNAVAIRPAC and COMNAVAIRLANT when soliciting interviews for those nurses who are in the process of or have recently left the aircraft carrier(s).

Also, the PI has obtained a letter of endorsement (see Appendix E) from the head of the division of Navy Medicine that governs health care on aircraft carriers (Director, Aerospace Medicine Programs [MED-23] at the Bureau of Medicine and Surgery [BUMED] in Washington, D.C.).

Finally, the PI has obtained a letter of endorsement (see Appendix F) from the Navy's Specialty Advisor for Operational Nursing. This Specialty Advisor will help the PI access the population of interest.

The PI has learned that there is no need to obtain permission from PERS-OOH (the Navy agency responsible for coordination and control of all surveys, including

Timeline for Conducting Study (Years 2000 – 2001)

	Aug.	Sept.	Oct.	Nov.	Dec.	Jan.	Feb.	Mar.	April	May	June	July
Query Population of Interest	▉	▉										
Data Collection (Interviews)		▉	▉	▉								
Data Analysis					▉	▉	▉	▉				
Literature Review									▉			
Preparation of Report										▉	▉	
Dissemination of Findings												▉

interviews) for this project because PERS-OOH is only interested in approving quantitative surveys involving Navy personnel. PERS-OOH communicated that asking one research question, which falls in the qualitative research domain, is of no concern to it. PERS-OOH recommended obtaining approval for the study through the IRB at one of the major medical centers in the Navy. At the time of this submission, this proposal is being considered by the IRB at the National Naval Medical Center, Bethesda, MD. The materials were submitted to the IRB in September 1999 for a preliminary review and the PI has been notified that a formal review will occur once this proposal is submitted to TSNRP for grant funding. Once approved, the endorsement letter will be forwarded to TSNRP to be incorporated in the grant application.

Sample and Recruitment Procedures

It is not possible to accurately determine the exact number of participants needed for this phenomenological study. After a careful review of qualitative research studies, it is anticipated that between seven and twelve aircraft carrier nurses will be necessary to obtain saturation. The PI will first try to contact those nurses who have left the aircraft carriers within the past two years—September 1998 to September 2000 ($n = 12$). If unsuccessful with getting seven to twelve out of that group, the PI will expand to the prior year of 1997 to 1998 ($n = 6$) and then the year preceding 1997 ($n = 6$). This provides a potential applicant pool of 24 for the designated period. The PI is confident that at least seven to twelve former aircraft carrier nurses from the group identified will agree to participate. If this is not the case, in a backwards year-by-year progression, former aircraft carrier nurses will be solicited. Incidentally, Taylor and Bogdan (1998) report that it is not too difficult to line up people for interviews because most people are willing to talk about themselves and that people are usually honored at the prospect of being interviewed for a research project.

In an attempt to limit the fears of coercion, subject identification, and possible retaliation (as suggested by the TSNRP reviewers in respect to the previous grant submission), the sample population will be those nurses who have already left the aircraft carriers instead of those nurses currently stationed aboard the aircraft carriers. This also addresses the concern that a nurse in an aircraft carrier billet for six months (who is considered a novice) cannot be compared to one who has been in the billet for two years (who is considered an expert).

Potential Benefit

Participants will not receive any compensation for participation. The potential benefit for the participants to partake in this study will come from the opportunity to share their experience with the researcher and to know that their unique perceptions may contribute to advancing nursing practice on board aircraft carriers.

Potential Risks/Inconveniences

The known risks associated with participating in this study are the unlikely prospect of awkward or embarrassing events during the interview and the possible loss of composure with emotional issues. Should the researcher recognize signs of stress or anxiety associated with the interview, the participant will be informed of the PI's desire for him or her to access the military health system and/or contact appropriate support organizations. In a telephone conversation, the PI learned that if the participant expresses an unwillingness to use available services, the PI is released from any liability.

Confidentiality

Participants will be assured that information shared with the PI will remain confidential. Code numbers will identify audiotapes and demographic data forms. All audiotapes will be erased once accurate transcription is verified. All data will be stored in a locked filing cabinet. A codebook containing code numbers and names and addresses of informants will be stored in locked file separate from all other data. Informants will be assured that their identities will not be revealed. Publications resulting from these data will be devoid of identifying information.

As discussed earlier, the PI has no obligation to report any revealed sensitive information because she will not be acting in an official capacity for the Navy when conducting the interviews.

Subject Rights

Participants will be given a copy of the consent form. The consent form will include the e-mail address, telephone number, and fax number of the researcher and all other required information as well as the statement that they may withdraw from the study at any time.

Literature Cited

Austin, A. (1993–1994). Nursing aboard a starship. *Minority Nurse, 42*–45.

Creswell, J. W. (1998). *Qualitative inquiry and research design.* London: SAGE Publications.

Greene, J. C. (1990). Three views on nature and role of knowledge in social science. In E. Guba (Ed.), *The paradigm dialogue* (pp. 227–245). Newbury Park, CA: SAGE Publications.

Lincoln, Y. S., & Guba, E. G. (1985). *Naturalistic inquiry.* Beverly Hills, CA: SAGE Publication.

Locke, L. F., Spirduso, W. W., & Silverman, S. J. (1993). *Proposals that work* (3rd ed.). London: SAGE Publications.

Munhall, P. L., & Boyd, C. O. (1999). *Nursing research: a qualitative perspective* (2nd ed.). New York: National League for Nursing Press.

Natanson, M. (1973). *Edmund Husserl: philosopher of infinite tasks.* Evanston, IL: Northwestern University Press.

Polit, D. F., & Hungler, B. P. (1995). *Nursing research: Principles and methods* (5th ed.). Philadelphia: J. B. Lippincott Company.

Sandelowski, M. (1986). The problem of rigor in qualitative research. *Advances in Nursing Science, 8*(3), 27–37.

Seidman, I. (1998). *Interviewing as qualitative research* (2nd ed.). New York: Teachers College Press.

Shiffer, S. W. (1990). Today's role of the Navy nurse. *Military Medicine, 155,* 208–213.

Sorrell, J. M., & Redmond, G. M. (1995). Interviews in qualitative nursing research: differing approaches for ethnographic and phenomenological studies. *Journal of Advanced Nursing, 21,* 1117–1122.

Streubert, H. J. (1991). Phenomenological research as a theoretic initiative in community health nursing. *Public Health Nursing, 8*(2), 119–123.

Streubert, H. J., & Carpenter, D. R. (1995). *Qualitative research in nursing: Advancing the humanistic imperative.* Philadelphia: J. B. Lippincott Company.

Streubert, H. J., & Carpenter, D. R. (1999). *Qualitative research in nursing: Advancing the humanistic imperative* (2nd ed.). Philadelphia: Lippincott.

Taylor, S. J., & Bogdan, R. (1998). *Introduction to qualitative research methods* (3rd ed.). New York: John Wiley & Sons, Inc.

Yonge, O., & Stewin, L. (1988). Reliability and validity: misnomers for qualitative research. *The Canadian Journal of Nursing, 20*(2), 61–67.

CRITIQUE OF FUNDED GRANT

Department of Defense
Triservice Nusing Research Program
Proposal Number: *N00–002*
Principal Investigator: *CDR Catherine Wilson Cox*
Title of Proposal: *The Lived Experience of Nurses Stationed*
                                Aboard Aircraft Carriers

EVALUATION CRITERIA

Scientific Approach and Technical Merit

This study seeks to elucidate the experiences of Navy nurses aboard ships, and as such, phenomenology is an appropriate methodology to use. The background information given about the demands of nursing practice aboard ship provide good context for the research question being addressed and reflect improvements form the previous proposal.

The initial lit review has been limited to studies or works about Navy nurses in general, and shipboard nursing in particular. Though it is understandable that there are few such studies, I believe there is more information in the literature about nurses who practice in isolation, for example nurses who worked for the Frontier Nursing Service. These narratives could add valuable context and insight to the initial problem description, as well as to the analysis and discussion later on.

It would be useful if the PI would state clearly what kind of phenomenology she is doing. Most likely it is descriptive or empirical, versus interpretive, but that distinction would be helpful to reviewers in making judgments about method-ological adequacy. A purposive sample will be used for the study, but it isn't clear how this might differ from a convenience sample, or a snowball sample. In some sense, all samples are purposive, it would be more useful to know how she chose this kind of sample, and how she sees it as better than other kinds of samples in getting the data she wants.

Data saturation is not particularly appropriate for phenomenology—it is a con-cept and technique that comes from grounded theory, and isn't useful here. The purpose of empirical phenomenology is to fully describe a lived experience—to identify its essential structures, as related by the participants. This description does not necessarily gain credence from a larger sample. The experience is the experi-ence, and has validity whether one person or 25 people are differences in the types of description that come from across case analysis, versus intra-case analy-sis, but the essence of each experience can stand on its own. In this methodology, more than any other, worries about sample size are mostly immaterial. Data satu-ration doesn't help assure the adequacy of a phenomenological study.

Sample size will most likely be adequate. There is a difference between brack-eting, as described by Natanson in this proposal, and the description of the researcher's interests in the project. (P28) Furthermore, though her description of what she will do to bracket, and when she will do it are very good, the notion of eliminating researcher bias in phenomenological inquiry is probably not achiev-able. Rather, how does one account for one's biases in the analysis—after all, they might be very useful or accurate.

Description of interview procedures is fine. Initial question may be a bit daunting. A better approach might be to ask the participants to tell the story of how it was to be a nurse aboard ship. Generally, this is a strong section. There is no good reason not to use pilot data in this study, if it helps elucidate the phenomenon.

·*Data Analysis*

This section has weaknesses. In general, the phases of data analysis are not very clear. How she will uncover essences is not made clear. What is an essence, and what mental actions does the researcher take to construct them? What is the difference between a theme (also characterized as some kind of commonality in qualitative data), and an essence? What is the difference between "Apprehending essential relationships" and identifying themes? In other words, what actions does a phenomenologist pursue with data that make this analysis different from content analysis? What are the usual features of a formalized, exhaustive description of the phenomenon? Though I firmly believe there are parts of qualitative analysis that do not lend themselves to a linear approach, I also know that any researcher should be able to say clearly what they plan to do to the data in their analysis. This is an instance where it would be helpful to look at more primary sources for phenomenological analysis—Moustakis and Giorgi among them.

It is not clear, beyond the brief description of using Atlas how data organization will be done (beyond reading the transcripts for general meaning). The rationale for waiting to complete interviews prior to in-depth analysis is weak. Since the PI is doing all the interviews, she will naturally impose meaning from one interview to the next in the act of doing them. If her plan is to describe this experience across participants, then she will eventually impose such meaning across cases anyway. The accumulation of many pages of transcript from these participants will make data analysis harder.

I am not opposed to discussions of evaluating the merit or worth of qualitative projects. I would point out that the originators of the credibility, dependability, etc. terminology—most notably Yvonna Lincoln, have moved on in their thinking about these things. In effect, these terms have devolved into concepts analogous to reliability/validity, etc.

Overall, the descriptions of processes to achieve dependability, auditability, and transferability are very weak. It is not quite accurate to say the responsibility for assessing transferability rests with the readers and not the researchers. It is a shared responsibility, and the researcher's job is to make a case for possible uses of the findings, so that readers can determine local usefulness.

Sources cited for all of the above are dated-newer work would shed some light on current thinking about assessing the worth of qualitative work that might be more specific to phenomenology.

Ethical considerations were nicely laid out and the lit review is appropriately placed.

Originality and Innovative Nature of the Proposal

This is an innovative proposal, and has the potential to expand our understanding of clinical nursing in a "service unique" environment.

Qualifications, Expertise and Research Experience of the Principal Investigator and Staff

The PI is a doctoral nursing student and has educational training in qualitative methods, as well as some supervised experience in conducting such studies. She does not have publications in the area of qualitative research.

Dr. Jeanne Sorrell is the PI's mentor and advisor in her graduate studies. She holds a PhD since 1987, has completed several qualitative research projects, and lists 9 publications on a variety of topics, including qualitative methods, philosophy of science, ethics, and writing. She coordinates the PhD program at George Mason, and teaches courses in research and the scholarship of writing.

Dr. Helen Streubert is a consultant for this project. She earned an EdD in 1989, and is known for her textbook on qualitative methods in general, and has two publications from phenomenological studies. Overall, I believe the expertise and experience are adequate to complete the study.

Availability of Institutional Resources and Adequacy of the Environment to Support the Project

Strengths: The resources of George Mason University are readily available to the PI, including libraries, administrative support, and faculty support. Weaknesses: No significant weaknesses noted.

Significance and Relevance to Nursing Research

This project has great potential, both as a means to gain understanding of important experiences in military nursing, and by demonstrating that phenomenological inquiry can be a most useful approach when little is known of these experiences. The constructions of experience and meaning that are produced could be immediately helpful in planning for nurses' deployment aboard aircraft carriers.

Reasonableness of the Budget and Duration of the Project in Relation to the Proposed Research

The budget seems reasonable—no category seems excessive, with the possible exception of the computer. Similarly configured computers are priced well below $2200 now.

SUMMARY

This study aims to describe the lived experiences of nurses stationed aboard aircraft carriers. The design is descriptive phenomenology, using open-ended interviews and written materials as data, with the purpose of constructing a "formalized, exhaustive" description of the phenomenon. The study has relevance to military nursing.

Strengths

- A useful topic for study—with the possibility of significant impact for manpower planning
- Aims clearly identified

- Appropriate permission to access participants is complete
- Appropriate assistance available to PI
- Study design matches research question

Weaknesses

- Use of data saturation as a method to determine when data collection should stop—doesn't match methodology
- Unclear description of data analysis phases
- Inadequate description of data organization methods
- Inadequate description of how merit and quality will be addressed

EVALUATION CRITERIA

Scientific Approach and Technical Merit

This qualitative study proposes a one-year phenomenological study design to describe the lived experiences of Navy nurses practicing aboard aircraft carriers. This will be done through personal interviews to explore the nurses' experiences aboard aircraft carriers. There is no explicit a priori hypothesis formulated. A strength of this proposal is the relevance of the topic to the TriService Nursing Research program priorities. Specifically, this proposal addresses clinical practice in service unique environments and is extremely relevant to military deployment and readiness. A study of this nature would provide important information to the Navy in particular for preparation of nursing personnel to be deployed in aircraft carriers. Some of the issues to be raised potentially include stress in performing nursing duties in a contained mostly male environment. Issues regarding separation over long periods of time from family and significant others can also influence perceptions of nurses assigned to these duties.

Appropriateness, Feasibility, Adequacy of Background/Significance Section
The PI provides detailed information (mostly textbook) and quotations of phenomenology and qualitative study design. Streubert's method guides the research. However from readings, the consultant name does not appear in the commonly used qualitative design books.

There is no literature review to speak of, merely a statement that "the intended research cannot build on what has already been done because there has been no research conducted on this aspect of Navy nursing." Although the statement may be accurate, there is research on some of the issues mentioned above. Some may not be in military life or in the Navy per se, but there is research related to occupational stress, female nurses working in a predominately male environment, and probably on female troop deployment and the impact of this activity on performance of individual.

The PI mentions 9 studies appropriate for review regarding shipboard nursing, yet only one short article dealing with aircraft carriers is mentioned in the Background and Significance section of this proposal. An in-depth literature review is appropriate and paramount to qualitative studies. Although this is an exploration of a phenomena [sic], there are still many related issues meriting review. Also from this literature review, is where some of the open-ended questions surface and help guide the inquiry.

Appropriateness, Feasibility, Adequacy of Preliminary
Studies Section

It is not clear to this reviewer whether any formal preliminary studies were conducted. The PI mentions "Anecdotal information expressed to the PI from nurses previously assigned to aircraft carriers." Although the information provided by the aircraft nurses is quite interesting and pertinent, the PI does not integrate this information in designing some guide of open-ended questions with areas that might be important to probe in more depth. There is no instrument guiding the interview, nor a set of questions regarding demographic information. The PI merely presents a list of demographic info. There is no listing to whether the nurse is married/lives with partner, has children, or the nurse's ethnicity. Some of this information may be critical to the perceptions and experiences of nursing aboard an aircraft carrier. Perceptions may differ and some nurses may experience stress, depression, etc. related to extended periods of separation from family.

Appropriateness, Feasibility, Adequacy of Methodology, including
sampling and data collection

Sampling is purposive and data collection is done until saturation, as is done in most naturalistic inquiry and phenomenological studies. However, after this is stated, the PI goes on to say she will only interview seven to twelve nurses.

There is discordant information as to who will be interviewed from the text and the support letters, as well as how many and for how long. Also, in the text is mentioned that participants will be contacted a second time to share the outcome to confirm the credibility of findings. However, there are opposite schools regarding this issue, I happen to agree with previous reviewers in the sense that participants may disagree with the researcher interpretation of findings. Another alternative is to have an expert panel to confirm credibility of findings.

Some methodological approaches are unclear to reviewer, specifically the concept of "bracketing" (p. 27) and "leaving an audit trail" are poorly described and appear mostly regurgitation from textbooks.

Originality and Innovative Nature of the Proposal

The proposal is very innovative in aiming at describing this particular form of nursing aboard an aircraft carrier. The methodology proposed is appropriate. However, the PI fails to submit a coherent, well-structured study.

Qualifications, Expertise and Research Experience of the Principal Investigator and Staff

The investigator is a doctoral student ready to embark on her dissertation. This study certainly would be ideally suited for a dissertation. She has gathered two experts in the area of qualitative research, one in-kind Dr. Sorrell, that will be her Dissertation Committee Chair, and Dr. Streubert who is a Co-Author in a book on qualitative research, where the methodology to be used in this research is published.

Availability of Institutional Resources and Adequacy of the Environment to Support the Project

These are all adequate for the proposed study. Letters of support are at issue, some are old, from previous submission and some contradict and limit the scope of the research proposed here.

Significance and Relevance to Nursing Research

The topic is very significant and relevant to nursing research.

Reasonableness of the Budget and Duration of the Project in Relation to the Proposed Research

The costs associated to this proposal are within needed expenses to carry out the research. The costs of transcription may have been somewhat underestimated.

SUMMARY

The purpose of this phenomenological research study is to describe the lived experiences of Navy nurses practicing aboard aircraft carriers. Using phenomenology, nurses previously stationed aboard aircraft carriers will be interviewed to explore their experiences as a ship's nurse. The question guiding this inquiry will be: "What is your experience as a nurse on an aircraft carrier?" Interviews will be conducted until data saturation is reached. The interviews will be tape recorded, transcribed, and analyzed in four steps following Streubert steps. The principal investigator is a doctoral student ready to embark on her research for her dissertation, should be prepared and able to conduct the interviews, and design "an interview guide and probes" to follow with the assistance of her research team.

Strengths

- Relevant topic
- Expertise of research team
- Availability of study population

Weakness

- Sample saturation (pre-conceived)
- Lack of substantive literature review
- Lack of open-ended question guide with probes
- Lack of form to collect demographic data
- Controversial support letters
- Ethical issues dealing with a small pool of individuals easily identifiable by other Navy personnel

TriService Nursing Research Program FY 2000 Scientific Review Discussion Summary

Proposal Number: N00–002
PI: CDR Catherine Cox
Title: The Lived Experience of Nurses Stationed Aboard Aircraft Carriers

Discussion: The purpose of this extremely relevant proposal, reported the primary reviewer, is to describe the experiences of nurses who are or have been stationed on 12 aircraft carriers deployed worldwide. The principal investigator (PI) will conduct interviews until data saturation is achieved. The reviewer noted that this proposal follows a training proposal submitted by the PI, and it is clear that the PI has made an effort to incorporate recommendations from the prior review into the current document. The reviewer felt that it was also clear that the proposed research could offer valuable insights into issues that are relevant to service-specific environments. The methodology proposed—a phenomenological approach—is appropriate. The literature review, however, does not offer relevant studies (focusing on exact phenomenology but not addressing other research into nursing in isolation) that would help support the kind of phenomenological approach (interpretive vs. empirical) that will be used. The PI cites references that are considered survey literature, when in the reviewer's opinion she should be referencing primary resources on phenomenology. Data saturation is unlikely to be useful, although the PI offers a clear explanation of how she will conduct interviews and a strong attempt to discuss her proposed use of the bracketing technique. Ethical considerations are addressed appropriately. Other strengths of the proposal include a highly qualified mentor who is well known in the field of qualitative research, a proposed consultant who will likely make a significant contribution, and excellent resources.

The primary reviewer argued that the proposal's data analysis section is the weakest. The PI lays out five analytical steps but does not describe how she will complete them (i.e., what is an essence and how does one uncover it?) She does not yet appear to understand that there is a difference between apprehending essential relationships and identifying themes. The PI also does not spell out how she will manage the data she obtains and analyzes.

The secondary reviewer agreed with many of the primary reviewer's comments, except that this reviewer felt that the preliminary data obtained during the training grant study was inadequately presented. The reviewer also found the literature review inadequate and suggested that the PI refer to literature on occupational stress. The letters of support limit the PI's number of interviews and access to carriers.

Panel members expressed their concern that the PI still needs to do more work in methodology—it appeared clear from the proposal that she is probably still in the development phase but that she is also getting the help she needs. As she is a student, 100 percent of her time will be devoted to the project. The panel agreed that her dissertation proposal is likely to be even stronger than this proposal.

Human Subject Protection: The panel ethicist was concerned about ensuring individual interviewees' confidentiality when their experiences may identify them. The sample has changed to nurses who are no longer aboard carriers, which will decrease identification threat. The PI includes consent for taping and transcription. She allows for review of information by subjects and plans for use of data in an aggregate confidential manner. There is little risk to participants. The investigator provides thoughtful, detailed information related to ethical considerations and human subject protection. Written consent will be obtained prior to the study (not attached) and IRB approval is pending (not attached).

Budget: The PI should be able to purchase the computer she proposes for less money than she has budgeted.

GLOSSARY

Action Research   A research method characterized by the systematic study of the implementation of a planned change to a system.

Actors   Individuals within a particular cultural group who are studied by ethnographic researchers.

Analytic Induction   A method of qualitative data analysis wherein the researcher seeks to refine a theory through the identification of negative cases.

A Priori   Form of deductive thinking in which theoretical formulations and propositions precede and guide systematic observation.

Archives   Contain unpublished materials that often are used as primary source materials.

Auditability   The ability of another researcher to follow the methods and conclusion of the original researcher.

Authenticity   Term used to describe the mechanism by which the qualitative researcher ensures that the findings of the study are real, true, or authentic. In historical research refers to assuring that a primary source document provides the truthful reporting of a subject.

Biographical History   Studies the life of a person within the context of the period in which that person lives.

Bracketing   A methodological device of phenomenological inquiry that requires deliberate identification and suspension of all judgments or ideas about the phenomenon under investigation or what one already knows about the subject prior to and throughout the phenomenological investigation.

Category   Classification of concepts into broader categories following comparison of one category to another. Broader categories serve as an umbrella under which related concepts are grouped.

Chat Rooms   A computer-mediated method of communication and data collection whereby individuals log on to the world wide web and can communicate back and forth in a synchronous manner.

Coding   The process of data analysis in grounded theory whereby statements are grouped and given a code for ease of identification later in the study.

Conceptual Density   Data generation that is exhaustive and comprehensive and provides the researcher with evidence that all possible data to support a conceptual framework has been generated.

Confirmability   This is considered a neutral criterion for measuring the trustworthiness of qualitative research. If a study demonstrates credibility, auditability, and fittingness, the study is also said to possess confirmability.

Constant Comparative Method of Data Analysis   A form of qualitative data analysis wherein the researcher makes sense of textual data by categorizing units of measuring through a process of comparing new units with previously identified units.

Core Variable   The central phenomenon in grounded theory around which all the other categories are integrated.

Covert Participant Observation   A method of data collection that involves observing participants however, the individuals are unaware that they are being observed.

Credibility   A term that relates to the trustworthiness of findings in a qualitative research study. Credibility is demonstrated when participants recognize the reported research findings as their own experiences.

Critical Theory   A philosophy of science based on a belief that revealing the unrecognized forces that control human behavior will liberate and empower individuals.

Cultural Scene   An anthropological term for culture. It includes the actors, the artifacts, and the actions of the actors in social situations.

Deductive   The process of moving from generalizations to specific conclusions.

Dependability   This is a criterion used to measure trustworthiness in qualitative research. Dependability is met through securing credibility of the findings.

Dialectic   A form of logic based on the belief that reality is represented by contradiction and the reconciliation of contradiction.

Dialectical Critique   A form of qualitative data analysis wherein the researcher engages in dialogue with research participants to reveal the internal contradictions within a particular phenomenon.

Discipline of History   Both a science and an art that studies the interrelationship of social, economic, political, and psychological factors that influence ideas, events, institutions, and people.

Dwelling   A term used to demonstrate the degree of dedication a researcher commits to reading, intuiting, analyzing, synthesizing, and coming to a description or conclusion(s) about the data collected during a qualitative study. Also called immersion.

Eidetic Intuiting   Accurate interpretations of what is meant in the description.

Embodiment (or Being in the World)   The belief that all arts are constructed on foundation of perception, or original awareness of some phenomenon (Merleau-Ponty, 1956).

Epistemology   The branch of philosophy concerned with how individuals determine what is true.

Essences   Elements related to the ideal or true meaning of something that gives common understanding to the phenomenon under investigation.

External Criticism   Questions the genuineness of primary sources and assures that the document is what it claims to be.

Field Notes   Notes recorded about the people, places, and things that are part of the ethnographer's study of a culture.

Fittingness   A term used in qualitative research to demonstrate the probability that the research findings have meaning to others in similar situations. Fittingness is also called transferability.

Free Imaginative Variation   A technique used to apprehend essential relations between essences and involves careful study of concrete examples supplied by the participant's experience and systematic variation of these examples in the imagination.

Genuine   When a primary source is what it purports to be and is not a forgery.

Grand Tour Question(s)   General opening question(s) that offer(s) overview insights of a particular person, place, object, or situation.

History   Webster's New International Dictionary defines history as "a narrative of events connected with a real or imaginary object, person, or career...devoted to the exposition of the natural unfolding and interdependence of the events treated." History is a branch of knowledge that "records and explains past events as steps in human progress..." [it is] "the study of the character and significance of events." Barzen and Graff (1985) describe history as an "invention" and as an "art."

Historiography   Historiography requires that historiographers study and critique sources and develop history by systematically presenting their findings in a narrative. Historiography provides a way of knowing the past.

Historian/Historiographer   Balances the rigors of scientific inquiry and the understanding of human behavior; develops the skill of speculation and interpretation to narrate the story.

Historical Method   Application of method or steps to study history systematically.

Holism   A belief that wholes are more than the mere sum of their parts.

Immersion   A term used to demonstrate the degree of dedication a researcher commits to reading, intuiting, analyzing, synthesizing, and coming to a description or conclusion(s) about the data collected during a qualitative study. Also called dwelling.

Induction   The process of moving from specific observations to generalizations.

Inductive Theory Building   Theory derived from observation of phenomena.

Informed Consent   When engaging participants in a research study, ensuring that they have complete information, that they understand the information, and that they have freely chosen to either accept or decline participation in the investigation.

Intellectual History   Studies ideas and thoughts over time of a person believed to be an intellectual thinker, or the ideas of a period, or the attitudes of people.

Intentionality   Consciousness is always consciousness of something. One does not hear without hearing something or believe without believing something.

Internal Criticism   Concerns itself with the authenticity or truthfulness of the content.

Interpretive Phenomenology/Hermeneutics   The interpretation of phenomena appearing in text or written word.

Intuiting   A process of thinking through the data so that a true comprehension or accurate interpretation of what is meant in a particular description is achieved.

Life History   A research method wherein the researcher listens to the telling of life story for the purpose of understanding a particular aspect of the individual's life.

Local Theory   A theory that describes a particular group or sample that cannot be generalized to a larger population.

Narrative Picturing   A data collection method whereby participants are asked to imagine or picture an event or sequence of events as a method of describing an experience.

Naturalistic Inquiry   A research methodology based on a belief in investigating phenomena in their natural setting free of manipulation.

Participant Observation   The direct observation and recording of data that require the researcher to become a part of the culture being studied.

Phenomenological Reduction   A term meaning recovery of original awareness.

Present-Mindedness   Use of a contemporary perspective when analyzing data collected from an earlier period of time.

Primary Sources   Firsthand account of a person's experience, an institution, or of an event and may lack critical analysis; examples include private journals, letters, records.

Process Informed Consent   Requires the same criteria as informed consent; however, is differentiated by the fact that this type of consent requires the researcher to re-evaluate the participants' consent to be involved in the study at varying points throughout the investigation.

Reflexive   This term refers to being both researcher and participant and capitalizing on the duality as a source of insight.

Reflexive Critique   A form of qualitative data analysis wherein the researcher engages in dialogue with research participants to reveal each individual's interpretation for the meanings influencing behavior.

Reliability   The consistency of an instrument to measure an attribute or concept that it was designed to measure.

Saturation   Repetition of data obtained during the course of a qualitative study. Signifies completion of data collection on a particular culture or phenomenon.

Secondary Sources   Materials that cite opinions and present interpretations from the period being studied such as newspaper accounts, journal articles, and textbooks.

Selective Sampling   In a grounded theory investigation, selecting from the generated data those critical pieces of information relevant to the current investigation, and avoiding incorporation of material that is not connected to the current investigation.

Situated   A term that reflects the position of the researcher within the context of the group under study.

Social History   Explores a particular period of time and attempts to understand the prevailing values and beliefs through the everyday events of that period.

Social Situation   The activities carried out by actors (members of a cultural group) in a specific place.

Symbolic Interactionism   A philosophic belief system based on the assumption that humans learn about and define their world through interaction with others.

Tacit Knowledge   Information known by members of a culture but not verbalized or openly discussed.

Theme   Used to describe a structural meaning unit of data that is essential in presenting qualitative findings.

Theoretical Sampling   Sampling on the basis of concepts that have proven theoretical relevance to the evolving theory (Strauss & Corbin, 1990).

Theoretical Sensitivity   Personal quality of the researcher that is reflected in an awareness of the subtleties of meaning of data (Strauss & Corbin, 1990).

Transferability   A term used in qualitative research to demonstrate the probability that the research findings have meaning to others in similar situations. Transferability is also called fittingness.

Triangulation   Method of using multiple research approaches in the same study to answer research questions.

Triangulation of Data Generation Techniques   The use of three different methods of data generation in a single research study for the purpose of generating meaningful data.

Trustworthiness   Establishing validity and reliability of qualitative research. Qualitative research is trustworthy when it accurately represents the experience of the study participants.

Validity   The degree to which an instrument measures what it was designed to measure.

INDEX

Note: Page numbers followed by *f* indicate figures; those followed by *t* indicate tables; those followed by *b* indicate boxed material.